Childhood Medical Guide

By the Editors of Time-Life Books

Alexandria, Virginia

Time-Life Books Inc.
is a wholly owned subsidiary of

Time Incorporated

FOUNDER: Henry R. Luce 1898-1967

Editor-in-Chief: Henry Anatole Grunwald
President: J. Richard Munro
Chairman of the Board: Ralph P. Davidson
Corporate Editor: Ray Cave
Group Vice President, Books:
Reginald K. Brack Jr.
Vice President, Books: George Artandi

Time-Life Books Inc.

EDITOR: George Constable
Director of Design: Louis Klein
Director of Editorial Resources:
Phyllis K. Wise
Acting Text Director: Ellen Phillips
Editorial Board: Russell B. Adams Jr.,
Dale M. Brown, Roberta Conlan,
Thomas H. Flaherty, Donia Ann Steele,
Rosalind Stubenberg, Kit van Tulleken,
Henry Woodhead
Director of Photography and Research:
John Conrad Weiser

PRESIDENT: Reginald K. Brack Jr.
Executive Vice Presidents: John M. Fahey Jr.,
Christopher T. Linen
Senior Vice Presidents: James L. Mercer,
Leopoldo Toralballa
Vice Presidents: Stephen L. Bair, Ralph J. Cuomo,
Neal Goff, Stephen L. Goldstein, Juanita T. James,
Hallett Johnson III, Robert H. Smith, Paul R. Stewart
Director of Production Services:
Robert J. Passantino

Library of Congress Cataloguing in
Publication Data
Childhood medical guide.
  (Successful parenting)
  Bibliography: p.
  Includes index.
  1. Children — Diseases — Treatment. 2. Pediatric
emergencies. 3. Sick children — Care and treatment.
I. Time-Life Books. II. Series.
RJ61.C549 1986   618.92   86-14507
ISBN 0-8094-5908-6
ISBN 0-8094-5909-4 (lib. bdg.)

Successful Parenting

SERIES DIRECTOR: Donia Ann Steele
Deputy Editor: Jim Hicks
Series Administrator: Norma E. Shaw
Editorial Staff for *Childhood Medical Guide:*
Designer: Cynthia T. Richardson
Picture Editor: Jane Jordan
Text Editor: Robert A. Doyle
Staff Writers: Janet Cave, Patricia Daniels
Researchers: Jean Crawford (principal), Mark Moss,
Myrna Traylor-Herndon
Assistant Designer: Jennifer B. Gilman
Copy Coordinators: Vilasini Balakrishnan,
Marfé Ferguson
Picture Coordinator: Bradley Hower
Editorial Assistant: Eileen Tansill

Special Contributors: Amy Goodwin Aldrich,
Lynne W. Bair, Sarah Brash, Lois Gilman, Donal
Kevin Gordon, Sandy Jones, Brian McGinn, Robert
Menaker, Carolyn Mooney, Barbara Palmer, Susan
Perry, Jane Ann Peterson, Brooke Stoddard, Robert
Stokes, David Thiemann, Laurie Baker Walden
(text); Laura Boudreau, Jill Denney, Melva
Holloman, Sydney S. Johnson, Brandi McDougall,
Marilyn Terrell Murphy (research)

Editorial Operations
Copy Chief: Diane Ullius
Editorial Operations: Caroline A. Boubin
(manager)
Production: Celia Beattie
Library: Louise D. Forstall

Correspondents: Elisabeth Kraemer-Singh (Bonn);
Dorothy Bacon (London); Maria Vincenza Aloisi
(Paris); Ann Natanson (Rome). Valuable assistance
was also provided by Christina Lieberman
(New York).

First printing. Printed in U.S.A.

Published simultaneously in Canada.
School and library distribution by
Silver Burdett Company, Morristown,
New Jersey 07960.

TIME-LIFE is a trademark of Time
Incorporated U.S.A.

Other Publications

HEALTHY HOME COOKING
UNDERSTANDING COMPUTERS
YOUR HOME
THE ENCHANTED WORLD
THE KODAK LIBRARY OF CREATIVE PHOTOGRAPHY
GREAT MEALS IN MINUTES
THE CIVIL WAR
PLANET EARTH
COLLECTOR'S LIBRARY OF THE CIVIL WAR
THE EPIC OF FLIGHT
THE GOOD COOK
WORLD WAR II
HOME REPAIR AND IMPROVEMENT
THE OLD WEST

*For information on and a full description
of any of the Time-Life Books series listed
above, please write:*
Reader Information
Time-Life Books
541 North Fairbanks Court
Chicago, Illinois 60611

This volume is one of a series about raising children.

The Consultants

General Consultants

Dr. Robert Johns Haggerty, chief medical consultant for this book, is an internationally recognized authority on children's health. A former president of the American Academy of Pediatrics, he currently serves as Clinical Professor of Pediatrics at Cornell University Medical School. He is also editor-in-chief of *Pediatrics in Review* and president of the William T. Grant Foundation, which sponsors research in children's mental health. During his career, Dr. Haggerty has held faculty and administrative positions at Harvard Medical School, Children's Hospital in Boston and the Harvard School of Public Health. He has written extensively in his field and coedited *Ambulatory Pediatrics,* a widely used pediatric text. Dr. Haggerty has served, as well, on the editorial boards of many leading medical journals.

Dr. Daniel W. Ochsenschlager consulted on the "Accidents and Emergencies" section and on other hospital-related issues in this volume. He is currently Medical Director of the emergency room at Children's Hospital National Medical Center in Washington, D.C., and Associate Professor of Child Health and Development at the George Washington University School of Medicine. Dr. Ochsenschlager has served on several committees and task forces dealing with trauma and emergency services for children. He is a contributor to *Pediatric Emergencies,* a comprehensive pediatric sourcebook, as well as to *Pediatric Emergencies Manual,* an instruction book for health-care professionals.

Special Consultants

Dr. Walter C. Allan, a pediatric neurologist, consulted on the "Nervous System" section of the *Childhood Medical Guide.* Dr. Allan has researched and published numerous articles on the subject of nervous-system disorders and their treatments in premature and newborn infants. He currently practices pediatric neurology in association with the Maine Medical Center in Portland.

Dr. Christopher Scott Conner developed the guide to children's medicines that appears in the closing pages of this volume. He was assisted by staff members at the Rocky Mountain Drug Consultation Center in Denver, Colorado, where he previously served as director. Dr. Conner is currently Assistant Professor of Medicine at the University of Colorado School of Medicine and the editor and author of Drugdex, a computerized drug information system used by hospitals around the world. He has written columns on medicine-related issues for the *Denver Post* and other Colorado newspapers.

Dr. Roma S. Chandra, who assisted in the preparation of the anatomical drawings in the book, is Chairman of Anatomic Pathology at the Children's Hospital National Medical Center in Washington, D.C., and Professor of Pathology at the George Washington University School of Medicine. She has participated in many seminars and conferences dealing with child pathology and has published more than 50 articles concerning her research on liver and other organ disorders.

Dr. Paul Louis McCarthy, an expert on fever in children, developed the chart in the "Fever" section of this volume to aid parents in judging the severity of illness in a feverish child. The information is based on extensive research Dr. McCarthy conducted with his associates at Yale-New Haven Medical Center, where he is Director of General Pediatrics. He also currently serves as Professor of Pediatrics at Yale University School of Medicine. Dr. McCarthy has written widely for books and pediatric journals on the subjects of fever and childhood illness.

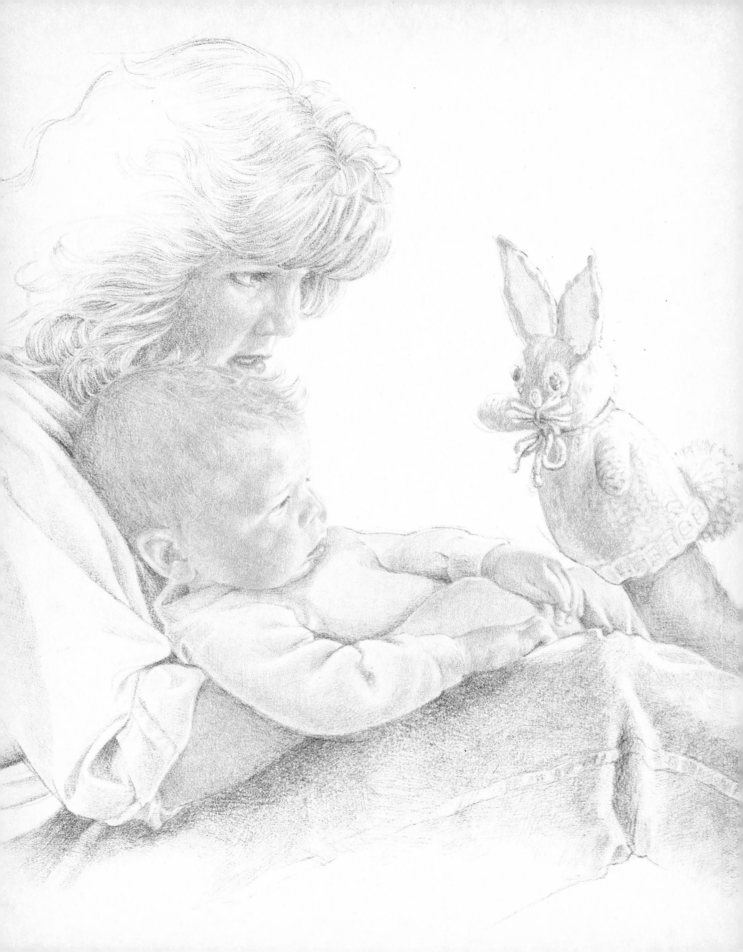

Using This Book

The sight of a sick or injured child arouses powerful protective instincts in parents. Perhaps this is one of nature's survival schemes, for the loving care of a mother or father is a powerful healer in itself. But caring alone is not enough; along with instinct, a parent needs information. Knowing what symptoms to look for and what to do while waiting for the doctor to return a call can help you face the ailments and accidents of early childhood with more confidence and competence. Providing that information is the aim of the *Childhood Medical Guide,* which deals with the accidents, emergency situations and medical conditions most commonly suffered by children from birth to six years of age. The bibliography suggests a number of medical books for those who would like to read more about a particular illness. The index lists every subject in the volume; among the entries there are many general symptoms, followed by listings of the various conditions and diseases that might cause those symptoms.

Although this volume is a valuable reference tool, it cannot and should not replace the advice of a doctor. Always consult your physician whenever you are concerned about your child's well-being.

Contents

Accidents and Emergencies   8

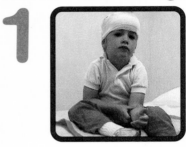

Illnesses and Disorders   42

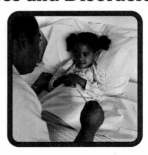

Keeping Children Healthy 128

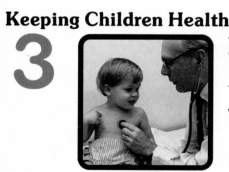

3

☐ indicates a chart or other supporting material

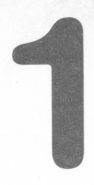

Accidents and Emergencies

Young children are creatures of much impulse and curiosity, with little awareness of danger. In the course of growing up, they are bound to have their share of accidents. In fact, the sobering truth is that accidents are the leading cause of death and disabling injury for children. But most life-threatening emergencies can be avoided if you take precautions with babies and toddlers and teach your older children about safety. One point to remember is that accidents occur most frequently in stressful situations — when a parent or child is tired, when parents argue, when the youngster moves to new surroundings.

Accident prevention must begin on day one. Infants ought never to be left alone outside the crib or playpen. Hazardous objects, such as drugs, cleaning supplies and sharp implements, must always be kept out of reach of the growing, exploring child. As your child's world expands, she is exposed to new adventures — and new risks — every day. You should begin to instruct her as well as protect her. A toddler must be told "no" when she touches the stove. A four-year-old must be reminded that crossing the street can be dangerous. As soon as possible, you will want to teach your youngster to swim. As time passes, she should learn to take ever more responsibility for her own safety.

Regardless of the care that you take, however, you cannot eliminate every risk. For your child's well-being and for your own peace of mind, prepare yourself and your home for emergency situations *(page 10)*. Have necessary medical supplies and information ready at hand, and take some time to familiarize yourself with the steps you can take in the event of an accident. All parents should be as adept at giving first aid as they are at preventing injuries in the first place.

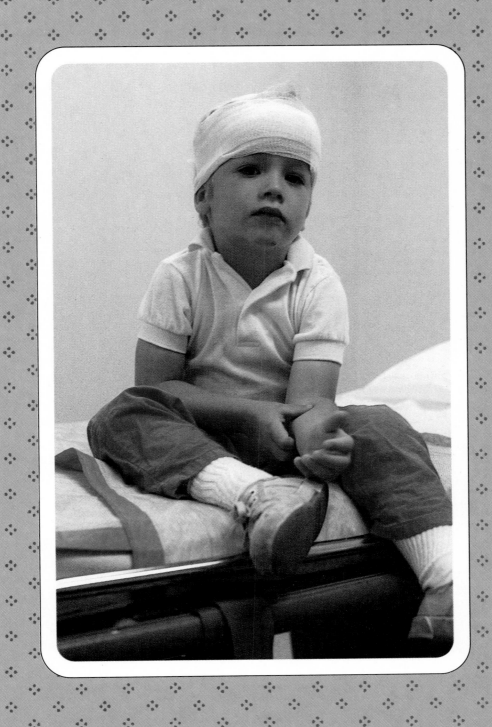

Handling a Medical Emergency

Although emergencies require immediate action, they can be divided into two levels of urgency: life-threatening emergencies and dangerous situations.

A life-threatening emergency occurs when one of the body's critical functions — breathing or circulation — fails. When this happens, the child is in immediate danger of death; you must respond with first aid at once, even before calling for assistance. Accidents which can be life-threatening include poisoning, drowning, electric shock, an obstructed airway, extensive burns and a wound with uncontrollable bleeding. Prolonged unconsciousness and shock are important signals that a youngster's life is in danger.

Dangerous situations are those serious accidents or illnesses — head injuries, wounds with controllable bleeding, or meningitis, for example — in which the child is imperiled but does not face imminent death. In these cases, your child is breathing regularly, has a pulse — although it may be fast or slow — and is usually conscious and not suffering from shock. Here your first priority is to call for emergency medical help or take your child to the hospital as quickly and calmly as possible. Concentrate on keeping your child comfortable and reassured until he can get professional care.

To be prepared for emergencies, you should learn to give artificial respiration *(page 16)* and should take a course in cardiopulmonary resuscitation, a method for restarting a stopped heart that requires hands-on training and practice to learn properly and to master. CPR courses are available through many hospitals and American Red Cross chapters. Learn also the techniques for stopping severe bleeding *(page 25)* and for treating shock *(page 38)* and choking *(page 23)*. Find the route to your local emergency room and make a trial run.

Finally, be sure to have a list of emergency telephone numbers at your fingertips. Before making a list, find out whether you can dial a single number — such as 911 — for centralized access to emergency services. You should keep your list of the following numbers on, or next to, your telephone:

- fire, police and ambulance
- regional poison-control center
- family doctor
- hospital emergency room
- a reliable local taxi
- nearest 24-hour pharmacy
- parents' workplace

You should also post clearly written directions to your house that can be given to emergency personnel over the telephone, as well as pertinent health information including: blood types, allergies, medication being taken and any special health conditions, such as diabetes or asthma.

The First-Aid Kit

Every home should have a first-aid kit reserved for emergency use only. The kit illustrated at right consists of nonprescription medicines and simple instruments and supplies used to treat injuries that do not require professional attention or to deal with more serious accidents until help arrives.

Label your kit clearly and keep it well out of children's reach — in a separate, lockable cupboard or on a high shelf in an adult's room. Take the kit with you on vacation and keep a duplicate in any place you spend a lot of time — a vacation home, a boat or the family car.

Resist the urge to raid your first-aid kit for everyday medical supplies; otherwise, you may find some crucial item missing in a real emergency. Keep duplicates of often-used items in your bathroom medicine chest *(pages 130-131)* and use those for day-to-day needs.

Replenish the contents of your first-aid kit as they are used and periodically check expiration dates for perishable items. Ipecac syrup, for example, needs to be replaced every year.

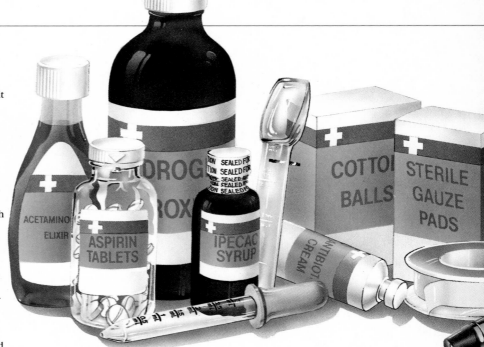

ACETAMINOPHEN ELIXIR, a liquid medication for pain and fever; ASPIRIN for fever, pain and inflammations; HYDROGEN PEROXIDE for cleaning small cuts; IPECAC SYRUP to induce vomiting; a calibrated DOSAGE DROPPER to dispense medication to younger children; a cali- *brated DOSAGE SPOON for older children; ANTIBIOTIC CREAM to prevent infection in cuts and minor burns; COTTON BALLS for bleeding from the nose or ear, or to absorb drainage from ear injuries; STERILE GAUZE PADS, two and four inches square, to cover cuts and burns;*

Priorities for Life-Saving Action

A parent's first task in any emergency is to stay calm: Your clear head and common sense can make the difference in your child's survival.

Your second task is to give emergency first aid according to the priorities listed below. If other people are on hand, have one of them call for emergency help. If you are alone with the child, attend to life-threatening problems first before making a phone call. Do not waste time leafing through a phone book if emergency numbers are not posted; simply call the operator, tell her "This is an emergency," and be prepared to give your name, address, and a calm assessment of the child's condition.

In an emergency situation, follow this sequence of actions:

- Check your child for consciousness. If he is conscious and breathing, then call for medical help.

- Check for breathing: put your ear to the child's mouth and nose while watching for his chest to rise and fall. If he is not breathing, begin artificial respiration at once *(page 16)*.
- Check the pulse at the upper arm or on the side of the neck *(page 17)*. If the heart has stopped, have someone trained in cardiopulmonary resuscitation respond.
- If the child appears to be choking, apply the rescue procedure appropriate for his age *(page 23)*.
- Stop profuse bleeding by applying direct pressure *(page 25)*.
- If you detect signs of poisoning — burns or stains around the mouth, pills or plants nearby — contact the poison-control center for instructions on appropriate treatment.
- Then, assess your child's condition and call for help.

While waiting for help:
- Remove the child from any source of immediate danger — flames, heavy smoke or threatening traffic.
- Treat your child for shock if necessary *(page 38)*.
- Check the child's breathing and pulse periodically.
- Continue to stem bleeding.

DO NOT:
- move the youngster unless he is in immediate danger.
- give anything to eat or drink.
- induce vomiting.
- attempt to remove an object from the child's throat if he can still breathe.
- leave the child unattended unless absolutely necessary.
- give up. Always assume he is alive and continue with artificial respiration or CPR until help arrives.

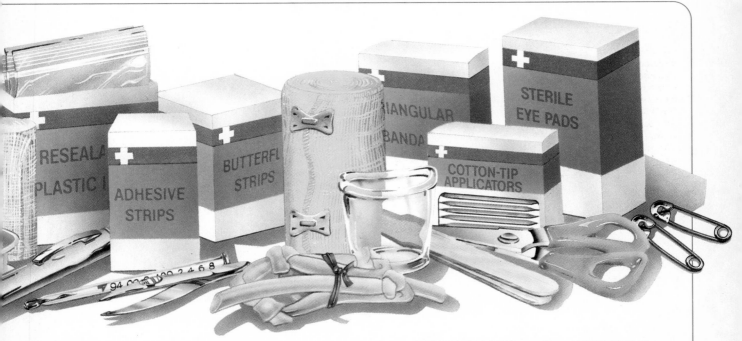

ADHESIVE TAPE to secure gauze over wounds; GAUZE BANDAGES for wrapping cuts and burns; a SMALL FLASHLIGHT to locate items in the dark and to check eyes for signs of concussion; RESEALABLE PLASTIC BAGS for ice packs; ADHESIVE STRIPS for small cuts and scrapes; a RECTAL THERMOMETER for children under five (include an oral one for older children); TWEEZERS to remove splinters and ticks; BUTTERFLY STRIPS to hold a cut together; ELASTIC BANDAGES for sprains; a TOURNIQUET — rubber surgical tubing with knots at one-inch intervals — for uncontrollable bleeding; an EYECUP to irrigate the eye; STERILE EYE PADS to cover the eye in an injury; COTTON-TIP APPLICATORS to hold eyelids open when removing foreign objects; TONGUE DEPRESSORS for finger splints; SCISSORS; a TRIANGULAR BANDAGE for a sling; SAFETY PINS to hold the sling together.

Bites and Stings

Read First

- After a bee or wasp sting, watch for signs of shock or allergic reaction — especially breathing difficulties, itchy eyes, nausea or cramps. See a doctor immediately if your child has any of these reactions.
- Call the doctor if a youngster suffers multiple stings.
- For animal bites, first control any serious bleeding, then seek medical care.
- Administer first aid and get to a doctor immediately after a youngster has been bitten or stung by a poisonous snake, poisonous spider, scorpion or any marine creature.
- If you are not sure of the source of a bite the child has received, follow treatment for the worst case.

Insect stings

Insects with stingers — including bees, wasps, hornets, yellow jackets and ants — inject minute quantities of venom beneath the skin. Though they may be painful, insect stings are seldom serious, and symptoms usually begin to subside after three or four hours. In rare instances, an acute, potentially fatal allergic reaction involving breathing difficulty and other symptoms may follow within a few minutes to an hour after an insect sting. If your child suffers from allergies or asthma, you should be especially alert to this possibility. In general, rapidly appearing symptoms indicate a more serious reaction — and a greater danger that your child will go into anaphylactic shock *(page 38)* or lose consciousness.

Symptoms:
- swelling around the sting
- redness
- burning pain and itching
- difficulty breathing or swallowing, flushed face, itchy eyes, nausea or abdominal cramps; in a severe case, shock or loss of consciousness

What to do:
- Scrape a honeybee sting with a knife or fingernail to remove the stinger and attached venom sac. (This bee is the only insect to leave its stinger in the skin.) Do not squeeze the stinger; it may release more venom.
- Wash the sting with soap and water. Apply ice or a cool, damp cloth for 20 to 30 minutes to minimize swelling.

What to do for allergic reactions:
- Keep the child still to limit the circulation of venom. If the sting is on an arm or leg, you should apply a constricting band between the sting and the heart *(page 14)*.
- If the youngster goes into anaphylactic shock *(page 38)*, seek emergency medical help immediately. If the child is not breathing, begin artificial respiration *(page 16)*.

Insect bites

Although a few serious diseases, including malaria, can be transmitted by biting insects, the most common bites — those inflicted by fleas, mosquitoes, gnats and chiggers — are usually no threat to health. If a child scratches a bite, however, there is a risk of infection and scarring.

Symptoms:
- small, round, red welts
- localized itching

What to do:
- Wash the bite with soap and water.
- Apply ice or a cold compress to the area for five to 10 minutes.
- Follow the compress with an application of calamine lotion in order to reduce the itching.
- Trim the child's nails short and keep them clean to reduce the risk of infection from scratching.

Tick bites

A feeding tick looks like a quarter-inch-long dark bag adhering to the skin or scalp. The insect pierces the skin with its head and a pair of pincers and holds on to its victim tenaciously as it sucks blood. Tall grasses, woodlands and shrubby areas may harbor ticks, which will feed on any warm-blooded creature. Pets may bring them into the house. These insects transmit several diseases, including Rocky Mountain spotted fever *(page 121)*. Remove a tick as soon as you discover it — the longer it remains in place the greater the chance of infection.

What to do:
- Cover the tick with petroleum jelly, salad oil, mineral oil, machine oil or alcohol to block its breathing pores and make it relax its hold. If the tick does not release its hold, remove it carefully, using tweezers.
- If no oil is at hand, grasp the tick as close to the skin as possible and pull it off gently, trying not to crush it.
- Examine the tick. If its head and pincers did not come out, soak the area twice a day with warm water until healing is complete.
- Scrub the area thoroughly with soap and water to remove any germs.
- For two to three weeks, watch for reddened skin around the tick bite and for fever, a rash around the ankles and wrists, headaches, and generalized pains and aches. If any of these symptoms occurs, take the youngster to your doctor immediately and tell him about the tick bite.

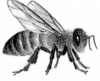

honeybee

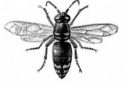

hornet

yellow jacket

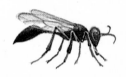

wasp

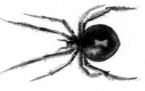

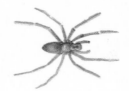

The shiny half-inch body of the black widow spider is marked with a bright red hourglass shape on its underside. The black widow, whose leg span is about two inches, spins its web in dark, sheltered spots such as sheds and woodpiles.

The brown recluse, a brown or tan spider with a body one half inch long and a leg span of one and a half inches, has a dark violin-shaped marking on its back and three pairs of eyes on its head and body. It lives in dark, protected places.

Nonpoisonous spider bites

Common house and garden spiders have venom so weak that their bites, while itchy and sometimes slightly painful, present no risk other than infection from scratching and subsequent scarring. Follow the treatment suggested for insect bites *(left)*.

Poisonous spider bites

Only two kinds of spiders native to the United States — the black widow and the brown recluse — have venom so toxic that their bites constitute emergencies. Seek medical help immediately.

The more dangerous of the spiders is the black widow, easily identified by the red hourglass-shaped marking on its underside *(above, left)*. Its venom, drop for drop, is more potent than that of a rattlesnake. Because of their low body weight, infants and toddlers are especially vulnerable to black-widow bites and may suffer respiratory arrest or even die if they are not treated promptly with antivenom. The venom of the brown recluse spider *(above, right)*, though less potent and slower acting than that of the black widow, is also potentially fatal.

The bites of these spiders produce different symptoms, but they are handled in the same way. If the spider is still in the vicinity, try to identify it before you kill it, taking care not to be bitten yourself. Until you can obtain medical help, take the steps described under "What to do" *(right)* to slow the spread of the venom through the child's system.

Symptoms of a black-widow bite:

- usually mild to moderate pain at the moment the bite is inflicted
- redness around the bite
- painful abdominal cramps, nausea and sweating
- pins-and-needles sensation in the hands and the feet

- in severe cases, breathing difficulty or convulsions

Symptoms of a brown-recluse bite:

- itching, pain, redness and blistering at the site of the spider bite; blister may develop into an open sore within one to two weeks
- chills and fever, nausea and vomiting, pain in the joints within several hours
- general weakness
- rash over much of the body within 24 to 48 hours
- in severe cases, difficulty breathing or convulsions

What to do:

- Call for medical assistance as soon as possible.
- Keep the child calm and still, positioned so that the wounded area is lower than the heart.
- Support a bitten limb with a pillow, coat or towel. Do not let it dangle.
- Place a constricting band between the wound and the heart *(box, page 14)*. Remove it after 30 minutes.
- Watch breathing closely. If it stops, begin artificial respiration immediately *(page 16)*.
- If convulsions occur, loosen the child's clothing but DO NOT restrain his movement. When the seizure subsides, turn the youngster on his side to aid his breathing.

Scorpion stings

Scorpions are close relatives of spiders and, like spiders, may be poisonous or nonpoisonous. The poisonous varieties produce venom that can be fatal to infants and small children. This poison, which is injected by the scorpion's stinger *(below)*, begins to take effect within an hour or two. Scorpion stings are not a widespread problem in the United States, however, since these arachnids are native only to areas of the Southeast and

Southwest; the most dangerous varieties are found in Arizona and New Mexico.

Symptoms:

- pain or tingling sensation at the site of the scorpion sting
- localized swelling
- difficulty swallowing or speaking
- nausea and vomiting
- convulsions or unconsciousness

What to do:

- Apply ice.
- Follow the first-aid procedures that are recommended above for poisonous spider bites.
- Seek medical help immediately.

Animal and human bites

The principal danger of a bite inflicted by an animal is rabies, a disease that is virtually always fatal once symptoms develop, but that can be prevented by inoculations during its incubation period. Many animals, from bats, raccoons and skunks to domestic dogs and cats, are potential rabies carriers. If your child is bitten, make every effort to capture the suspect animal; a medical examination of the animal is the fastest and surest way of determining how the child should be treated.

Bites inflicted by nonrabid animals or by humans may cause profuse bleeding and may become infected.

What to do:

- Taking care not to be bitten yourself, try to confine the animal. Immediately call the local animal-control authorities or the police.
- If the skin has been broken, seek medical help immediately.
- Control the bleeding *(see Cuts and Wounds, page 25)*.
- Wash the wound with soap and water.
- DO NOT apply an antiseptic, ointment or other medication.
- Apply a sterile dressing and secure it with adhesive tape or a bandage.

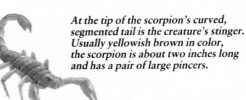

At the tip of the scorpion's curved, segmented tail is the creature's stinger. Usually yellowish brown in color, the scorpion is about two inches long and has a pair of large pincers.

Snake bites

Four kinds of snakes in the United States and Canada are poisonous — copperheads, rattlesnakes, water moccasins and coral snakes. The bites of other snakes are actually no more dangerous than a painful pinch. However, a bite from one of these poisonous snakes constitutes a medical emergency that could result in death and therefore requires immediate action. It is wise to carry along a snakebite kit for emergency use whenever you are in areas that are inhabited by poisonous snakes.

If your youngster is bitten by a snake, examine the wound for fang marks. If there are rows of small tooth marks only, the bite was in all likelihood inflicted by a nonpoisonous snake. Poisonous varieties of snakes have relatively large fangs through which they inject their venom, and the fang marks are usually evident. Baby poisonous snakes, however, may leave tiny fang marks that are difficult to detect, although their bites, too, can be fatal to victims.

If you believe your child may have been bitten by a poisonous snake, get her immediately to a hospital or other medical facility where antivenom can be administered. If you can kill the snake quickly and without endangering yourself, take it with you for identification. Until professional help is at hand, you should follow the steps that are de-

copperhead

rattlesnake

water moccasin

coral snake

Of the poisonous snakes native to the United States, rattlesnakes are scattered most widely. They thrive in many parts of the country, usually in arid regions. Copperheads inhabit rocky, swampy and wooded areas in the central and eastern states. Coral snakes are found throughout the southern states, while water moccasins primarily live in marshy lowlands in the southeastern region.

scribed under "What to do" *(below)* to limit the spread of the snake's venom through the victim's body.

Symptoms of a rattlesnake, copperhead or water-moccasin bite:
- intense pain at the site of the wound
- rapid local swelling
- localized discoloration of the skin
- rapid pulse, shortness of breath and general weakness
- nausea and vomiting
- blurred vision
- shock

Symptoms of a coral-snake bite:
Symptoms may not appear until 12 to 24 hours after the bite.
- slight burning pain at the site of the wound, mild local swelling
- blurred vision, drooping eyelids, speech that is slurred, mental confusion, drowsiness
- increased salivation and sweating
- nausea, vomiting, abdominal pain
- difficulty in breathing
- shock
- paralysis
- convulsions
- coma

What to do:
- Seek emergency medical assistance immediately.
- Keep the youngster calm and still, positioned so that the wound is lower than the heart.
- Immobilize a bitten arm or leg with a splint *(page 17).*

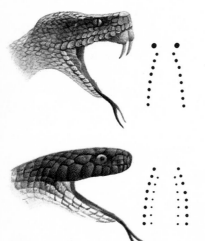

The bite of a poisonous snake (top left) often leaves a pair of large fang marks and two converging rows of small tooth marks in the victim's skin. The bite of a nonpoisonous snake (bottom left) lacks fang marks and is distinguished by four rows of small tooth marks in the victim's skin.

- Treat for shock *(page 38).*
- If the child is not breathing, begin artificial respiration *(page 16).*
- Apply a constricting band *(box, below)* if the bite is on an arm or leg and the youngster develops mild swelling, skin discoloration, moderate pain or tingling sensations around the site of the wound, nausea, vomiting or shortness of breath.
- DO NOT give any medication for pain unless a physician approves it.
- DO NOT apply ice or cold compresses to the bite.

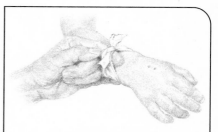

A Constricting Band for Snake or Spider Bites

To make a constricting band that slows the spread of venom from a wound inflicted by a poisonous snake or spider, use a strip of cloth or rubber three quarters to one inch wide. Wrap this band twice around the limb, two to four inches above the wound, and tie a square knot, leaving just enough slack to slip your finger under the band. Loosen the constricting band if the area around it starts to swell. Check the pulse of the area below the band frequently to make sure that you do not cut off blood circulation. DO NOT under any circumstances use a constricting band on the head, neck or trunk.

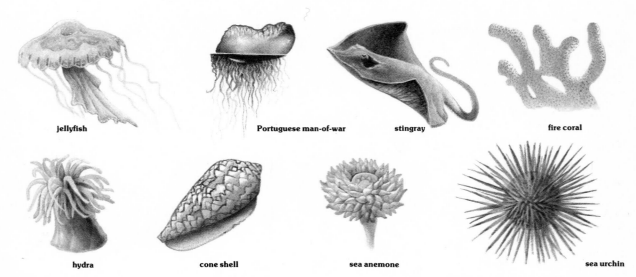

jellyfish   Portuguese man-of-war   stingray   fire coral

hydra   cone shell   sea anemone   sea urchin

Marine stings

Children at the beach may step on or brush against marine creatures that protect themselves with poisonous stings. Reactions to these stings are normally mild but can sometimes be very severe, particularly if the child has an allergic response to the toxin. Always seek a doctor for these stings, if only as a precaution.

In most cases, first aid will include applying an antidote to the venom from the sting. Alcohol and ammonia are antidotes for the venom of jellyfish and the Portuguese man-of-war. Heat inactivates the poisons from sea anemones, hydroids and stingrays. After a stingray attack, you may also have to cope with wounds from the ray's lashing tail or stinging spike.

There are no antidotes to the toxins from cone shells, sea urchins or fire coral. With the first two, you simply slow the flow of toxin to the child's heart and get medical help. Your primary concern with a fire-coral injury will probably be the bleeding that the coral causes, rather than the effects of the venom.

Symptoms of jellyfish or Portuguese man-of-war sting:
- intense, burning pain
- swelling and reddening of the skin
- in a severe case, chills, nausea, backache, breathing difficulty or anaphylactic shock

What to do:
- Gently brush away any clinging tentacles with a towel, taking care to protect your fingers.
- Wash the injury with ocean water.
- Apply alcohol or diluted ammonia.
- If necessary, treat the victim for anaphylactic shock *(page 38)* or breathing difficulty *(page 16)* and seek immediate medical attention.

Symptoms of cone-shell or sea-urchin sting:
- swelling and pain
- dizziness
- in a severe case, numbness around the mouth, difficulty swallowing, shock, temporary paralysis or total collapse

What to do:
- Have the child lie still with the wound positioned lower than the heart.
- Apply a constricting band *(box, left)* above the wound.
- Soak the wound in hot water for 30 minutes, then remove the band.
- For a sea-urchin injury, remove the spines if they come out easily.
- If necessary, treat the child for shock *(page 38)*.
- Seek medical help at once.

Symptoms of sea-anemone or hydroid sting:
- burning pain around the sting
- chills

- stomach cramps and diarrhea

What to do:
- Soak the affected part in hot water for 30 to 60 minutes.
- Seek medical aid at once. Keep soaking on the way to the hospital.

Symptoms of stingray sting:
- lacerations or puncture wounds
- excruciating pain around the sting
- in severe cases, victim may experience dizziness, nausea, muscle spasms, breathing difficulty, convulsions, temporary paralysis or shock

What to do:
- Control the bleeding *(see Cuts and Wounds, page 25)*.
- Remove any visible fragments of the creature's stinger.
- Soak the wound in hot water for 30 to 60 minutes.
- Be prepared to give artificial respiration or treatment for shock.
- Seek emergency medical aid. Keep soaking on the way to the hospital.

Symptoms of fire-coral injury:
- cuts, scrapes and bleeding
- burning pain

What to do:
- Control the bleeding if it becomes heavy; light bleeding may help to remove the toxin.
- Wash with soap and water.
- Seek medical attention. ❖

Breathing Difficulties

Read first

- If the youngster is gasping for air, gagging or coughing, see Choking *(page 23)*.
- If breathing has stopped, give artificial respiration; if the heart has stopped, CPR should be applied at once. Get emergency medi-cal aid for stopped breathing or acute breathing distress.
- Perform resuscitation efforts until victim revives or medical help appears: DO NOT STOP.
- For minor breathing difficulty, contact your physician.

Every parent should be prepared to react quickly to a child's breathing when it is distressed or when the youngster has stopped breathing altogether; this is often the most serious aspect of an emergency situation.

Breathing failure can result from accidents such as drowning *(page 28)*, electric shock *(page 29)* and choking *(page 23)*. If respiration ceases and is not provided artificially, a child can suffer brain damage in four minutes or so and die within about six minutes. Restarting the youngster's breathing, therefore, should take priority over any other form of first aid that you administer.

Long before the need arises, it is important that you learn the technique of artificial respiration *(right)*. A course in cardiopulmonary resuscitation, which is available through your local hospital or American Red Cross chapter, will teach a method for restarting the heart if it has stopped beating.

In an emergency situation, you should check breathing right away: Listen with your ear near the youngster's mouth and nose, and watch for the child's chest rising and falling.

If possible, have another person telephone for help while you try to resuscitate the child. If you are alone, give the youngster artificial respiration or cardiopulmonary resuscitation for several minutes before telephoning for emergency medical help. Then continue your efforts until the victim breathes or medical assistance arrives. If no telephone is nearby,

you should keep trying to revive the child and simultaneously attempt to attract the attention of a passerby.

Stopped breathing is the most critical respiratory emergency, but labored breathing, shortness of breath, or stridor — a harsh whistling or crowing sound — can also become serious enough to require emergency action. These problems accompany some illnesses, such as croup *(page 77)* or pneumonia *(page 81)*, and in these cases you will probably have time to call your doctor for advice. But if the breathing problem comes on quickly, or if the youngster's distress is severe, you should call for an ambulance.

A disease that may create sudden breathing problems is epiglottitis *(page 78)*, a potentially fatal throat infection — marked by fever, sore throat and swelling of the epiglottis — that can block the child's airway within a few hours. If epiglottitis is suspected, the youngster should be taken immediately to a hospital emergency room.

If your child has not been ill but suddenly exhibits stridor, gasps for air, gags or drools, his airway may be obstructed by an object that he has inhaled. If the blockage is severe, however, the youngster may make little or no noise. In either case, you should follow the treatment for choking on page 23.

If the child inhales a small object into the lower airway — the larynx, trachea or

Artificial Respiration

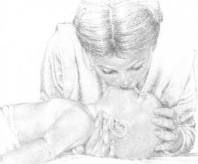 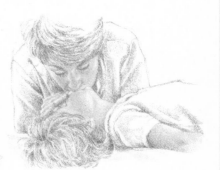

Lay a child younger than a year on his back. Gently lift the neck and tilt the head slightly backward. Check for breathing; if there is none, cover the infant's mouth and nose with your mouth and quickly blow in four puffs of air. If the chest does not rise, retilt the head and give puffs again. If the airway seems blocked, see Choking, page 23. If the chest rises, the airway is clear. Check for a pulse (opposite, top). If there is a pulse, give the infant one puff of air every three seconds; if none is detected, begin CPR.

For a child older than a year, tilt the head back until the chin points straight up. Check for breathing; if there is none, pinch the child's nose closed, then cover the child's mouth with yours and quickly blow in four puffs of air. If the chest does not rise, retilt the head and give puffs again. If the airway seems blocked, see Choking, page 23. If the chest rises, the airway is clear. Check for a pulse (opposite, top). If there is a pulse, give the child one puff of air, just enough to move the chest up and down, every four seconds. If there is no pulse, begin CPR.

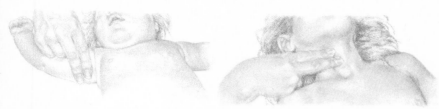

To check the pulse of a baby up to 12 months old, place the tips of two fingers on the inside of his arm between the elbow and the armpit, with your thumb on the outside of the arm; squeeze gently. For an older child, place two fingers on the Adam's apple, then slide them into the groove between the trachea and the neck muscles; press gently. Check for at least five seconds, but no more than 10 seconds, before resuming resuscitation.

lungs — he may seem to recover from the choking episode but then later exhibit pneumonia-like symptoms. In this event, consult your doctor.

Symptoms of stopped breathing:
- no feeling of exhaled breath from the child's mouth and nose
- no rise and fall of the chest
- unconsciousness, bluish gray skin

What to do:
- Begin artificial respiration. Check for a pulse *(page 17)*. If there is no pulse, have someone trained in cardiopul-

monary resuscitation respond.
- Call for emergency medical help; continue rescue efforts until victim revives or help arrives: DO NOT STOP.

Symptoms of distressed breathing:
- labored or shallow breathing, shortness of breath, a whistling or crowing sound when breathing
- breathing difficulty with drooling, gagging, wheezing, leaning forward to breathe, barking cough, agitation

What to do:
- For acute breathing distress, call for

emergency medical assistance. If the youngster's breathing stops, artificial respiration should be administered immediately.
- If symptoms of epiglottitis are present — fever, sore throat, shallow breathing, muffled voice, drooling — the child should be taken to a hospital emergency room.
- If the youngster has trouble breathing but does not appear to be in any immediate danger, you should telephone your physician. ⋮

Broken Bones

Read First

- If there is a possibility of a back or neck injury or if the child is unconscious, do not try to move her. Call for an ambulance.
- Treat life-threatening conditions, such as breathing problems, severe bleeding or shock, first.
- Before moving the child, immobilize injured area without changing its position.
- Do not give the child anything to eat or drink.

Considering their high energy levels and daring natures, it is not surprising that many children suffer broken or dislocated bones sometime during their early years. Fractured wrists, elbows and collarbones, and dislocated elbows and fingers are among the most common.

Fortunately, the softness of children's growing bones means that few of these

injuries are serious and that the vast majority heal quickly. Nonetheless, they do require the care of a doctor, who may have to X-ray the bone to determine the damage and then set it in a cast so it will heal properly.

Symptoms of a fractured bone commonly include pain, swelling, discoloration and, occasionally, visible crookedness. In some cases, however, symptoms will not be obvious: Be alert for other clues, such as the child's reluctance to use the injured limb.

In general, it is best to immobilize the injured limb or joint in the position you find it, using splints or slings fashioned from simple materials *(below and page 18)*. This prevents further damage to nerves and blood vessels while you await medical help. It is also important to keep the child as calm as possible to minimize both pain and the chance of shock.

Naturally, you cannot guard against every potential accident, but anticipating trouble and taking extra precautions may help prevent some. Do not leave an infant

unattended on a bed or changing table, and always make sure your toddler's activities are adequately supervised and that any child is properly secured when riding in a car.

Fractures

Broken bones fall into several categories, but buckling fractures and greenstick fractures are the most common in small children. In a buckling fracture, the bone's outer surface is dented. In a greenstick fracture, the bone bends and cracks but does not break all the way through, because a child's bones are soft and pliable, like the green wood of young trees.

Other categories of broken bones include closed, or simple, fractures, in which the bone is broken but the skin remains intact, and open, or compound, fractures, in which the bone is broken and there is an open wound on the skin caused either by the injury itself or by a piece of bone piercing through.

A broken or dislocated leg bone can be tied to the uninjured leg if a splint is not available. Place padding between the legs and tie them together with cloth strips above and below the injured joint and at intervals from hip to ankle.

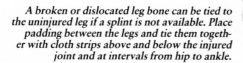

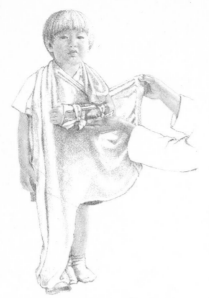

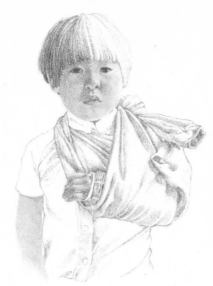

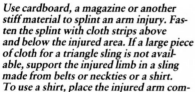

Use cardboard, a magazine or another stiff material to splint an arm injury. Fasten the splint with cloth strips above and below the injured area. If a large piece of cloth for a triangle sling is not available, support the injured limb in a sling made from belts or neckties or a shirt. To use a shirt, place the injured arm com-

fortably across the chest (above, left), then hold it in place by tying the shirt sleeves together at the child's shoulder. Fold excess fabric forward at the elbow and secure it with a safety pin (above). Periodically check for numbness in the fingers to make sure the splint is not too tight. Loosen the ties if necessary.

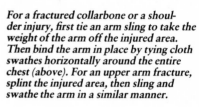

For a fractured collarbone or a shoulder injury, first tie an arm sling to take the weight of the arm off the injured area. Then bind the arm in place by tying cloth swathes horizontally around the entire chest (above). For an upper arm fracture, splint the injured area, then sling and swathe the arm in a similar manner.

Symptoms:
- inability to move the injured limb or digit normally or to put weight on it
- intense pain, numbness or tingling, or loss of pulse in the injured area
- swollen, misshapen or bluish black appearance of affected area
- a snapping sound at the time of the accident, or the child's report that she felt or heard something snap

What to do:
- Treat emergencies first. If the child is bleeding profusely, gently cut away clothing and try to stanch the flow by applying a thick layer of gauze to the wound *(page 25)*.
- Immobilize the injured area in the position you found it with splints or a sling *(above and page 17)*.
- If a fracture is open, or compound, and the bone is protruding through the skin, DO NOT touch it. This may cause infection. Cover the injury with sterile gauze and call an ambulance.
- If the area of a simple, or closed, fracture is swollen, apply a bag of ice wrapped in a towel.

- DO NOT give the child anything to eat or drink.
- Call an ambulance or take the child to a hospital emergency room.

Dislocations

A dislocation occurs when a bone is pulled out of its socket by a sudden, wrenching movement. Ligaments connecting the bone to the socket may also be torn. Many young children suffer dislocated elbows when someone picks them up or swings them by the arm. Or they may dislocate an elbow or finger by falling off playground equipment.

As with fractures, dislocations require prompt medical treatment to realign the bone in its normal position.

Symptoms:
- pain and an inability to move the limb or digit normally
- a swollen or deformed appearance of the injured area

What to do:
- Immobilize the injured area.
- Apply a bag of ice wrapped in a towel.
- Take the child to an emergency room.

Back and neck injuries

In a serious accident, there is the possibility of a back or neck injury. Moving the child is extremely hazardous because damage to the spinal cord could cause paralysis. If the child is unconscious, assume there is a back or neck injury.

Symptoms:
- numbness or weakness in injured area, or trouble moving arms or legs
- loss of bladder or bowel control

What to do:
- Leave the victim where she is and in the bodily position in which you find her. Try to calm the child.
- Immobilize the child's head in the position you find it by placing pillows or rolled-up towels or blankets around the child's neck and shoulders. Do not put anything under the head.
- Call an ambulance.

Splints and slings

Immobilizing an injured body part in the position you find it can help relieve a child's pain and prevent further injury, particularly if she must be transported to the doctor's office or hospital.

Many common household objects can be used as makeshift splints and slings. To splint a broken leg or knee injury, for instance, you can use a broomstick, an umbrella or a piece of cardboard; wrap the object in foam rubber or a towel for padding. Just make sure the splints are long enough to extend past the joints at both ends of the injured part.

Place the splint on the inside of the leg and tie strips of sterile gauze or clean cloth around it just above and below the injured area and then at intervals along the length of the splint. To make sure the ties are not so tight that they constrict circulation or cause nerve damage, you should periodically check to see if the youngster can move her fingers or toes. If she cannot, or if she complains of tingling or numbness, the ties should be loosened immediately.

If no rigid object is available, you can at least partially immobilize an injured leg by splinting it to the other leg *(page 17)*.

Ankles, wrists and knees can be wrapped in pillows or several layers of newspaper and tied in a similar manner. If a knee joint is bent after sustaining an injury, gently try to straighten it. But if this is very painful for the child, it is better to splint it in a bent position.

After splinting an arm injury, tie it in a sling, which can be made by folding a large scarf or handkerchief into a triangle. Place the child's arm at a right angle across her chest and slip the widest part of the scarf under the forearm. Then pass the two ends around the child's neck and tie them in a knot near her shoulder. If no cloth triangle is available, a sling may also be improvised from a belt or necktie. •:•

Bruises

Bruises, the most common of injuries, are usually harmless side effects of an energetic childhood. The baby starting to crawl, the toddler taking her first eager steps, the preschooler running to meet a friend — all are going to meet with bumps and bangs.

When the impact is hard enough to crush tissues beneath the skin, small blood vessels rupture and bleed, and a bruise forms. Since blood under the surface of the skin appears purplish blue, the wound soon develops its familiar black-and-blue color. Within the next two weeks, the blood coagulates and the body absorbs the clot. The bruise then fades to a greenish yellow mark.

While the vast majority of bruises require no more than home care, some do call for medical attention. A child who bruises unusually easily or for no apparent reason may have an illness affecting bleeding and should be examined by a physician. A child with a bruised head should be checked for signs of head injury *(page 32)*. And you should contact your doctor immediately if a fever coincides with a bruise, since this may be a sign of joint or bone infection. Rapid medical attention is also helpful when a fingernail or toenail is pinched and the digit is bruised *(see Finger and Hand Injuries, page 31)*.

Most bruises, however, need little attention. If the collision hurt enough to distract a child from play, you can relieve the pain — and limit the severity of the bruise — by applying a cold cloth or an ice bag and elevating the bruised limb. These measures help because they reduce the flow of blood to the wound.

Symptoms:
- red area on skin from impact, turning black-and-blue within 24 hours
- swelling, tenderness or pain
- greenish yellow color for 10 days to two weeks

What to do:
- Apply cold pack — cloth-wrapped ice or ice bag — for 20 minutes; DO NOT use uncovered ice.
- Raise injured limb above level of child's heart for 10 to 15 minutes for minor bruise; one to two hours for large or severe bruise.
- If skin is broken, treat the wound *(see Cuts and Wounds, page 25)*.
- For bumps to head, apply cold pack and see Head Injuries *(page 32)*.
- If the eye area is bruised (if the child has a black eye), apply cold pack or cloth soaked in cold water.

Call the doctor if:
- the child experiences acute pain.
- moderate pain lasts more than a day.
- a bruised joint becomes swollen.
- the victim has difficulty moving an injured limb, finger or toe *(see Broken Bones, page 17)*.
- the bruise is extensive or severe or if it is near an eye.
- the youngster's fingernail or toenail is damaged *(page 31)*.
- the child's vision is affected.
- a fever coincides with the bruise.
- the child bruises easily, out of proportion to the severity of the blow or for no apparent cause. •:•

Burns

Burns damage or destroy living tissue. The damage can range from superficial injury to destruction of both the skin's surface and its underlying layer, a network of tissues containing blood vessels and nerves. On rare occasions a burn will penetrate to the muscle layer. Heat, certain chemicals and electrical current can all cause burns, opening up the body to infection, one of the chief perils of damaged skin. Burns may also cause loss of body fluids and — if they are extensive — jeopardize vital functions.

The deeper the burn, the more serious it is. First-degree burns affect only the skin's outer layer, healing in a few days. Second-degree burns harm underlying tissues, damaging blood vessels and cells containing water; they heal in one to three weeks. Third-degree burns, which will not heal without medical care, kill all layers of skin, including nerves and regenerative cells. If a child has been badly burned but does not complain of pain, he may have a third-degree burn.

But a large first-degree sunburn can be more serious than a small third-degree burn because so much body fluid is lost to the sun's rays. And burns in certain locations — the hands, feet, face and genitals — can lead to complications unless treated by a doctor. Sometimes extensive burns can stop a child from breathing. So can inhalation of smoke or of gases from burning plastics or other common materials. Always check to determine if an unconscious child who has been involved in a fire is breathing.

Most first- and second-degree burns respond well to prompt treatment. Cold water is the best first aid. By cooling the skin — or washing off harmful chemicals — the water stops further damage to tissues. It also soothes smarting flesh. Immerse the burn at home, and — if medical care is needed — keep the burn moist with cold cloths on the way to a hospital emergency room. Do not immerse third-degree burns unless they are very small. Instead, cover them with cool, wet, sterile compresses.

Butter and margarine, along with other old-fashioned kitchen remedies, may contaminate burned skin and should never be applied to a burn. For a very small, first-degree burn, antibiotic cream provides some protection against infection and alleviates pain.

All burns to babies under two merit at least a call to the doctor. If your toddler or preschooler has a first- or second-degree burn larger than his hand, call your doctor. Even the mildest burn covering more than 10 percent of a child's body — roughly the area of one arm — should be seen by a doctor, as should all burns to critical areas such as the face and genitals. And any child with burns from chemicals or electricity should receive medical care. Whenever a burn is severe — or if you have doubts about how to treat it — get medical help.

Heat Burns

Since running a home involves stoves, irons, boiling liquids and other sources of extreme heat, you naturally take special precautions to protect your young children. Until a child understands that certain things are too hot to touch, she should not be left unattended in a room with anything that can burn her. Keep pot handles turned inward on the stove top, out of the reach of grasping hands. Tell toddlers clearly and often that hot things burn, and illustrate by bringing a child's hand close enough to the stove or radiator so she can feel the heat without being harmed by it.

Most first-degree burns that small children suffer are caused by scalding liquids carelessly left within reach or from a hot-water faucet turned on by a toddler playing unattended in his bath. When contact is prolonged, the hot liquids burn deeper, causing the characteristic blisters and oozing skin of a second-degree burn. You can set the thermostat of your water heater lower to avoid bathtub and hand-washing scalds — but in any case, a very young child should never be left unattended in a bathroom. Matches and flammable substances such as turpentine, of course, must be kept out of the reach of young children. Remember that preschoolers are more mobile and resourceful than toddlers in their quests for forbidden objects.

Safety measures can also prevent sunburn. Although sunburns are caused by ultraviolet rays rather than heat, the skin reacts as it would to burning heat. Most sunburns are superficial, first-degree burns: The skin reddens and is tender, but it does not blister and it does not require a doctor's attention. There are times, though, when a widespread sunburn of this type will cause fever, chills and nausea. And although first-degree heat burns do not cause loss of fluid, sunburn does, because the body loses moisture during exposure to the sun's warmth. Prolonged exposure to strong sunshine can cause second-degree burns, especially in southern latitudes and on fair-skinned children; it can also cause heatstroke *(page 33)*.

Children should be guarded against the sun's rays by a sunscreen lotion and a hat. Infants are particularly vulnerable and should receive no more than 15 minutes of exposure to the hot summer sun in a day. Should a child get too much sun, call your doctor right away. Medication given soon after exposure to the sun can reduce the pain of the burn and speed the healing process.

Symptoms of first-degree burns:
- reddened, tender skin

What to do:
- Quickly remove any clothing that hot liquid has soaked.
- Cool the burn under cold running water, in a basin of cold water or with cold cloths, until the pain stops.
- Pat the burned area dry and protect it with a loose, sterile bandage, if necessary *(right)*.
- For sunburn, have the child soak in a tepid bath and give her plenty of fluids to drink. *(For severe sunburn, see Second-degree burns, below and Heat Exposure, page 33).*
- Give aspirin if a burn is painful, but if the child has recently been exposed to any viral infection, such as chicken pox, flu or a cold, DO NOT use aspirin *(see Reye syndrome, page 105):* Give acetaminophen instead.
- Get medical help if a burn is larger than the child's hand.

Symptoms of second-degree burns:
- reddened, blotchy or streaked skin
- severe pain
- moist, oozing or blistered skin appearing within several hours

What to do:
- Remove wet clothing unless it adheres to the burn. Cool the burned area with water. If it is so small that it does not need medical treatment, bandage it as for a first-degree burn *(above)*. Keep a larger burn covered with a cold, wet compress while taking the child to a physician.
- Give the child plenty of fluids.
- For pain-relief advice, refer to the what-to-do instructions for first-degree burns *(above)*.
- Do not break blisters.
- Seek medical help for burns larger than the child's hand or for burns that blister extensively.

Symptoms of third-degree burns:
- no pain or sensation after initial burn
- blanched or charred skin, looking mottled and pale, red, or blackened

When a child is burned, immediately hold the burned area under cold running water or immerse it in a filled basin until the pain subsides. The cold liquid not only eases the pain by numbing nerve endings, but reduces the damage by removing heat from the body tissue. Bandage small first- and second-degree burns with gauze. Never use fluffy material that might stick to the burn. Wrap the bandage gently but firmly around a burned limb. If the burn is on an area too large to wrap, tape gauze over the burn, making sure the tape is far enough away from the burn that it will not damage the skin when being removed.

- pale, clammy skin; rapid pulse; irregular breathing or any other symptoms of shock

What to do:
- If the child is not breathing, begin artificial respiration *(page 16)* at once. Call for emergency medical help; continue your rescue efforts until the assistance arrives.
- If there is no pulse, have someone

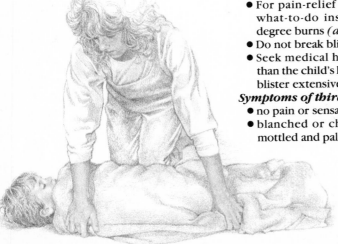

To extinguish blazing clothing, quickly lay the child flat on the ground and smother the fire with a rug, blanket or heavy coat, or with your own body, if necessary. Do not roll the child around. Do not let a panicked child run about, since this will fan the fire.

trained in cardiopulmonary resuscitation respond immediately.
- If necessary, treat the youngster for shock *(page 38)*.
- Remove any constricting clothing that has not stuck to the burn.
- Keep the burn covered with cold, wet cloths while awaiting the arrival of emergency medical personnel or driving to the emergency room.
- DO NOT allow the burned youngster to walk around.
- Avoid giving the child any food, drink or pain-relieving drugs in case surgery is necessary.
- Get emergency medical help as quickly as possible.

Chemical Burns
Chemical burns have much the same effect as heat burns, reddening and blistering the skin. Common household products such as drain cleaner and oven cleaner are caustic chemicals that will burn skin. So will paint stripper and battery acid. If such substances get onto your child's body, flush the affected skin area with water immediately and thoroughly. The chemical will continue to damage the skin as long as any residue remains. Standing the youngster under a running shower is a good way to flush his skin. Powdered lime and other dry chemicals should be brushed off first, since they may do more damage when mixed with water.

To prevent young children from burning themselves with chemicals, avoid keeping harsh compounds around. Buy small containers and read the instructions carefully for warnings. Then use the product immediately and dispose of the container. When you must keep a caustic chemical in the house or the garage, store it out of children's reach.
Symptoms:
- reddened, painful skin
- blisters

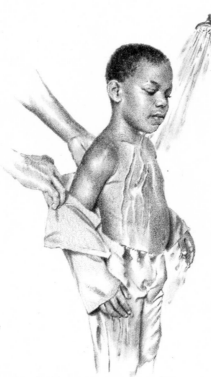

To flush a caustic substance from a child's skin, hold him under a cool shower or spray him with a garden hose. Take care that water mixed with the chemical does not splash into his eyes. Fast action arrests further burning, so remove clothing only after starting the shower. Keep flushing the area with water until all traces of the chemical are gone.

What to do:
- If a chemical has splashed into the child's eye, immediately flush the eye with water *(see Eye injury, page 30)*.
- Rinse the affected skin area by holding it under cool, running water for at least five minutes. If a large area is affected, use a shower. Remove the victim's clothing while flushing the burn.
- DO NOT try to neutralize the chemical without specific instructions from your local or regional poison-control center or a doctor's advice. The infor-

mation on containers is often out of date or incorrect.
- While traveling to the emergency room, keep the wound covered with a clean, moist cloth and continuously douse the cloth with cold water.
- Get emergency medical help for all chemical burns.

Electrical Burns
Anything electrical can produce a burn as well as a shock. As the electric current enters the body, it turns into heat and scorches the skin. Small and harmless-looking burns commonly appear at two sites: the entry and exit points of the current, such as a hand and the feet if the child grasps an electricity source while standing barefoot on a damp floor or other grounding surface. Although the burns may appear superficial, internal tissues may be badly injured. Any child who has been burned by electricity should see a doctor. Burns to a child's mouth, which can occur if a youngster chews a cord that is plugged in, should be examined very carefully. Their appearance — little burns at the corner of the mouth, or chapped-looking lips — can be dangerously deceiving; a major artery in the mouth may be damaged, resulting in profuse bleeding some time later.
Symptoms:
- small, round burns — sometimes, larger burns — at two sites
- chapped-looking lips, when the mouth is involved

What to do:
- If the child is not breathing, begin artificial respiration *(page 16)*. Call for emergency medical help; continue rescue efforts until help arrives.
- If there is no pulse, have someone trained in CPR respond.
- Cover burns loosely with moist, sterile pad or clean cloth.
- Call an ambulance or go to a hospital emergency room right away. ❖

Choking

Read First

- DO NOT interfere if the child can cough, breathe, speak or cry. Coughing is more effective than any help you can give.
- If the child is younger than 12 months and cannot cough, use the rescue procedure shown below.
- If the child is one year or older and cannot cough or speak, use the Heimlich maneuver shown below, right.

- DO NOT pound the back of a choking child who is in an upright position. The object could lodge deeper.
- If the child is not breathing, begin artificial respiration (page 16). Call for emergency medical help; continue rescue efforts until help arrives.
- If there is no pulse, have someone trained in cardiopulmonary resuscitation respond.

Symptoms:
- grasping of throat, gestures of distress
- coughing, high-pitched wheezing
- in more serious cases — inability to breathe, speak, cry or cough; bluish lips, nails or skin

What to do:
- If the child is coughing, do nothing for one minute. Wait to see if the cough gets rid of the obstruction.
- If a child older than 12 months continues coughing uncontrollably or cannot cough or speak, use the child's version of the Heimlich maneuver *(below)*. Use back blows and chest thrusts *(left)* for a younger child.
- If breathing stops, open the child's mouth. If you can see the obstructing object, try to remove it, but be extremely careful not to push it deeper.
- Continue the Heimlich variation or the back blows and chest thrusts until the airway is opened. Then, if breathing does not resume after the object is dislodged, begin artificial respiration.
- Have someone call for emergency help. If alone, call only after several minutes of artificial respiration.
- If heartbeat stops, have someone trained in CPR respond. ❖

Choking, one of the body's defense mechanisms, is triggered by any threat to the airway — such as a piece of food, a toy or some other small object that has lodged in the windpipe. The muscles surrounding the windpipe reflexively contract and the child begins to cough in an effort to dislodge the obstruction. In most cases, the choking mechanism functions smoothly and the child expels the blockage on his own. But sometimes coughing is not enough, and the child requires immediate assistance.

If the child is coughing, watch him for a full minute. He may cough up the object. You should be prepared to act quickly with an antichoking technique, however, if the child continues to cough uncontrollably or if he stops coughing or making sounds altogether.

And if breathing stops, begin artificial respiration *(page 16)* immediately, alternating it with antichoking techniques if necessary. Continue for several minutes before calling for help. If the child is breathing but unconscious, see page 41.

The best treatment for choking is prevention. Keep small objects, plastic bags, balloons and toys with removable parts out of youngsters' reach. Grapes, peanuts, popcorn, hard candy and gum are also potential hazards. Hot dogs — perfect plugs for tiny throats — choke more children than any other food and are best avoided by those under five. When your baby is sick and vomiting, place him on his stomach to reduce the chance of his accidentally choking on vomit.

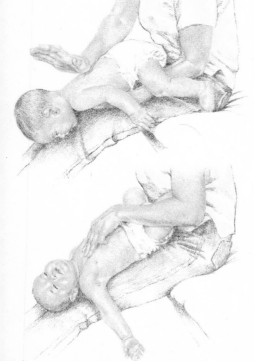

To assist a choking child under 12 months old, tilt the baby face down on your lap and one forearm (top left). With the heel of your other hand, give four sharp blows between the shoulder blades. If choking continues, turn the baby over. Place two or three fingertips on the breastbone and press down smoothly but quickly four times (bottom left). If the object is not expelled, turn the baby over and give four more back blows. You should repeat the sequence until the object is dislodged.

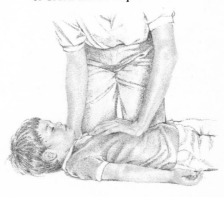

For a child over one year old, use this variation of the Heimlich maneuver: Lay the child on his back, then put the heel of your hand on his midsection between the navel and the rib cage (below). Give six to 10 rapid thrusts — pressing sharply inward and upward — until the object is expelled. Then administer artificial respiration if the child is not breathing or CPR if there is no pulse.

Convulsions and Seizures

Read First

- Remain calm. A seizure can be serious, but it is rarely a life-threatening condition.
- Clear an area around the convulsing child.
- DO NOT restrain the child except when necessary to prevent serious self-injury.
- DO NOT put anything in the youngster's mouth.

- DO NOT give the child anything to eat or drink.
- DO NOT throw water in the youngster's face.
- DO NOT put the child in the bathtub, even if the purpose is to lower a fever.
- If you suspect the child's convulsion is caused by poisoning, see page 36.

A seizure, or convulsion, is a series of involuntary muscle spasms caused by a short circuit in the brain. It can be frightening for a parent to watch, but a seizure is rarely life-threatening and often is not even serious. Most seizures last only five minutes and usually have no permanent effect on the youngster.

Your help for a convulsing child is limited to preventing the youngster from injuring herself or choking. Once the seizure is over, you should call your doctor, who will probably ask you for a complete description of what happened and may want you to bring the youngster in for an examination.

Most seizures in children under the age of six are brought on by fever. Such episodes are called febrile seizures and can be triggered by a temperature as relatively low as 101° F. Occasionally, the fever is an indication of a potentially serious infection of the brain or spinal cord, such as encephalitis or meningitis. Other things that cause seizures in children include poisoning and head injuries. Or the youngster may suffer from a recurrent seizure disorder for which the cause is not clear — a condition that is referred to as epilepsy.

Most febrile seizures are of the grand mal, or generalized, variety and present the classic symptoms *(right),* including falling to the floor, eyes rolling back and uncontrolled shaking. When the sei-

zure is over, the youngster may fall into a deep sleep; when she awakes later, she may feel confused. As long as the child's breathing is normal, the sleep is not a cause for concern and you should not attempt to rouse the child. Instead, gently place the youngster in the recovery position *(below)* and notify your physician immediately.

Petit mal seizures, on the other hand, are characterized by brief lapses of consciousness, usually lasting less than 15 seconds. Unless you are watching closely, you might not even know the youngster is having a seizure. She may only drop whatever she is holding or stop talking in mid-sentence and stare blankly ahead. A susceptible child may suffer many such disturbances in a day, or she may experience only one or two a month. There is nothing you can do to help the youngster during such a seizure, but you should call it to the attention of your physician. Some petit mal seizures can be traced to various neurological disorders, while the causes of others remain unknown. Nevertheless, the condition usually disappears by the time a youngster reaches puberty. *(See also Seizure disorders, page 106.)*

Symptoms of grand mal seizures:
- a collapse of the child to the floor
- eyes rolling upward
- foaming at the mouth
- stiffness that is followed by uncon-

trolled, jerking body movements
- sometimes, the loss of bladder or bowel control
- in febrile seizures — temperature of 101° F. or higher
- in more serious cases — breathing impairment, signaled by blue lips and heavy breathing

What to do:
- Clear away any objects that could injure the convulsing child.
- Loosen any tight clothing around her neck and waist.
- Turn the youngster's head to one side to keep the airway open and to prevent her from choking on saliva or vomit, but DO NOT restrain the child's movements in any way.
- If the child is not breathing, begin artificial respiration *(page 16).* Call for emergency medical help; continue rescue efforts until help arrives.
- Once the seizure is over, place the youngster in the recovery position *(below).* She will probably want to sleep and you should let her as long as her breathing is not impaired.
- If the seizure was caused by fever, undress the child and sponge her off with tepid water to lower her temperature and prevent a second seizure. DO NOT put the child in the bathtub, where another seizure could result in the aspiration of water.
- Notify your doctor that the child has suffered a seizure. ❖

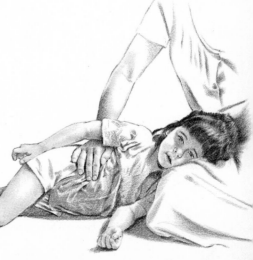

Once a seizure is over, turn the child on her side, in what is called the recovery position, with her head in your lap. This will keep her from choking on saliva or vomit. Allow her to sleep if she is breathing normally.

Cuts and Wounds

Read First

- Stop the bleeding by applying direct pressure on the wound. If bleeding does not stop after 15 minutes, press harder.
- Check for additional injuries to the child, including fractures and internal bleeding.
- NEVER remove an object that has impaled the body. Immobilize the object and take the child to a hospital emergency room.
- NEVER use a tourniquet unless every other method for controlling bleeding has failed.
- Treat for shock (page 38), if necessary. Lay the child on his back with his legs higher than his head and wrap him in a coat or blanket while waiting for emergency help to arrive.
- careful not to stop the circulation.
- Treat the youngster for shock (page 38) if necessary.
- Seek medical attention.

Symptoms of internal bleeding:
- frothy blood that is coughed up from the lungs
- vomited blood that is dark or bright red and that has the consistency of coffee grounds
- blood in the child's stools or urine
- shock, signaled by cold, clammy skin; pallor; restlessness and rapid pulse

What to do for internal bleeding:
- Treat for shock (page 38).
- Turn the child's head to one side to keep the airway open.
- Seek emergency medical attention.
- DO NOT give anything to drink.

Severe bleeding

For nearly all children, occasional cuts and scrapes are an inevitable part of growing up. Such injuries will involve a small amount of bleeding, which should stop by itself in a short time. But a large laceration or puncture wound can cause severe bleeding and, if untreated, can lead quickly to shock and unconsciousness. Fortunately, in almost every case you can stop the flow of blood.

Simply apply direct pressure until the bleeding stops, then bandage the wound and seek medical attention. In some cases, you can help matters by elevating the wound above the level of the heart (near right). Only in the most critical emergency — when life is imperiled and every other effort has failed — should you apply a tourniquet to a bleeding limb, because it may cause the loss of the limb. After any laceration or puncture wound, make sure your child's tetanus shots are up to date: He will need a booster if it has been five years since his last injection.

A child who suffers a sharp blow or has part of his body crushed by something heavy may experience internal bleeding as well, and this calls for immediate medical attention. Warning signs are blood coughed up from the lungs or blood that is vomited or passed in the urine or bowel movements. A child who has had a serious accident and is bleeding from the nose or ears may have suffered a frac-

tured skull (page 32). DO NOT move the child; call for emergency help.

What to do for external bleeding:
- You should press a sterile gauze pad or any clean cloth against the wound until the bleeding stops. Press hard for 15 minutes. If the bleeding continues — or if blood soaks through the cloth — add more gauze or cloth and press harder until the bleeding stops.
- Elevate the wound above the level of the heart; maintain direct pressure.
- Only if the situation is critical — such as a severed limb or sustained gushing bleeding that will not slow under direct pressure — should you apply a tourniquet (below, right). Then note the time, to keep track of how long circulation is cut off, and get the child to a hospital immediately.
- Once you have the bleeding under control, bandage the wound firmly enough to maintain pressure but be

Abrasions

In falls, a child often experiences injuries that rub off the top layer of skin, leaving a raw area exposed underneath. Normally, there is not much bleeding from these scrapes, or abrasions, although the wound can be painful, since millions of nerve endings may be left exposed. A

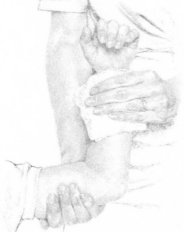

To stem severe bleeding in an arm or a leg, hold the injured limb higher than the heart and apply direct pressure to a pad of gauze or a clean cloth held on the wound. Do not lift a limb if a bone is broken.

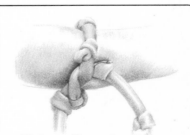

Using a Tourniquet

A tourniquet should only be used when bleeding is so profuse that it threatens the child's life and all other methods of stopping it have failed. Use rubber surgical tubing or rope that has been knotted every inch along its length. Wrap the tubing or rope around the injured limb ½ inch above the wound, tie a half-knot and pull tight until the bleeding stops. Note the time that you apply the tourniquet. Leave it in place until you reach the hospital.

scrape seldom requires a doctor's attention and it is easily treated at home. Make sure, however, that you remove any dirt or grit from the scrape to prevent subsequent infection or scarring.

Symptoms:
- superficial injury that scrapes off the upper layer of skin
- little bleeding, perhaps no bleeding at all from some parts of the abrasion

What to do:
- Wash the wound with soap and water to remove any dirt or other debris.
- Stop any bleeding by applying direct pressure over the wound.
- Apply an antibiotic ointment, then cover with a sterile bandage.
- Watch for signs of infection, including fever or pus, swelling, tenderness or reddening around the scrape.

Call the doctor if:
- you notice any signs of infection.
- the injury bleeds profusely or is deeper than the full thickness of the skin.
- your child needs a tetanus booster.

Cuts and lacerations

Cuts and lacerations are injuries that slice

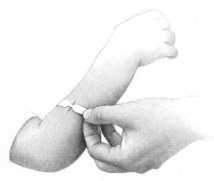

Butterfly strips are helpful in treating many cuts. To use them, draw the edges of the cut together and place one or more strips across the wound, holding it closed. You should keep the injury bandaged until it has completely healed.

To remove a fishhook that is not deeply imbedded in the skin and is not on the face, push the hook through the flesh in the direction it entered until the barb protrudes from the skin. Use wire cutters or pliers to snip off the barb, then pull the shank back out. Clean and dress the wound, then consult your doctor.

or tear the skin, often causing bleeding and tissue damage beneath the skin. Broken glass, knives, razor blades and other sharp objects are typical culprits.

Most minor cuts can be treated safely at home. However, if the cut is more than superficial or involves severe bleeding, you should seek medical attention. Any cut on the face or a wide, gaping laceration elsewhere on the body also should be seen by a doctor. Suturing may be necessary in such cases to close the wound, prevent undue scarring or repair damaged muscles and tendons.

Cuts usually heal within a week. If stitches are necessary, they usually have to be removed in three to 14 days, depending on the size and location of the cut. (Some stitches are self-dissolving.)

A cut should not be painful for longer than 12 to 18 hours. If it is — or if you notice any signs of infection — contact your doctor promptly.

Symptoms:
- a break in the skin of any size or depth
- bleeding

What to do:
- Stop the bleeding using direct pressure on the wound.
- Thoroughly wash the area surrounding the wound with soap and water.
- Apply hydrogen peroxide to further cleanse the wound and then use butterfly strips, if necessary, to close the wound *(left)*.
- Cover the cut or laceration with a sterile bandage.
- Watch for such signs of infection: fever; pus, swelling or tenderness; red-

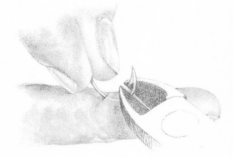

dening around the wound; or red streaks branching out from it.

Call the doctor if:
- the cut is on the face, or if it extends through the full thickness of the skin to the bone or tissue beneath.
- the cut involves serious bleeding.
- any signs of infection appear.
- the child needs a tetanus booster.

Puncture wounds

Puncture wounds, small holes that penetrate to the tissue underlying the skin, are caused by sharp objects. For children, the most likely offenders are nails, knives, needles, splinters and fishhooks. Animal bites *(page 12)* are another common cause of puncture wounds and should be seen by a doctor.

Shallow puncture wounds and many fishhook injuries can be treated at home. You should always be alert for signs of subsequent infection, however. A puncture wound in the chest, abdomen or any of the joints — or a fishhook injury to the eye or face — should be considered an emergency requiring immediate medical attention. In such cases, do not move or remove the puncturing object — this might cause additional damage or bleeding. Instead, immobilize the object by padding it into place with bulky wrappings of gauze or cloth and take the child to the nearest emergency room. Puncture wounds in the hands must also be treated with special caution because here they pose a greater risk of infection, which can sometimes permanently impair the use of a hand.

The kinds of objects that cause puncture wounds may harbor the bacteria that are responsible for tetanus. You should make certain that your child's inoculations are up to date.

What to do for shallow puncture wounds:

- Encourage bleeding with gentle pressure to help clean the wound.
- Wash the wound thoroughly with soap and water, or soak the affected limb in a bowl of warm, soapy water.
- Inspect the wound to see that no foreign matter remains under the skin, then cleanse with hydrogen peroxide and cover with a sterile bandage.

- Check the wound at least twice a day for signs of infection, including pus, swelling, tenderness, reddening or red streaks around the affected area.
- To keep the wound clean, soak it in warm water two or three times a day for 15 minutes. Continue this treatment for a couple of days.

What to do for deep wounds:

- DO NOT remove the object that has caused the wound. Immobilize it with wrappings of gauze or cloth, then apply pressure to the area around it to stop the bleeding.
- Go immediately to an emergency room. En route to the hospital, keep the wounded part of the body elevated above the level of the heart.
- Make sure the youngster's tetanus shots are up to date.

- Notify a physician if any signs of infection appear later.

Severed digit or limb

Accidental amputations of toes, limbs or fingers — though rare — are frightening. But try to stay calm: If you can get the victim and the severed part to an emergency room quickly enough, doctors may be able to reattach the limb or digit and restore its use. First, stop the bleeding. Then wrap the severed part in a clean dressing and put it in a plastic bag. Place that bag inside a second one packed with ice, or wrap the bag containing the body part in towels and place it in a container of ice. Do not freeze the severed part or immerse it in water, alcohol or any other liquid. Call an ambulance or take the child to a hospital emergency room. ❖

Delirium

When your child has a fever or is taking strong medication, her brain's metabolism may become temporarily disturbed, causing delirium — a condition in which the victim suddenly becomes disoriented and confused and sometimes suffers some loss of judgment and memory. Delirium itself is not harmful to a youngster, but the condition may be a symptom of an underlying ailment that requires the attention of a doctor.

In children, one common cause of delirium is high fever from an infection — pneumonia or meningitis, for example. Certain medicines, such as those doctors prescribe for asthma and hay fever, can trigger a reaction resulting in delirium. So can lead poisoning and ingestion of household solvents (see Poisoning, page 36). Reye syndrome (page 105), a serious complication of some viral infec-

tions, can also cause delirium. Another cause of the condition is sudden, acute pain, such as the kind that comes from breaking a bone. And occasionally a head injury (page 32) is severe enough to produce delirium.

If your child shows signs of delirium, contact your doctor immediately. Depending on the underlying cause, he will decide whether you should take the youngster to the hospital. Whatever the reason for the disturbance, you should stay with your child and remain calm and reassuring. A treasured stuffed animal or a favorite blanket may also help the youngster feel secure.

Symptoms:

- slipping in and out of contact with the real world
- incoherence, difficulty remembering and understanding, limited attention

- nervous, aimless or excited activity
- disrupted sleep pattern
- trembling, lack of coordination
- hallucinations
- exaggerated emotional reactions

What to do:

- Get in touch with your child's physician immediately.
- If the child has a high fever, try to reduce it (page 94).
- Note any medication that the youngster is taking.
- Attempt to determine if the youngster has ingested a nonprescribed drug or a poison, such as a household solvent.
- Avoid giving anything by mouth; this can cause choking.
- Remain with the youngster, remind her that she is safe and assure the child that she will soon stop feeling strange and confused. ❖

Drowning

Drowning, in which water in the lungs deprives a victim of life-sustaining oxygen, is a major cause of accidental death among children. Most drownings occur in backyard swimming pools, but they can also take place in wading pools, bathtubs or any other place where water is a few inches deep.

When a child takes in enough water that it halts breathing, you must immediately get air into his lungs, rather than worry about getting the water out. Refer to page 16 for detailed instructions on mouth-to-mouth resuscitation. If the interruption of breathing causes the heart to stop as well, have someone trained in cardiopulmonary resuscitation apply that procedure, and summon emergency help immediately. Once breathing is restored, get the child to a hospital. Complications such as pneumonia can follow a near-drowning incident.

The only effective protection against drowning is close and constant supervision of children near water. If small children play unattended by a pool, one of them is likely to fall in sooner or later.

What to do:

- Watch the child's chest, and place your ear near his mouth and nose to feel and listen for breathing: If he is gasping for air, lay him face down to let the water drain from his mouth.
- If the child is not breathing, begin artificial respiration *(page 16)*. Call for emergency medical help; continue rescue efforts until help arrives.
- If the youngster has no pulse, have someone trained in cardiopulmonary resuscitation respond.
- When the youngster's breathing resumes, place him on his side to let the water drain from his mouth. Cover the child with a blanket or coat.
- If the water was very cold, treat the child for hypothermia *(page 33)*, a lowering of body temperature. Take off his wet clothing and wrap him in blankets in a warm room.
- Call for emergency assistance. ❖

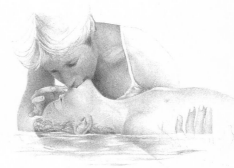

Begin mouth-to-mouth resuscitation as soon as you reach the child, even while still in the water, if you can manage it there. Give one puff every three seconds to an infant, one every four seconds for an older child.

Ear Injuries

Cuts on the ear

Cuts and lacerations on the ear are common in small children. Control the bleeding with direct pressure on the wound *(page 29, top)*. Keep the child sitting up or raise his head with pillows. A detached piece of the ear flap should be treated in the same way as a severed finger or toe *(see Cuts and Wounds, page 27)* and taken to the hospital with the child.

Discharge from the ear

Discharge from the ear always requires a doctor's attention. The most serious possible cause — and the least likely — is a heavy blow to the head that fractures the skull and sends blood or a clear fluid out the ear canal *(see Head Injuries, page 32)*. More often, the discharge is white or yellow and signals that an eardrum has been ruptured by the pressure of pus from a middle-ear infection. The rupture probably will heal on its own, but the infection should be treated promptly. A

To stop bleeding from a cut or laceration on the outer ear, apply light, even pressure with a pad of gauze on the wound. Hold the compress in place with one bandage over the top of the child's head and a second bandage around his forehead. Do not attempt to stop bleeding from the ear canal itself; instead, get medical help.

white, cheesy discharge usually means an outer-ear infection.

If the discharge is yellow to brown in color and has a foul-smelling odor, it may be caused by an insect or some small object that has become trapped in the youngster's ear canal.

What to do:
- Place a cotton ball or a wad of gauze loosely in the youngster's ear. DO NOT block the drainage.
- Have the child lie on his side with the affected ear down or have him sit up with the ear cushioned on his shoulder, and take him to see a doctor.

Foreign objects in the ear
Some toddlers like to put things in their ears. They seem inspired by the discovery of objects just the right size for the opening: peanuts, raisins and beads, for example. Insects, too, occasionally get into an ear — and drive the child to distraction with their buzzing.

You can quiet a bug by dripping a few drops of oil into the ear — mineral oil, baby oil, even cooking oil will do. But unless the insect or other object is in plain view, where it is easy to grasp, ask your doctor to remove it. Otherwise you might make matters worse by pushing the object farther into the ear or by damaging the eardrum.

Symptoms:
- pain in the ear
- a movement or buzzing inside the ear
- sometimes, a foul-smelling discharge

What to do:
- In most cases, take the child to a doctor to have the object removed.
- DO NOT try to flush an object out of the ear using copious amounts of liquid. Flushing is dangerous if the child's eardrum has been perforated by an infection; in addition, the fluid you use to flush the ear may cause a trapped object to swell.
- DO NOT allow the child to thump her head to dislodge the object. ❖

Electric Shock

Read First
- Before touching the child, cut off the current or separate the youngster from its source *(below)*. If the child has stopped breathing, give artificial respiration *(page 16)*. If the heart has stopped, cardiopulmonary resuscitation should be applied immediately.
- Treat for shock *(page 38)*, keeping the victim warm with a blanket or coat.
- Seek emergency medical help for the child immediately.

If an electric current passes through a child's body, it may just knock the youngster down, but it can also leave him unconscious or even halt his breathing or heartbeat. And though signs of electrical burns may be minor on the skin, there is sometimes widespread burn damage to underlying tissue *(page 22)*.

Before you touch the child, be certain his body is no longer conducting live current. If he is still touching an electrical cord or appliance, quickly pull out the plug, turn the current off at the circuit-breaker panel or fuse box, or otherwise break the child's contact with the current. Be aware of the possibility of electrical shock if you discover your child collapsed; look first before helping.

What to do:
- Turn off the current or move the child away from its source without putting yourself at risk; use a nonmetallic object to move the victim.
- If the child is not breathing, begin artificial respiration *(page 16)*. Call for emergency medical help; continue rescue efforts until help arrives.
- If there is no pulse, have someone trained in CPR respond.
- Treat for shock *(page 38)*.
- Treat any burns as a serious third-degree injury. Wrap the area lightly with gauze and seek medical help. ❖

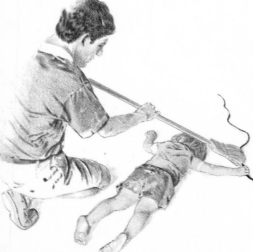

Separate an electric-shock victim from the source of the current by pushing the two apart with a broom or any other dry, nonmetallic implement. Be careful not to touch the child in the process.

Eye Injuries

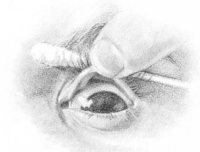

To expose the top portion of the eye, place the stem of a cotton-tip applicator across the upper eyelid. With a thumb or finger, carefully pull the upper eyelid up and over the stem of the applicator.

Chemical burns

Most chemical burns to the eye result from splattered cleaning fluids and detergents. Keep children well out of the way when you are using these substances. If a chemical does get splashed into a child's eye, the eye will usually look watery and red. In severe cases the cornea — the clear surface over the colored portion of the eye — may turn a dull white.

What to do:

- Immediately flush the eye with generous amounts of tap water *(below)*. Continue flushing for 10 minutes. If you are unable to calm the child, you may have to restrain her while washing the eye: It is essential that the chemical be completely removed.
- Cover the eye with a pad of gauze taped loosely in place.
- Take the child to an emergency room.
- DO NOT let the child rub the eye.

Cuts and blows

Cuts and bruises on the eyes or the face around the eyes are not always as serious as they look, but they should be treated with caution. A black eye should always be seen by a doctor. To assess the severity of an injury, first quiz the child about loss of vision — the surest sign of a serious problem. Then examine the eyeball itself, looking for cuts on its surface. Never force open an eye that is swollen shut.

What to do for cuts:

- Cover the injured eye with a gauze pad taped loosely in place.
- Take the child to a doctor or an emergency room, keeping him in a semi-reclining position en route.
- DO NOT let the youngster touch or press on the eye.

What to do for blows to the eye:

- Have the youngster lie on his back with his eyes closed.
- Cover the eye with an ice pack or a washcloth soaked in cold water.
- Consult the child's doctor.

Foreign objects in the eye

When your child gets something in his eye, you should remove the foreign matter promptly or it may become embedded or scratch the surface of the eyeball. The usual mishaps — stray eyelashes, or cinders, dust or sand in the eye — will often take care of themselves as tears form and wash the foreign matter away. If not, remove such loose objects by dabbing them out with the corner of a clean handkerchief; sometimes you will need to lift the top eyelid as shown above. Other techniques for cleansing an eye are listed at right. Always wash your hands before examining or treating an eye. And do your best to be calm, since you will need to have your child's cooperation.

If the object cannot be removed easily, it may already be embedded in the eye's surface. In that case, take the young-

ster to a doctor or an emergency room.

Symptoms:

- teary eyes, redness
- a burning sensation
- blurred vision
- sensitivity to light

What to do for a loose object:

- Ask the youngster to blink repeatedly to produce tears.
- Pull the upper lid down over the lower lid and hold it for a few moments.
- If these steps fail, wash the eye with water from an eyecup or eyedropper.

What to do for an embedded object:

- To protect the eye, cover it with a gauze pad taped loosely in place.
- DO NOT try to remove the object. Let a doctor do it.

Heat burns

Heat burns to an eye can be caused by spattered grease from the stove or by a cinder from an open fire. Unless the burn is obviously deep, flush the eye quickly with water *(left)*. If the burn was caused by a cinder, examine the eye and, if necessary, dab the cinder out with the corner of a clean handkerchief. Cover the eye with a gauze pad, then take the child to a doctor. If the burn is deep, do not put water in the eye. Cover with gauze and go immediately to an emergency room. •:•

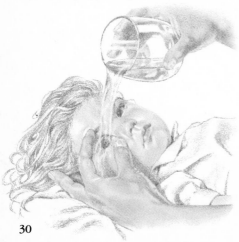

For chemical or heat burns, bend the youngster sideways over a sink so that the injured eye is lower than the healthy eye. Hold the injured eye's lids open with your fingers and flood the eye continuously with cool water for at least 10 minutes.

Finger and Hand Injuries

Treat most hand and finger injuries at home as you would any other cut, bruise or burn. But bear in mind that the nerves, muscles and blood vessels of the hand are so important and vulnerable that hand injuries need special scrutiny.

Probably the most common hand injury is a smashed fingertip followed within hours by a painful bruise beneath the nail. A small bruise less than a quarter of the size of the fingernail will disappear within a few weeks. If painful pressure builds up under the nail, a doctor can relieve it by making a hole in the nail. A torn nail should be trimmed, then taped in place until the new nail grows in. Treat toenail injuries the same way.

Compare the appearance and range of motion of a hurt finger or hand to the uninjured one. Discrepancies such as swelling, a slightly bent finger or restricted motion should be evaluated by a doctor. Because the growth of a child's bones and tendons magnifies any disability, even apparently minor injuries to a hand or finger may require a cast.

Infections can travel along tendon sheaths from the fingers into the wrist and forearm. If diffuse pain, redness, heat or swelling extends up a finger or into the palm, visit the doctor within the day, before the infection can erode the tendons or bone. Also see a doctor if the fingertips or the cuticle areas around the fingernails become swollen and infected: They must be drained promptly. ❖

Frostbite

Frostbite is the freezing of skin tissue. It usually affects extremities, such as the hands, feet, ears and nose. It ranges from relatively minor first-degree frostbite to third-degree frostbite, which can lead to permanent death of tissue, or gangrene. In rare cases, this requires amputation of the affected tissue.

In cold weather, dress your child warmly and supervise his outdoor play — especially in high winds. Children are more susceptible than adults to frostbite because they have poorer circulation .

Symptoms:
- First-degree frostbite — red skin and a stinging or burning sensation

- Second-degree frostbite — mottled or blistered gray skin; pins-and-needles sensation leading to numbness
- Third-degree frostbite — waxy-white skin, hard to the touch and numb

What to do:
- For third-degree frostbite, seek emergency assistance immediately.
- For first- or second-degree frostbite, gradually thaw the area in warm water (not over 110° F.).
- If you cannot get indoors, warm the frozen area by holding it in your hand or tucking it into your armpit.
- Do not let the child sit by a radiator or a fire. If the affected area is numb, he may be burned without realizing it.
- Separate frostbitten toes and fingers with gauze; cover broken blisters.
- Keep in mind that as the skin thaws it may become swollen and painful.
- Offer warm drinks.
- After warming the frostbitten area, call your doctor. ❖

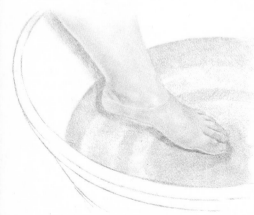

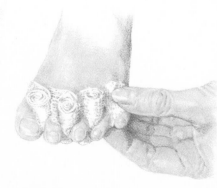

Treatment for frostbitten hands or feet includes soaking them in warm water and separating the digits with sterile gauze.

31

Head Injuries

Your immediate concern in the case of a head injury is whether the child has been hit hard enough to cause a skull fracture or a concussion — injuries that might cause damage to the brain itself. But try to keep in mind that the vast majority of head injuries turn out to be minor. You will probably be amazed at how resilient your child's head is. And if the damage is serious, your child will look and act unmistakably sick.

Cuts and bruises

Head wounds tend to bleed profusely because there are so many tiny blood vessels just under the skin. Bruises that do not break the skin may swell up quickly into goose eggs because of bleeding under the scalp. As a result, such injuries often look more serious than they really are. A youngster who suffers a blow to the head may vomit or be sleepy or irritable for a while. If his behavior returns to normal within a few hours, chances are the child is fine.

Symptoms:
- bloody cut or large goose-egg bump
- temporary headache, dizziness, drowsiness or vomiting

What to do:
- Gently apply pressure to the wound to stop the bleeding.
- Apply ice to reduce swelling.
- If a cut on a youngster's head is gaping or if it does not stop bleeding after several minutes, call the doctor. The wound may need stitches.

Concussion

A concussion occurs when the brain strikes the inside of the skull hard enough to leave the child dazed or even unconscious. In most cases of concussion, the damage is relatively mild and the youngster recovers within a day or two. In other cases — sometimes called contusions — tiny blood vessels inside the brain can break, forming a clot underneath the skull. Then the child may require medication or surgery to remove the clot. If the doctor is uncertain about the extent of damage, she may hospitalize your youngster for observation.

Symptoms:
- possible loss of consciousness
- repeated vomiting, pale appearance, severe headaches
- sleepiness, difficulty in rousing
- inability to walk
- loss of memory about the accident
- pupils that appear uneven in size and do not shrink when you shine a penlight at them *(right)*

What to do:
- Call the doctor immediately if your child presents any of the above symptoms after banging his head.
- Observe your youngster closely for at least six hours after the accident, since signs of concussion do not always show up right away.
- If the child goes to sleep, rouse him every hour. If he does not awaken, make sure he is breathing and call for emergency help.

- Do not give the youngster food or drink for several hours, since this may cause him to vomit.

Skull Fracture

Like concussions, skull fractures may be minor or serious. Many small fractures go undetected and heal themselves within a few months. In others cases, however, the crack may be severe enough for cerebrospinal fluid to escape. Or a piece of skull bone may have been dented into the brain. Such cases may require surgery, and the doctor may prescribe antibiotics to prevent infection of the brain itself. It is next to impossible to positively determine whether the skull has been fractured without getting an X-ray. When in doubt, call the doctor.

Symptoms:
- same as for concussion, plus:
- secretion of fluid from the ears or from the nose
- bruised appearance around the eyes or behind the ears
- indentation in the skull

What to do:
- Contact the doctor immediately if your child exhibits any of the above symptoms of a skull fracture.
- If no symptoms appear right away, watch the youngster closely and follow the other instructions for a concussion *(previous entry).* ❖

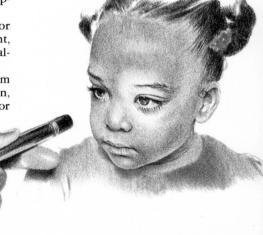

One way to check for a possible concussion is to shine a penlight at your child's eyes in a darkened room. If the pupils do not contract normally, the youngster may have suffered a concussion.

Heat Exposure

Read First

- Check for symptoms of heat-stroke: a temperature higher than 104° F.; dry, flushed skin; and a strong, rapid pulse.
- If these symptoms appear, you should immediately take steps to lower your child's temperature. Remove the youngster's clothing and either place him in a tub of cool water; spray him with a hose; wrap him in a cool, wet sheet; or sponge him down with cool water until his temperature drops to 102° F.
- Then get the child to a hospital. Continue to fan the child or cool him with air conditioning on the way there.

The effects of heat exposure range from cramps and dizziness to heatstroke, which is a life-threatening emergency. Heat cramps — pains in the lower extremities and abdomen — and the more serious heat exhaustion, marked by dizziness and pale, clammy skin, are caused by the loss of water and salt through sweating. The best treatments for these ailments are rest, a cool environment and drinking fluids — water, juice or a glucose drink such as Gatorade ®.

These milder forms of heat exposure are characterized by sweating and a normal body temperature, while heatstroke — much more dangerous — is signaled by dry, red skin and a drastic climb in the body's temperature. Heatstroke occurs when the body's temperature-regulating mechanism is overwhelmed. Heatstroke can lead to brain damage or death if it is not treated quickly. If your youngster exhibits symptoms of heatstroke, you should cool the child immediately by any means available.

Symptoms of heat stroke:
- very hot, dry, red skin
- body temperature over 104° F.
- no sweating
- strong, rapid pulse
- fainting, convulsions or unconsciousness

What to do:
- Lower the child's temperature immediately. Remove his clothing and either place him in a bathtub of cool water; spray him with a hose; wrap him in a cool, wet sheet; or sponge him down with cool water.
- Call an ambulance or take the youngster to the hospital, continuing to cool him on the way there.
- If the child is thirsty, give him plenty of fluids, but not anything containing alcohol or caffeine. ❖

Hypothermia

Read First

- Remove wet clothing and wrap the child in blankets.
- Always try to warm up a child afflicted by the cold, even if he appears dead.
- Seek medical help at once.

Extremely low body temperature (hypothermia) is a life-threatening emergency that requires immediate medical help. Prolonged exposure to cold air or water can lower body temperature dangerously, especially in small children, who are more susceptible to hypothermia than adults. A hypothermia victim may not feel cold and may claim to be fine. However, he will suffer a gradual physical and mental deterioration as his respiratory and circulatory systems slow down. Since advanced hypothermia can mimic death, never give up if you come upon a child who seems lifeless; continue efforts to warm him until you can get help.

Symptoms:
- body temperature below 95° F.; skin cold to the touch
- slow or slurred speech, no control of hands and feet, drowsiness, confusion
- in infants — no crying; red color appearing in cheeks, nose and limbs; weak sucking action when baby is fed
- in advanced stages — muscle spasms or rigidity, inability to use arms or legs, sometimes unconsciousness

What to do:
- Remove wet clothing and wrap the child in blankets and warm clothes. Cover the head but not the face. Use plastic, aluminum foil or a sleeping bag for extra insulation.
- DO NOT plunge a cold youngster into hot water.
- DO NOT move the child unnecessarily. Too much handling of the youngster could cause heart failure.
- Continue efforts to gently warm the child on the way to the hospital. ❖

Mouth Injuries

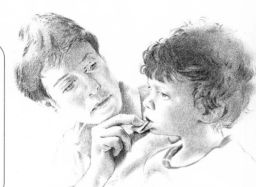

You can stop a cut lip from bleeding by pressing gently on both sides of your youngster's lip with sterile gauze or a clean cloth.

If your child's mouth is injured, check for injuries to the head and neck *(see Head Injuries, page 32)*. Control bleeding in the mouth by pressing tightly on the wound for a few minutes with sterile gauze or a clean cloth. If the tongue or lip is cut, squeeze the gauze-covered wound gently between your thumb and finger until the bleeding stops.

Sometimes injuries to the teeth appear more alarming than they are; a child's dental structure, deformed by an accident, can often be realigned with a relatively simple dental procedure. Keep a knocked-out tooth in a container of cold water in case the dentist can reimplant it. For a large or persistently bleeding cut, call a physician; stitches may be needed. And although infections in the mouth are rare, remember to keep all wounds clean.

Symptoms:
- cuts, bleeding or bruising of the lips, tongue, palate or gums
- crooked, broken or missing teeth

What to do:
- Check for a head or neck injury.
- Have the child lean forward so he does not inhale or swallow blood.
- Call a doctor if the wound is large or bleeds persistently.
- Wipe the wound gently with gauze dipped in hydrogen peroxide or, if external, wash with soap and water.
- To control bleeding, press gently on the wound with sterile gauze.
- Apply an ice pack or have the child suck on an ice pop to reduce swelling.
- After the first day, rinse with warm salt water to promote healing.
- Give acetaminophen for pain. ❖

Nose Injuries

With the important exception of a nosebleed following a blow to the skull, few nose injuries require immediate medical attention. Nosebleeding that follows a skull blow may indicate an internal head injury, and emergency aid should be summoned at once. Other nosebleeds are rarely serious.

The most common nose injuries are spontaneous nosebleeds and nosebleeds that result from picking the nose. A fall or a blow to the nose may also cause bleeding, and in addition may break the bony upper part of the nose or damage the softer cartilage of the lower part. Other problems may arise when young children stick foreign objects such as beads, nuts, beans, or paper balls into their noses. These can become very difficult to remove and may cause infection.

Nosebleeds
Nosebleeds result from the rupture of tiny, fragile blood vessels in the lining of

the nose — nearly always on the septum, the wall between the nostrils. Picking is by far the most common cause, so keeping the fingernails cut and discouraging your child from picking are good preventive measures. Nose-blowing and irritation by a virus, as during a cold, also cause nosebleeds. If the membranes of the nose are dry, bleeding is more likely. In winter, using a humidifier and keeping the heat down inside the house can help to prevent dryness of the nasal membranes.

Many nosebleeds will simply stop by themselves. If bleeding persists, it can almost always be stopped within five to 10 minutes by applying firm pressure to the nostrils just below the bone. When you apply pressure, the blood vessels squeeze closed and a clot forms. The clot can form only when bleeding slows down, because steadily flowing blood will wash away components in the blood that make it clot. This is why pinching the nose helps speed the clotting.

The child should lean forward slightly so he does not swallow the blood and so you can tell whether the bleeding has stopped. Leaning forward will not cause the bleeding to increase. Try to calm and reassure the child, because crying does increase the blood flow. Aspirin, which inhibits clotting, should not be given to a child with a nosebleed.

You should call the problem to a doctor's attention if the youngster has frequent nosebleeds, or if you are unable to stop a nosebleed on your own after 30 minutes. The doctor may use medicines that help shrink the blood vessels, or as a last resort the doctor may pack the nose or cauterize the bleeding point chemically or electronically.

What to do:
- Have the youngster sit down and lean slightly forward.
- Pinch the youngster's nostrils together gently but firmly just below the bony bridge of the nose.

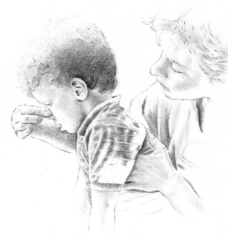

To stop a nosebleed, pinch the nose just below the bridge, the bony upper part of the nose. Have the child lean forward while you apply pressure for five to 10 minutes. Cold compresses on the nose or face may also help stop bleeding.

- Apply pressure for five to 10 minutes.
- Apply cold compresses or ice across the bridge of the nose and on the face.
- If pressure does not work at first, try again for up to 10 minutes.
- If bleeding still does not stop, insert a gauze pad (not absorbent cotton) into the youngster's nostril and apply pressure again. Let part of the pad stick out for easy removal, but do not hurry to remove it. It may be helpful to moisten the gauze pad with nose drops, which will shrink the membranes lining the nose.
- If bleeding persists after 30 minutes, seek medical help.
- A child must not blow his nose for several hours after a nosebleed. Discourage sniffling, too.

Foreign objects in the nose

If a child has an object in his nose that does not belong there, you may not detect it right away. After a day or two the nose may become infected or the child may have trouble breathing through the affected nostril. Even if you cannot see anything in the nostrils, you should suspect a foreign object if the following symptoms are present.

Symptoms:
- difficulty breathing, especially through one nostril
- a foul-smelling, sometimes blood-tinged discharge, which indicates the presence of a nasal infection

What to do:
- Calm the child and tell him to breathe through his mouth.
- Have him blow his nose several times.
- If you can see the object and easily grasp it with your fingers, try to remove it yourself, but if not take the child to a doctor.
- DO NOT use tweezers or other instruments to try to remove the object. You may accidentally push it farther into the youngster's nose and make it more difficult to remove.

Blow to the nose

Because a broken nose is not always obvious and can go undetected, a doctor should examine your child's nose after any hard blow to it. It is perfectly safe, however, to defer treatment of a nasal fracture for several days if there is no significant bleeding or deformity. The doctor will probably wait until the swelling subsides, even as much as four to eight days, to realign bones or cartilage. The bones of the nose heal very quickly, but if they do not heal in their correct positions, they may cause breathing problems in the future or alter the child's appearance. The doctor may splint or tape a broken nose in order to reposition the bones. Plaster casts for nose fractures are rarely necessary.

What to do:
- Have the child lean forward so that he will not swallow blood.
- Reduce swelling with cold compresses or an ice pack.
- Give the child acetaminophen for pain relief, if necessary.
- See a doctor if the nose appears particularly misshapen. ❖

Poisoning

A Quick Guide to Poisoning Emergencies

One of the first steps in treating a poisoned child is to call your regional poison-control center. You should keep that number posted by your phone. If you do not know it, dial 911 and ask for the number, or call a hospital emer-gency room. Do not begin first aid until you are certain of the proper course of treatment. Above all, you should not induce vomiting unless counseled to do so by the poison-control center or a doctor.

If the child is unconscious:
- Turn him on his side.
- Check repeatedly for breath-ing and pulse *(pages 16-17)*. If necessary, perform artificial respiration or have someone trained in CPR respond.
- Have someone call for an ambu-lance; if no help is available, make the call yourself after one or two minutes of resuscitation. Then continue resuscitation until the ambulance arrives.

If the child is convulsing:
- Quickly clear a space around him so he cannot injure himself.
- Call for an ambulance.
- If the child vomits, turn him on his side to prevent choking.
- DO NOT put anything in the youngster's mouth or give him anything to eat or drink.

If the child has swallowed any poison — either a prescription or over-the-counter drug or a nondrug poison:
- Do not give food or drink.
- Call the poison-control center.
- If he vomits spontaneously or if the poison-control center in-structs you to induce vomit-ing, collect the vomit in a pan; also collect any urine the child passes. Such samples may help the center identify the type and amount of poison ingested.

If the youngster's skin or eyes have been in contact with a poisonous substance:
- Immediately remove any con-taminated clothing and continu-ously flush the skin or eyes with cool water, as you would for a chemical burn *(page 22)*.
- Call the poison-control center.

If the child has inhaled poison:
- Carry the child to fresh air, but be careful not to breathe the poi-sonous fumes yourself.
- Summon emergency medical help if the child has painful breath-ing, shortness of breath or any other signs of lung injury.
- Call the poison-control center.

Poisoning is the fourth leading cause of accidental death among children — and one of the most preventable *(box, oppo-site)*. To forestall such accidents, bear in mind that from the time your child can crawl, he explores the world by putting things in his mouth. This oral phase is strongest in one- and two-year-olds, who comprise two thirds of all childhood poi-soning victims. Only by the age of four or five are children fully able to understand that drugs and chemicals can make them sick. So your prevention program must begin before your baby's first birthday and continue until he is at least five. Your poison-control center or hospital can provide warning labels and other materi-als to help you identify, lock up or discard potential poisons.

Should a poisoning occur despite your precautions, the key to effective treat-ment is immediate action. If you find evi-dence that your child has touched a poi-son or consumed any nonfood substance, call the poison-control center at once. On your way to the phone, question the child or bystanders. Remember that chil-dren sometimes ingest several poisons at once and that more than one child may be poisoned. Try to establish quickly what the poison was, when the poisoning occurred and how much poison was in-volved. Make a fast search for containers, pills and other evidence. Take them to the telephone with you and, if necessary, to the hospital.

In some circumstances you may have to deduce that your child has swallowed poison without finding any physical evi-dence, judging only by his symptoms. The most common symptoms include:
- vomiting or diarrhea
- excessive sweating, drooling and watery eyes
- hot, dry skin and mouth
- lethargy or unusual behavior
- dilated or constricted pupils
- flickering, sideways eye movement
- racing or irregular pulse and rapid breathing
- headache, agitation, hallucinations, tremor and convulsions

If you suspect poisoning, do not waste time searching for proof. Even if you can-not identify the substance, telephone your regional poison-control center. If the child is convulsing or unconscious, begin the first-aid measures described in the box above.

Regional Poison-Control Centers

Regional poison-control centers are staffed day and night by specialists who provide advice to parents, pediatricians and emergency-room physicians. Using computer data banks, these experts can instantly assess a poison's toxicity and decide whether hospital treatment is required. If so, the center can arrange for emergency transportation and forewarn the hospital personnel. But in most cases, home treatment is sufficient, with periodic follow-up telephone calls from the poison-control center to make sure that no problems arise.

Using the poison-control center is particularly important because the immediate measures that you take at home can be the most critical phase of the treatment. Only in about 10 percent of all cases is there a specific antidote that will help once the poison is absorbed through the skin, lungs or stomach.

Ingested poisons

Nearly 90 percent of all poisonings involve substances that a child swallows. Most often these are drugs: Chewable vitamins alone account for 14 percent of the emergencies. But the list of ingestible poisons is extensive. It includes not only household chemicals but many other nonfood substances that a child might suck on or swallow: batteries, cosmetics, perfume, shoe polish, insecticides, fertilizers, cigarette butts and the dregs of liquor in nearly empty glasses.

For many of these accidents, the key to treatment is syrup of ipecac, which induces vomiting, thoroughly emptying the stomach within 20 minutes. A one-ounce bottle of ipecac, available without prescription, should be in your first-aid kit. Replace the bottle if opened or if its expiration date lapses. Be aware, however, that ipecac is not appropriate treatment for all types of poisonings and should be used only at the direction of the poison-control center or a doctor.

Inhaled and absorbed poisons

Although less common than poisoning by ingestion, poisoning from fumes or sub-stances that are absorbed through the skin or eyes can be just as dangerous. The most frequently inhaled poison is carbon monoxide. In recent years, the childhood death rate from this gas has multiplied two and a half times, mostly as a result of poorly vented kerosene space heaters and wood stoves. The only measure you can take when a poison is inhaled is to rush the child into fresh air, then call for an ambulance. Contact poisoning of the skin or eyes often requires only minute amounts of the toxin to cause profound damage. Pesticides and herbicides are the usual culprits. Treatment for these accidents is the same as the treatment for chemical burns (*page 22*).

Lead poisoning

Unlike most poisoning hazards, lead poisoning is a gradual process that develops imperceptibly over months or years. Despite a 1977 ban on lead-based paints and the phase-out of leaded gasoline, the danger of lead poisoning has not been eliminated: One of every 25 American children between six months and five years old still has high levels of lead in his blood. Lead poisoning can occur wherever children inhabit old buildings layered with lead-based paints or live in proximity to heavy automobile traffic or industrial wastes. Children typically ingest lead while eating pieces of dirt, plaster or paint — a habit that is not uncommon among toddlers.

Lead poisoning during the preschool years may cause nausea and headaches; prolonged or repeated poisoning can cause learning disabilities, personality changes and retardation. If you suspect that your house contains high levels of lead, ask a doctor to screen your child for lead levels. You can minimize the hazard by scraping off loose paint and plaster, vacuuming the house often to remove dust and particles of lead, and wallpapering walls that children can reach. ⋮

How to Prevent Poisoning

- Never leave a poison unattended while it is in use. If you are interrupted even momentarily, cap the poison and take it with you.
- Buy all medicines and household products in child-resistant containers, and never transfer them to other bottles or jars.
- Get Mr. Yuk or Dr. Ugh stickers from your hospital or poison-control center, then teach your child what they mean and apply them to all poison containers.
- Survey your house for possibly accessible poisons.
- Store all potential poisons, including liquor, household cleaning products, vitamins and medicines, out of reach of your children and preferably under lock and key.
- Never underestimate a toddler's agility or ingenuity. Many two-year-old children can climb to countertops to explore high cupboards and medicine cabinets.
- Do not leave women's purses within reach; they frequently contain medicines.
- Teach your children that they should not eat plants, leaves, berries, paint chips or dirt.
- Never refer to medicine as candy, and do not take medication in front of very young children.
- Before giving your child medicine, be sure that your spouse or babysitter has not already done so; and you should never dispense medicine in a darkened room. About 10 percent of childhood poisonings are caused by such mistakes.
- Be vigilant for poison hazards during periods of family stress and while meals are being prepared — times when children tend to be active and parental supervision may be stretched thin.
- Pay special attention to children who have previously poisoned themselves; about 25 percent of these youngsters repeat the experience within a year.

Shock

Read First

- If a youngster displays symptoms of shock *(below)*, call for emergency medical assistance immediately.
- Treat whatever injury has caused the condition of shock.
- If a neck or back injury is suspected, you should not move the child.
- Keep the youngster prone, with her feet elevated higher than her heart, if there is no head injury. Cover with a coat or blanket to prevent chilling.

The term "shock" describes the state of the body when the supply of blood to the vital organs, including the brain, heart, liver and kidneys, is inadequate. Shock can be caused by a variety of factors, including an allergic reaction to drugs or insect venoms and a significant loss of blood or other body fluids.

If an accident gives your youngster a bad fright but she has sustained no injuries, the child is not suffering from true medical shock. She needs to be kept warm, comfortable and calm, but the youngster does not necessarily need medical treatment.

Real shock is a medical emergency that can be fatal if not treated promptly. It is characterized by rapidly falling blood pressure and progressive deterioration of the body's condition. The goal in treating shock is to restore the victim's normal blood pressure and stabilize the body's vital functions.

Only medical personnel with the proper equipment can actually treat shock, but parents can administer helpful first aid while they wait for emergency medical assistance to arrive. It is essential to check for signs of shock in any youngster who has had a serious accident. Even if the child shows none of the symptoms of shock, such as pale, clammy skin or rapid, shallow breathing, it is a good idea to have her rest quietly for a period as a preventive measure.

Hypovolemic shock

Hypovolemic shock is shock caused by loss of blood or other body fluids. It may occur in children after any serious injury, such as a fractured bone, a severe burn or a wound that bleeds heavily. Hypovolemic shock can also result from severe dehydration caused by prolonged vomiting, diarrhea or heat exhaustion.

Symptoms:
- pale, cold and clammy skin
- rapid but faint pulse
- shallow breathing
- either restlessness and overactivity or lethargy and decreased activity
- dull or sunken-looking eyes
- perspiration on forehead or palms
- nausea and vomiting
- severe thirst

What to do:
- Call the doctor.
- Keep the youngster lying down with her feet raised higher than her heart in order to improve circulation to vital body organs, as long as there is no possibility of head injury.
- If the child is having trouble breathing, you should gently prop up her head and neck with a pillow.
- Loosen the youngster's clothing and place a coat or blanket over her to prevent a chill. But do not make her too warm, or you might increase her circulatory problems.
- Keep the child quiet and continue to reassure her.

Anaphylactic shock

This kind of shock occurs when a child has an extreme allergic reaction to a drug, such as penicillin, or to an insect toxin, such as a bee sting. The allergens enter the child's bloodstream and pass quickly through the body, causing an overwhelming reaction that can be fatal if not treated immediately.

Children with drug allergies should wear medical ID bracelets to alert medical personnel in emergencies. Children known to have severe allergic reactions to insect bites or stings should be evaluated by a doctor, who may prescribe a kit containing epinephrine (adrenaline), which a parent can administer to the child in an emergency.

Symptoms:
- wheezing, coughing or extreme difficulty in breathing
- tingling sensation around the mouth or around the face
- difficulty in swallowing or a feeling of tightness in the chest
- excessive itching of eyes
- cramps, nausea or vomiting
- convulsions or unconsciousness

What to do:
- Call an ambulance or take the child to the nearest emergency room.
- Give the child epinephrine if your doctor has prescribed the medication for such emergencies.
- Keep the youngster calm and do your best to reassure her. ⋮

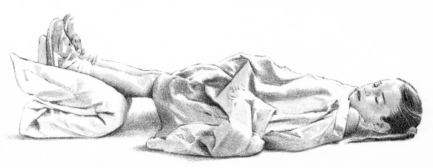

If the child is conscious and there is no head, neck or back injury or impaired breathing, have her lie on her back with her feet lifted higher than her heart. If breathing is difficult, prop a pillow under her head. If the child is vomiting, turn her on her stomach or side with her top knee bent forward to keep her from rolling over.

Splinters

In most cases, you should remove a splinter as soon as possible, using the following steps. The most difficult part of the task may be calming a child who panics at the anticipation of pain.

Do not try to remove tiny splinters, even painful ones. They probably will work their way out on their own, and by trying to extract them you may irritate the surrounding tissue.

If the splinter is metal, dirty, large or very deep, see the doctor, who can numb the area before removing the splinter and may want to give your child a tetanus shot. Also call the doctor if the wound is infected or if the splinter is glass, which might break off if you try to remove it.

What to do for a protruding splinter:
- Sterilize tweezers by soaking the tips

in rubbing alcohol or by holding them in the flame of a match. Cool the tweezers before use.
- Grasp the splinter with the tweezers and pull it back along its line of entry.
- Wash the area with soap and water.
- A small remnant probably will work its way out on its own. Soaking the area in warm water and Epsom salts for half an hour several times a day will reduce inflammation and help bring the remnant out.

What to do for an embedded splinter:
- Rub the skin around the splinter wound with ice to numb the area.
- Sterilize a needle and tweezers by soaking the tips in rubbing alcohol or by holding them in the flame of a match. Cool before use.

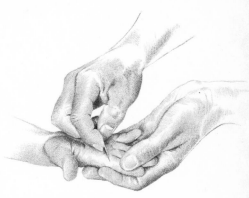

To remove a splinter embedded just beneath the skin's surface, gently tear the skin above the splinter with a sterilized needle. Then nudge the splinter free with the needle and pull it out with tweezers.

- Slip the needle under the skin above the splinter and tear the skin by pulling the needle up. Then slip the needle under the splinter to raise it so you can grasp it with the tweezers.
- Wash area with soap and water. ❖

Sprains and Strains

Read First

- Check the child first for a possible broken or dislocated bone *(page 17)*.
- Try to determine whether the injury is a sprain or a strain, as the two call for opposite treatments: heat for a strained muscle, ice packs for a sprained ligament.
- Call the doctor if pain or swelling is severe and persists after using ice packs.
- Do not let the youngster put any weight on the injured joint until the pain and swelling subside.

In the rough-and-tumble of their normal play, young children frequently turn an ankle or fall in a way that wrenches a knee or wrist. Thanks to the elasticity of their growing joints and muscles, most of these mishaps are minor. The child recovers quickly with nothing more than a little comforting.

Once in a while, however, a child may severely sprain a wrist or ankle or strain a muscle. Sprains occur when a joint is twisted into an unnatural position so that it causes damage to the ligaments that connect the bones. The joint may swell and become black-and-blue because of bleeding under the skin. Strains occur when muscles are stretched or torn from overexertion. Strains are often painful. But, unlike sprains, they do not usually result in much swelling or bruising.

These same symptoms might indicate the child has broken or dislocated a bone — even if he does not have any other symptoms, such as obvious crookedness of the limb or deformity at the joint. If you suspect a fracture or dislocation, see page 17. If the pain or swelling is severe and does not ease up after a few hours, have the injury checked by a doctor, who can determine whether a bone has been broken or dislocated.

Symptoms of sprains:
- pain or tenderness in the injured joint
- swelling or bruising of the area affected by the injury
- inability to bear weight on the joint or to move it normally

What to do for a sprained wrist or ankle:
- Elevate the injured joint on a pillow

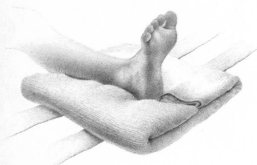

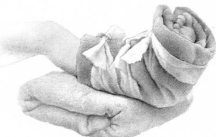

To immobilize a sprained ankle, place a folded towel or small pillow under it (far left) and bring the edges forward. Fasten with two cloth ties above the ankle. Then fold the bottom of the towel or pillow up over the foot and tie again, this time around the arch (near left). Elevate the foot above the heart and check the toes for numbness periodically to be sure the ties are not too tight.

and apply ice. To avoid cold burns, never apply ice directly to the skin; instead, place ice in a plastic bag and wrap the bag in a towel.
- Do not allow the child to put weight on the joint. Wrap the wrist or ankle in an elastic bandage, or, if there is a possibility of a fracture, immobilize it with a splint *(pages 17-18)*.
- As the joint heals, have the youngster move it in different directions in order to relieve stiffness.

What to do for a sprained knee:
- Elevate the leg and apply a bag of ice wrapped in a towel.
- If the knee moves from side to side or if the child cannot straighten it, immobilize the knee with a splint *(pages 17-18)* and call the doctor. This may indicate torn ligaments or cartilage.
- Do not let the youngster put any weight on the injured leg until the swelling and pain have subsided.

What to do for a sprained elbow:
- Elevate the arm on a pillow and apply a bag of ice wrapped in a towel.
- If there is a possibility of a fractured or chipped bone, immobilize the elbow with a splint and sling *(page 18)* and call the doctor.

Symptoms of strains:
- stiffness of a muscle
- pain when the muscle is used

What to do:
- Rest the injured muscle.
- Apply warm compresses. ❖

Swallowed Objects

Read First

- If the youngster cannot breathe, cough or speak see Choking, page 23.
- Seek medical aid if the child is coughing. DO NOT try to dislodge the object.
- Call a doctor if the child swallows a sharp or large object or one that causes persistent discomfort.

Most toddlers, if given the chance, will swallow almost any small item they can get their hands on. Some of their favorite indissoluble treats include teddy-bear eyes, marbles, coins, safety pins and needles. Fortunately, most small objects easily pass through the digestive tract to the

bowels with no adverse effects on the child. Within a few days, the object usually winds up in the child's stools.

Sometimes, however, an object gets stuck in a child's windpipe, esophagus or intestines, with symptoms ranging from an inability to breathe to slight stomach pains. A blocked windpipe poses the most immediate danger to your youngster, since a child who cannot breathe may die within six minutes.

The preferred treatment for a child who has swallowed an object will depend on the size and type of object and the child's symptoms. In general, smooth, small items will cause fewer problems than sharp, large ones.

Symptoms:
- violent coughing
- breathing difficulties
- chest, abdomen or neck pains

- vomiting
- drooling

What to do:
- If the child is choking, see page 23 for methods to dislodge the object.
- If the child is coughing, which indicates that his windpipe is partially obstructed, DO NOT try to dislodge the object. You risk moving it to a position that completely blocks the windpipe. Instead, encourage the youngster to cough up the item. If unsuccessful, seek medical assistance.
- Call a doctor when a child swallows a sharp, large item or exhibits the symptoms listed above.
- If the child has swallowed a smooth object that has caused no adverse effects, check his bowel movements for the next few days to make sure the item has been eliminated. ❖

Unconsciousness

Read First

- If a possible source of electric shock, such as a frayed electric cord, is evident, follow the guidelines in Electric Shock *(page 29)* for separating the child from the source of electricity before touching him.
- Tap the child on the shoulder and ask him loudly if he is all right. If he does not respond, he is probably unconscious.
- If breathing has stopped, give artificial respiration *(page 16)*. If heart has stopped, cardiopulmonary resuscitation should be applied immediately.
- Seek emergency aid.
- DO NOT move a child if you suspect he has any head, neck or back injuries.
- DO NOT splash cold water on the youngster's face. DO NOT use stimulants such as smelling salts or give anything to drink.

Unconsciousness, a sleeplike state of unresponsiveness, occurs in many forms. It can range from a brief loss of consciousness brought on by fainting to a long-lasting, very serious condition known as a deep coma. The causes of unconsciousness are varied: They include head trauma, shock, heatstroke, poisoning, severe infections, epileptic seizures, blood loss, drug overdoses and allergic reactions.

If unconsciousness is accompanied by life-threatening problems such as severe bleeding or breathing difficulties, treat them immediately. If the child has fainted, see that entry *(right)*.

Symptoms:
- lack of response to touch or voice; inability to hear, see, talk or move
- sometimes, drowsiness, confusion and lack of awareness of surroundings
- loose, floppy limbs

What to do:
- If the child is not breathing, begin artificial respiration *(page 16)*. Call for emergency medical help; continue rescue efforts until help arrives.
- If there is no pulse, have someone trained in CPR respond.

- If you suspect head, neck or back injuries, DO NOT move the child. However, if he is lying face up and starts to vomit, shift him into the recovery position *(below)*, so he will not choke on the vomit. Get help and handle the child very carefully, always keeping his head and back in the same position relative to each other. CAUTION: Move the victim only if it is absolutely necessary. You could cause serious, permanent damage to his spinal cord.
- Put an unconscious youngster without head, back or neck injuries in the recovery position *(below)*, so mucus and vomit can drain from his mouth.
- Loosen clothing around the neck.
- If you can see mucus or other debris in his mouth, sweep it out with your fingers. However, keep your fingers out of his mouth and all objects away from him if convulsions occur.
- Put a coat or blanket over the child.
- Treat external wounds.
- Seek medical assistance.
- DO NOT leave the child alone. Stay with him until help arrives and watch closely for changes in his behavior.

Fainting

Fainting is a temporary loss of consciousness that is caused by an insufficient supply of blood to the brain. Receiving a sudden fright, for instance, can cause a child's blood vessels to dilate reflexively, his blood pressure to drop and the youngster to faint.

Symptoms:
- dizziness and nausea
- pale, chilled and sweaty skin
- blurred vision
- tingling or numbness in hands or feet

What to do to forestall fainting:
- Seat your child in a chair and have him bend forward until his head is positioned between his knees.
- Tell him to wiggle his toes: This helps get blood circulating.
- Calm and reassure the child.

What to do to revive a child who has fainted:
- Turn the child on his back and elevate his legs eight to 12 inches.
- If the child starts to vomit, turn his head to the side.
- Place your finger in his mouth to remove visible mucus, vomit or other material. However, if convulsions occur, keep your fingers out of his mouth and all objects away from him.
- Loosen clothing around his neck.
- Keep him warm by covering him with a coat or blanket.
- Wipe his forehead and face with a cloth dipped in cool water, but do not pour cold water on his face.
- Treat injuries caused by the fall.
- Seek emergency medical assistance if recovery does not take place within five minutes. Even if the child recovers completely, promptly report the incident to his doctor. ❖

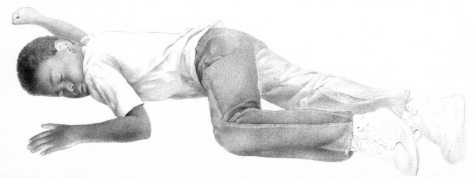

Put an unconscious child into the recovery position by rolling him onto his stomach or side and turning his head to the side. This will facilitate breathing and prevent him from choking on vomit or other debris. Move his chin forward and up so his tongue does not block his throat. If possible, raise his legs slightly above head level to increase the blood flow to his heart and brain.

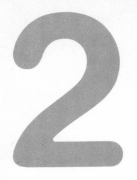

Illnesses and Disorders

Predictably, adults and small children have entirely different views on the causes of illness. While mothers and fathers fret and sometimes blame themselves, children tend to see sickness — and the shots and medications associated with it — as a form of punishment. A youngster comprehends little about how her body works and usually cannot grasp the reasons for the medicines, thermometers and extra naps that add aggravation to the discomfort of illness. For her part, the child may assume that she will always be sick.

Many parents also lack sufficient knowledge about physiology and medical matters, and they may unknowingly pass along their insecurities about a particular illness to the afflicted child. Evidence suggests that parents can improve their child's condition simply by learning more about it. In one experiment, for example, children whose mothers were briefed in advance about surgical procedures recovered more quickly and suffered fewer complications. The reason is simple: Knowledgeable parents are more confident, more relaxed — attitudes that they transmit to their children.

The lesson is a good one with regard to any of the illnesses and disorders discussed in this section of the book. Learn about their causes and effects, so you will know what to expect should they occur.

With the exception of a few broad topics such as allergies and fever, which are treated on their own, the illnesses have been grouped according to the systems of the body that they affect. Anatomical drawings accompany each of these subsections to help you understand why the body responds as it does. For an overview, begin with the whole-body anatomies of an infant and older child presented on the following pages.

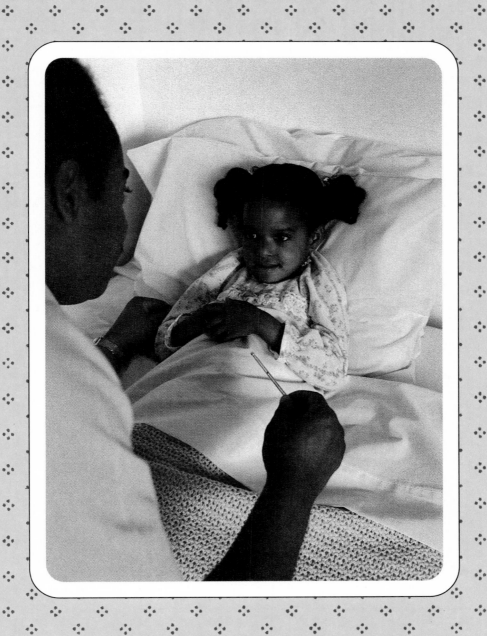

A Child's Changing Body

A basic awareness of your youngster's anatomy will help you to understand her illnesses better and also to make sense of the treatments that cure them.

The anatomical drawings throughout this section of the book isolate various subsystems of a child's body — the structure of bones and muscles, the circulatory and glandular systems, or the digestive tract, for example — so that you can see how disease affects each part. The illustrations on this and the facing page show how all those subsystems fit together and how they evolve as the youngster grows and matures.

At first glance, some infants resemble miniature adults, but a closer examination will reveal distinctly babyish qualities. For one, infants are notably top-heavy: Their heads make up fully one quarter of their length, while their legs are disproportionately short. In addition, they have oversized bellies and soft spots on their heads called fontanels.

These external differences point up the fact that an infant's body is still in a state of becoming what it one day will be — and not just in terms of inches or pounds. The development of bodily systems that begins in the womb continues for some years after birth. The infant's top-heaviness, together with the immaturity of her muscles and nervous systems, will limit her mobility and steadiness for a few years, until her legs lengthen proportionately and she grows more coordinated. Her belly protrudes for a while, until her still-developing abdominal muscles strengthen enough to hold her intestines firmly in place. And the soft spots on her scalp are places where the bones of her skull have not yet fully knitted together: The gap that remains there allows for rapid growth of the brain during the early months of life.

Other differences are concealed beneath the skin, some of them relating to the child's ability to fight off illness. But most of these differences — both visible and invisible — are short-lived. Even in the span between birth and six years, the ages of the children depicted below and at right, there are dramatic advances in physiological maturation. That ongoing process, which begins in the womb with the union of egg and sperm, eventually produces the graceful body of a six-year-old, which bears more resemblance to its future adult form than to the chubby shape of babyhood.

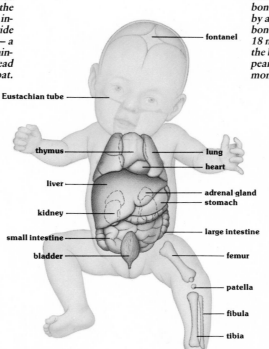

Eustachian Tubes
During an infection, the Eustachian tubes drain fluids from the middle ear into the back of the throat. In an infant the tubes are short, wide and almost horizontal — a shape that slows fluid drainage and facilitates the spread of germs from the throat.

Thymus
The thymus, an organ that produces infection-fighting cells, plays a key role in establishing an immune system for the vulnerable newborn. Disproportionately large at birth, the thymus will shrink by adulthood to a small bit of connective tissue.

Liver
During pregnancy, the liver is a delivery point for blood entering the fetus from the placenta, carrying oxygen and nutrients. Because of this vital role, the liver is oversize in newborns, accounting for 1/18 of an infant's total body weight.

Fontanels
The soft spots on a baby's head are gaps between the bones of the skull, protected by a tough membrane. The bones will grow and fuse by 18 months. The fontanel at the back of the head disappears first — usually by six months of age.

Adrenal Glands
The adrenals, which are overly large at birth, produce hormones that regulate blood pressure and help control metabolism. The glands shrink during the first three weeks, as the portions that aided in fetal development give way to mature tissue.

Bones
At birth the skeletal system is composed of about 350 segments made of cartilage and bone. The cartilage is pliable enough to pass through the birth canal. It grows quickly, letting the skeleton keep pace with the child's development.

fontanel

Eustachian tube

thymus

liver

kidney

small intestine

bladder

lung

heart

adrenal gland

stomach

large intestine

femur

patella

fibula

tibia

metatarsals

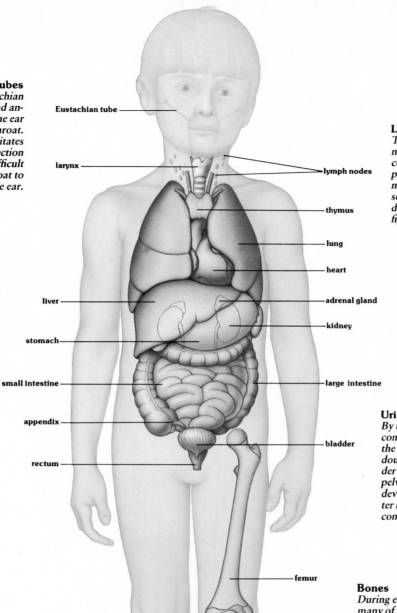

Eustachian Tubes
By school age the Eustachian tubes are narrower and angle downward from the ear to the back of the throat. The steeper angle facilitates drainage during an infection and makes it more difficult for germs in the throat to move up into the middle ear.

Liver
While still the largest internal organ, the liver has not grown as fast as other organs in the body. Its primary functions since birth have been to metabolize foods and to secrete bile to aid in the digestion of fats.

Lymph Nodes
The immune system's lymph nodes play an active role in combating the diseases that prey on young children. The nodes are easily felt and seen when swollen — an indication that the body is fighting infection.

Urinary Tract
By the age of six, the ureters connecting the kidneys to the bladder have more than doubled in length; the bladder has also settled into the pelvis, increased in size and developed a stronger sphincter muscle, making bladder control possible.

Bones
During early childhood, many of the infant's 350-odd bones fuse together as they grow and harden. The process continues throughout childhood and adolescence. Eventually, the skeletal system will have only 206 to 209 bones.

Eustachian tube

larynx

lymph nodes

thymus

lung

heart

liver

adrenal gland

kidney

stomach

small intestine

large intestine

appendix

rectum

bladder

femur

patella

fibula

tibia

metatarsals

Allergies

The itching eyes of hay fever, the hives induced by some foods and all the other annoying effects of allergies can be traced to faults in the immune system. This bodily mechanism is meant to be an automatic defense against disease. When it is working properly, the immune system recognizes a substance in or on the body that does not belong there — a dangerous foreign attacker.

It then mobilizes the white cells of the blood to release a chemical, called an antibody, that destroys the attacker. The immune system makes a unique type of antibody to neutralize each type of attacker. This process generates the symptoms that indicate the body is fighting off a disease: The sniffles of a cold, for example, result from the reaction between a cold virus and the immune system as it produces the antibodies to fight that particular cold virus.

In 80 percent of all children, the immune system operates with precision and restraint, eliminating harmful invaders and ignoring harmless ones. But in the other 20 percent, the system is overly sensitive: It reacts to a food, a plant pollen, dust or any of a huge variety of other natural and synthetic substances, called allergens, that ordinarily are benign.

This inappropriate response, or allergy, summons the same process as an appropriate one. The white blood cells are stimulated to manufacture a supply of the antibodies for the allergen, setting off the symptoms that ordinarily accompany a disease. Once the antibodies for a particular allergen have been made, some of them remain in the body after the allergen has disappeared. These serve as models to speed up production in future attacks by the same allergen. They sensitize the body so that it responds more quickly — and in some cases with more severe symptoms. Once a child has developed an allergy to a particular food or an insect sting, later attacks may become worse,

although most allergies become less severe in adult life.

The strength and persistence of a particular allergy can vary. For some people, sensitivity to a substance may be permanent. In others — especially very young children — the allergy may last a few months only. Dose also affects a reaction: A child may be able to tolerate small amounts of an allergen without trouble. And an allergic attack may be worse if the child is suffering from an infection, fatigue or emotional upset. Even sudden changes in temperature or humidity can make a difference.

If a baby is born into an allergic family, his own chances of developing an allergy are greater than average. You may be able to forestall the first attacks by breastfeeding the youngster rather than using a bottle formula.

Different allergies cause reactions in different parts of the body. Airborne allergens such as pollen usually affect the eyes, nose and throat, causing what is commonly known as hay fever. Less often, these allergens cause partial closure of passages leading to the lungs, which results in the condition called asthma *(page 74)*. Food and oral medicines usually react in the digestive system, but allergic responses to them can produce breathing difficulty, headache, eczema or hives. Other allergens cause irritation only when they come in direct contact with the skin. Allergens that enter the blood directly — injected medicines or a stinging insect's venom — also circulate to cause far-ranging symptoms. In rare cases an allergen can trigger anaphylactic shock *(page 38)*, an extremely dangerous condition in which air passages swell nearly closed and blood pressure may drop drastically.

There is no cure for allergies, although the symptoms of an attack can be relieved by a variety of drugs, such as oral antihistamines, nose drops and eye

drops. In most cases, the best treatment is avoiding the allergen as much as possible. When the allergen is an unavoidable one, such as pollen or insect venom, and the symptoms are intolerable or dangerous, your doctor may recommend a course of medical therapy that neutralizes the immune reaction to certain allergens.

Allergic contact dermatitis
When an allergen comes in direct contact with the skin, the results may be hives or a rough, red, itchy rash that looks like eczema. One way to distinguish this contact dermatitis from eczema is its distribution. Eczema can show up anywhere on the body, although it is most commonly found in the creases of the elbows and knees. Contact dermatitis is limited to the spots the allergen has touched.

A small group of plants — poison ivy, poison oak and poison sumac — is responsible for most contact dermatitis. For symptoms and treatments of these cases, see page 119.

Other common contact allergens are drugs, cosmetics, metal alloys containing nickel, and chemicals used in processing leather and fabric. A skin test may be required to pin down the cause. As with other allergies, the best treatment is avoidance of the offending substance. Use cool compresses, oral antihistamines or calamine lotion to reduce itching and soothe the inflamed skin.

Drug allergies
In general, children are less likely than adults to be allergic to drugs. The major allergenic offender among medicines is penicillin. Other medications that frequently generate allergic reactions include sulfa drugs and insulin, as well as local anesthetics such as novocaine. The most common symptom of a drug allergy is hives or a very itchy skin rash beginning as faint pink spots that enlarge and become red. If a sulfa drug is the allergen,

Dust-Proofing a Child's Room

Curbing the dust in an allergic child's bedroom can greatly relieve the severity of his symptoms, since the youngster probably spends more time there than in any other place. With the furnishings and cleaning procedures described here, exposure to pollen, dander, mites and other dustborne allergens will be substantially reduced.

- For a thoroughgoing initial cleaning, empty the room and closets of all objects, including any carpet or curtains. Clean all surfaces with damp cloths, an oil mop and a vacuum cleaner. Similarly, clean everything that will be returned to the room.
- Select a bedframe of wood or metal

and a mattress and pillow made of foam rubber or other synthetic material, rather than animal hair, feathers or down. Use open metal springs instead of a box spring.

- For bedding, use cotton sheets, cotton or synthetic-fiber blankets, and a cotton or synthetic-fiber bedspread with a smooth finish. Do not use comforters or quilts.
- For window coverings, you should use washable curtains or drapes only, and they should be laundered at least once every two weeks.
- Keep the floors bare or lay down small cotton rugs, which should be laundered weekly.

- Eliminate upholstered furniture and stuffed animals from the room.
- Close heating registers or cover with triple-density fiberglass filters.
- Keep the windows and doors closed as much as possible.
- Store the youngster's clothes in plastic garment bags.
- Wash the walls and floors frequently, giving dust-collecting areas such as bookshelves special attention. Use damp cloths, a vacuum cleaner and an oil mop. Avoid brooms and dry cloths, and clean only when the child is out of the room.
- Do not use insecticides or air fresheners in the bedroom or closet.

---

a rash may appear only on the skin exposed to direct sunlight. Other reactions to drugs are asthma, other breathing difficulties, prolonged fever or, rarely, anaphylactic shock *(page 38)*. The timing of symptoms varies: Hives or anaphylactic shock usually occurs within hours of the offending dose, while a skin rash may not appear until days after a youngster has stopped taking the drug. It may be difficult to determine whether a rash is caused by an allergic reaction to a drug such as penicillin, or whether it is a symptom of the infection being treated. It is important to find out, because penicillin may be needed to treat another infection at some later date.

If you think your child may be having an allergic reaction to a drug, report it to your doctor promptly. A skin test can help diagnose an allergy to penicillin or insulin; the results are less conclusive for other drugs.

Food allergies
Babies less than three months of age may show symptoms of food allergies, usually

in reaction to cow's milk. Breast-fed babies avoid this risk. Other highly allergenic foods are fresh fruits, egg whites, corn, wheat, chocolate, pork, seafood, nuts, berries and legumes. Of course, not all problems caused by foods are allergies. A food may be contaminated by bacteria *(see Food Poisoning, page 67)*, or it may contain a substance that for some reason the child is unable to digest properly, such as wheat products in the case of children with celiac disease *(page 64)*.

There are many symptoms of food allergy and they are often confusing. The easiest to connect with a food are abdominal pain, vomiting and diarrhea. Food can also produce sneezing, headache, hives, a rash, eczema *(page 114)* or, especially in very young children, an asthmatic attack *(see Asthma, page 74)*. Less frequent symptoms are insomnia and angioedema — large, hivelike swelling of the lips or the skin around the eyes or, more dangerously, in the mouth or throat. On rare occasions, a food causes severe anaphylactic shock *(page 38)*. Symptoms may develop a few minutes af-

ter the child has eaten the offending food or as much as a week later. Raw foods generally provoke the strongest reactions; cooking or processing can weaken allergic properties.

Tracing the particular food that causes an allergy may be tricky. The first suspect when allergic symptoms arise is any newly introduced item in the diet, although attacks can begin after a child has safely eaten a food for months or years. The skin tests used in diagnosing some allergies are not very useful with foods. If symptoms are mild, a better test is temporary avoidance: Remove the suspected food from the diet completely for seven to 10 days, then give the child a serving and watch for symptoms for a week. Repeat this procedure two more times, discussing any symptoms with the child's physician. Of course, if you think the suspect food might cause a potentially dangerous reaction, skip such a trial; instead simply eliminate the food from the child's diet.

Infants and small children often outgrow food allergies. After a food has been avoided for three to six months, you may wish to test it again, checking first with your physician.

Hay fever

Hay fever is the popular name for allergic rhinitis, an allergic condition that affects the upper respiratory tract, especially the nose. Symptoms include sneezing, watery nasal discharge, nasal congestion, coughing, and an itchy nose, ears, palate and upper throat. There may also be dark, puffy bags under the eyes, which are often red, teary and itchy. The child may try to relieve unscratchable itches by wrinkling his nose or rubbing his tongue against the palate. Pushing the end of the nose upward may be an attempt to open the blocked nasal passages.

It is easy to confuse allergic rhinitis with a cold. A cold often brings fever and a thick nasal discharge, and it generally goes away in about a week. If symptoms last longer than two weeks and include itchy eyes, the problem is more likely to be an allergy.

Allergens responsible for rhinitis are airborne and can be anything from industrial pollutants or tobacco smoke to specks of powdered detergents. More of-

ten, however, they are tree and grass pollens, mold spores and dander — flakes shed by furred or feathered animals. Any of these substances can be in house dust, which also contains microscopic mites that some children react to.

If a pollen is the allergen, attacks will be limited to the period of the plant's pollination. Some molds are also seasonal, but others grow and produce spores year round in damp spots such as basements or shower stalls. By keeping track of the time and place of attacks, you and your physician may be able to pinpoint the cause. Often, however, the cause can be identified only through a skin test. In this test, a physician places a solution of a possible allergen on a small scratch in the skin. If a small hivelike swelling then appears at that spot, the child is probably sensitive to the allergen. Unfortunately, skin tests are not one hundred percent reliable. A reaction to a substance during a test does not necessarily mean there will be a reaction when the exposure occurs naturally.

The principal technique for managing allergic rhinitis is avoiding the allergens. You can, for instance, limit pets to ani-

mals without dander-producing fur or feathers. Other allergens, such as pollens and mold spores, cannot be avoided altogether, but you can take steps to limit exposure. During pollen season, keep your child indoors as much as possible, especially on hot, dry, windy days. Keep the windows closed — especially in the child's bedroom, where he may spend 12 or more hours a day — and use air-conditioning as often as possible. Do not allow plants or cut or dried flowers in the house. To help your child avoid molds and their spores, limit play in areas where damp, decaying vegetation harbors spores and keep him out of basements and sheds. Children with allergic rhinitis tend to be extremely sensitive to house dust. You can limit dust in a child's bedroom by taking the steps on page 47.

Medicines such as antihistamines and nasal decongestants are effective and relatively safe drugs for treating hay fever. In very severe cases, the doctor may prescribe steroid drugs. Because they can produce serious side effects, steroid drugs are for short-term use only. If these measures are insufficient, your doctor may advise immunotherapy. ⁘

Bones and Muscles

Virtually every conscious motion your child makes — whether walking, jumping or crawling — depends on a healthy framework of bones, muscles, joints and connective tissue. Muscles also control the involuntary motions of the heart, lungs, digestive system and almost every other body system.

At birth, this internal structural system is only partially developed. The infant has some 350 "bones," but most of them are not really bones at all. Instead they are pieces of soft cartilage. During childhood, most of that cartilage will be turned into true bone as new blood vessels tunnel into the cartilage, and the surrounding tissue is seeded with bone cells — a process called ossification. At the same time, many of those 350 separate pieces will fuse together to form the 206 to 210 bones of the adult body. Exercise and a diet rich in calcium, phosphorus and vitamin D will help the process of ossification along.

Far from being a handicap, the softness of a child's bones works to his advantage. During birth, the flexible plates of a baby's skull and his pliable limbs and ribs help ease the infant's passage through the narrow birth canal. This same resilience protects the toddler from injury from the spills and tumbles that mark yet another rite of passage: learning how to walk. Even such birth defects as dislocated hips and clubfoot are easily corrected if detected early, when supple young bones respond best to manipulative therapy.

An additional advantage young children have is that their small, relatively weak muscles do not place much stress on their joints. Later, as a child reaches adolescence — a time when his muscles grow faster than his bones — the joints will be subjected to greater stress, with a greater likelihood of injury.

Only when it comes to infection is the child's skeletal system at a disadvantage, since any infection has the potential to damage bone growth plates, small areas of cartilage at the ends of bones. Here cartilage cells divide and eventually are replaced by bone cells, lengthening the bone. If the growth plates are damaged, this process is severely hampered, adversely affecting a child's growth. The danger increases with the younger child who is unable to communicate exactly where it hurts, setting the stage for a silent infection that could fester undetected. You should be alert, then, for any sign of joint infection — a limb that does not seem to move normally, a limp, a joint

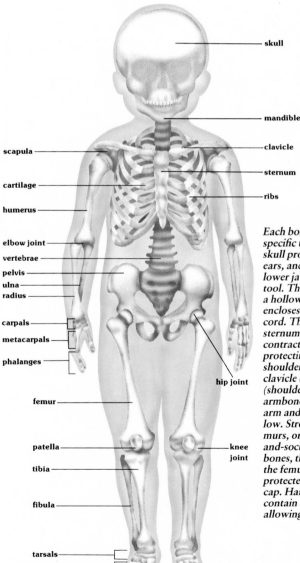

skull

mandible

clavicle

sternum

ribs

scapula

cartilage

humerus

elbow joint

vertebrae

pelvis

ulna

radius

carpals

metacarpals

phalanges

hip joint

femur

patella

knee joint

tibia

fibula

tarsals

metatarsals

phalanges

Each bone in the skeleton has a specific task. The hard plates of the skull protect the brain, eyes and ears, and the hinged mandible, or lower jaw, is an ideal crushing tool. The vertebrae of the spine form a hollow, flexible column which encloses and protects the spinal cord. The ribs, connected to the sternum by cartilage, expand and contract to allow breathing while protecting the internal organs. The shoulder girdle, made up of the clavicle (collarbone) and scapulae (shoulder blades), supports the armbones: the humerus in the upper arm and the radius and ulna below. Strong pelvic bones join the femurs, or thighbones, at a ball-and-socket hip joint. The lower-leg bones, the tibia and fibula, meet the femur at the knee, a delicate joint protected by the patella, or kneecap. Hands, feet, wrists and ankles contain dozens of small bones, allowing a wide range of movement.

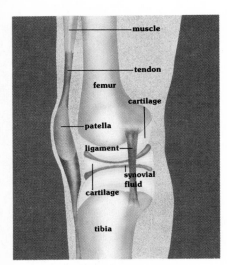

A diagram of the knee shows the complex workings of this hinged joint. Upper- and lower-leg bones, the femur and tibia, are connected by fibrous ligaments and buffered by cartilage. A tendon attaches the front thigh muscle to the tibia; built into it is the patella, or kneecap — a small, oval bone strategically placed to protect the delicate inner parts of the joint. The knee is cushioned by synovial fluid, a lubricant secreted by the membrane enclosing the joint.

swelling or any indication of pain near a joint — and contact a doctor promptly.

Arthritis

Arthritis is a general term used to describe an inflammation of the joints. There are more than a hundred different kinds of the disease, among them septic arthritis and osteoarthritis, although the most prevalent chronic form among children is juvenile rheumatoid arthritis, or JRA. The cause of this ailment remains unknown, despite research linking it to an infection by microorganisms and other evidence pointing toward a failure of the body's immune system.

JRA seldom occurs in children under the age of two and is four times more common among girls than boys. The disease causes pain and swelling in one or more joints, coupled with a characteristic blotchy red rash that spreads over the trunk and limbs. Since there is no specific cure, treatment is aimed at relieving symptoms and preventing deterioration of the joints. The most common therapy is aspirin, together with adequate rest and a home exercise program designed to strengthen muscles and to maintain or improve the range of joint motion. Some cases, however, need to be treated with prescribed anti-inflammatory drugs. Although some young victims of JRA will develop the adult form of the disease, the outlook is bright for the vast majority of afflicted children. With treatment, they should go on to lead normal adult lives with little or no disability.

Symptoms:
- pain, swelling, or redness of affected joints — most often the neck, knees, ankles, elbows and wrists, usually worse in the morning or after a nap
- brief bouts of fever of up to 105° F., occurring once or twice a day
- blotchy red rash over the youngster's trunk and limbs, appearing and disappearing with the fever
- swollen lymph glands
- fatigue
- loss of weight

What to do:
- If JRA is diagnosed, administer aspirin or other medication as directed by your physician and follow his instructions regarding exercise, rest and diet for the child.

Call the doctor if:
- your child suffers at any time from persistent joint inflammation or pain.

Gait problems

The most important thing to know about gait problems — peculiarities in the movement or shape of feet or legs — is that most are not problems at all. Such apparent abnormalities as flatfeet, bowlegs and knock-knees are actually normal developmental phases through which nearly all children pass. In most cases, the conditions are self-correcting and seldom require medical attention. You should, however, consult your doctor if you suspect that your child's legs or feet are developing abnormally or if she is experiencing unusual difficulty in walking. Treatment, when necessary, may be a simple matter of exercising or of changing the child's sleeping position. Nowadays, most doctors do not recommend the use of corrective shoes for these kinds of gait problems.

Appearances can be deceptive when it comes to flatfeet. A baby's naturally chubby feet may only seem to be flat, largely due to the presence of a fat pad lying just below the arch; an X-ray of the baby's feet would reveal the hidden structure of the arch. Even the feet of a preschooler may appear flat while the youngster is standing or walking, since the ligaments binding the bones of the feet together are still too loose to support the child's standing weight. Within a few years, these ligaments will tighten up, and by the age of six the youngster's arches should be well developed.

Walking duck-footed (toeing-out) or pigeon-toed (toeing-in) is also common during childhood. Many children will toe out during the early stages of walking. This condition is a reflection of the awkward balancing act that is a toddler's walk. In time the problem usually corrects itself. Later, many children develop knock-knee, and often toe in to keep their balance. This, too, is almost always self-correcting. When treatment is necessary for toeing-in, it may consist of changing a child's usual sleeping position, sometimes with the aid of a brace that keeps the feet and knees properly aligned.

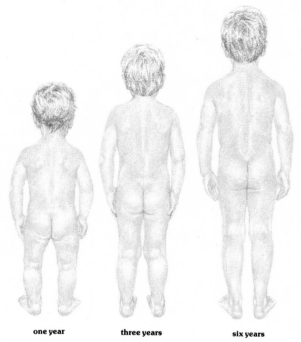

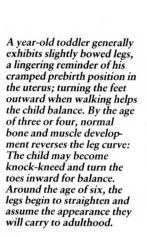

A year-old toddler generally exhibits slightly bowed legs, a lingering reminder of his cramped prebirth position in the uterus; turning the feet outward when walking helps the child balance. By the age of three or four, normal bone and muscle development reverses the leg curve: The child may become knock-kneed and turn the toes inward for balance. Around the age of six, the legs begin to straighten and assume the appearance they will carry to adulthood.

one year   **three years**   **six years**

Most children will tend to be bowlegged (when the ankles touch, the knees do not) until the age of 12 to 18 months. As the child learns to walk and the muscles gain strength, this tendency is gradually reversed — so much so that by the age of three or four, the child has become knock-kneed (when the knees touch, the ankles do not).

There is no reason to be concerned about this condition, either, unless the distance between the ankles when the knees are together is excessive. It should measure no more than one inch for each year of age up until the age of four. A four-year-old, for instance, may have as much as four inches between the insides of the ankles when standing with knees together. If the distance is greater than that, there may be a problem. But for most children, the knees and ankles begin to align at about four years of age and the legs will appear normal by the time the youngster is eight.

One orthopedic problem that should be detected and treated as early as possible is clubfoot. The condition may affect one or both feet and is the result of abnormally stretched or shortened muscles and tendons that twist the foot out of its normal position. Doctors are trained to look out for it during a newborn's first examination. Treatment — consisting of gentle manipulation, plaster casting and special shoes — should begin within the first few hours after birth, when the baby's bones are still extremely flexible. Occasionally, a surgeon's touch is needed to lengthen an offending tendon, but today, unlike in former times, a child born with a clubfoot can expect to run and walk normally.

Another condition physicians check for immediately is congenital dislocation of the hip — in which the ball-like head of the thighbone is not properly sited in the socket of the pelvis. At birth, the dislocation is usually only partial and can go unrecognized, so physicians keep checking by manipulating the baby's legs throughout the first year. In a very young infant, treatment is easy. A brace can hold the infant's thighs wide apart to force the ball into the socket. In an older infant, rectifying the problem is more difficult and can involve traction and spending several months in a plaster cast.

Joint pain

The most common cause of joint pain in children is trauma, an injury resulting from an accident. Happily, children heal quickly and with proper care will recover without impairment from all but the most serious injuries.

A simple, temporary joint pain without other symptoms usually does not require a doctor's attention. Often, such pain is merely the result of playtime overexertion and will disappear after a few hours of rest. Swelling, extensive bruising or constant pain may signal a more serious injury, such as a fracture or torn ligament, and you should summon medical help at once or go immediately to an emergency room. Pain accompanied by such symptoms as inflamed or swollen joints, fever or limping may indicate a bacterial or viral infection *(see Arthritis, page 50; Limp, below); Rheumatic Fever, page 82).* General viral infections such as influenza *(page 80)* can also cause limbs to ache. In general, you should call your doctor promptly at any sign of joint infection in your child or if joint pain persists for more than 24 hours.

Limp

A limp is caused by a child favoring one leg or by stiffness in a leg joint. It is a natural response to an injury or infection, and it may occur with or without pain. In a child too young to voice his complaint, limping may be the only indication of an underlying problem.

Among toddlers and young children, the leading causes of limping are trauma and hip disorders. Specifically, one- to three-year-olds are more likely to limp due to a fracture, sprain or other injury, while four- to six-year-olds are more prone to a hip inflammation called toxic synovitis — also known as transient synovitis or irritable hip syndrome. The cause of toxic synovitis is not known, although the ailment often occurs in the aftermath of an injury or a cold or sore throat. Pain and limping are the most frequently noted symptoms, and rest and warm baths are usually enough to get the youngster back on her feet.

Another hip disorder, Legg-Perthes disease, also afflicts children, most commonly boys between the ages of four and 10. It is due to an interruption of the blood supply to the round head at the upper end of the thighbone, which softens the bone. The disease develops slowly. The child may begin limping, then complain of vague pains in the joint *(see Joint Pain, page 5)*. Treatment consists of rest and a special brace that allows weight-bearing without further damaging the diseased bone end. Although therapy often must continue for several years, the outlook is for a complete recovery once the disease has run its course. Limping may also be a sign of more serious disorders, including arthritis *(page 50)* and rheumatic fever *(page 82)*.

As a general rule, contact your doctor whenever your child is limping but is too young to communicate the problem. An older child who is limping because of a bruise or minor injury will benefit from rest and applications of ice or heat to the affected area. However, if the limp persists for more than two days, the child should be taken to a doctor for medical evaluation. You should contact your doctor immediately if your child is limping and shows signs of fever or infection.

Muscle pain

Muscle pain is a common occurrence during childhood and is most often the result of overexertion during play. In such cases, the best cure is rest. Many children between three and six years old will occasionally complain of pains in the shins at night after a day of vigorous activity. Parents often call these aches, which are no cause for worry, "growing pains." The pains can be relieved by massage, heat application or aspirin. Do not give aspirin to a child who has, or has been recently exposed to, flu or chicken pox or other viral infection *(see Reye syndrome, page 105)*.

Everyday viral infections can also cause aches and pains *(see Influenza, page 80)*, while muscle pain associated with limping can be a sign of toxic synovitis *(see Limp, page 51)*. You should contact your doctor immediately if pain is coupled with a high fever or a rash *(see Arthritis, page 50; Rheumatic Fever, page 82)*. Depending on the underlying disorder, treatment may involve rest, special exercises or antibiotic therapy.

Spina bifida

Spina bifida is a birth defect that occurs second in frequency only to heart defects. It is a malformation of the spine that may affect the central nervous system. The bony rings of one or more vertebrae fail to close properly, and the spinal cord itself may also be defective. In most cases, spina bifida produces no symptoms other than a slight dimple over the affected area of the spine; mild cases of the disease may go undetected until a chance X-ray reveals the defect. In the most serious cases — when the delicate nerves of the spinal cord are covered only by a thin, bulging membrane — an afflicted child may suffer paralysis of the legs and lack of control of the bowel and bladder. Screening for spina bifida is part of every newborn's first examination, since early detection of the more severe form of this birth defect is crucial, and treatment, usually involving surgery, must be started immediately. ❖

Circulatory, Lymphatic and Glandular Systems

The circulatory system is composed of the heart and a network of veins and arteries through which blood is pumped. The blood shuttles oxygen and nutrients to every part of the body, while returning carbon dioxide and other waste products to the organs that dispose of them. Blood also forms a vital part of the body's defenses because its white cells trap and then destroy germs.

The lymphatic system, too, works to rid the body of wastes and helps protect it from infection. In this system, a network of vessels carries the excess fluid, called lymph, from body tissues, filtering it through lymph nodes, which remove and destroy bacteria and other invaders. Finally, the lymph is drained into veins near the heart, where the fluid enters the bloodstream. The spleen, which manufactures infection-fighting white blood cells and antibodies, and filters impurities from the blood, is also part of the lymphatic system. So are the thymus, the tonsils and the adenoids, all of which act as antibody-producing barriers against infectious agents invading the body.

The endocrine system consists of a number of glands, including the pituitary, thyroid, parathyroids, pancreas, adrenals, ovaries and testes. Each of these glands manufactures and secretes one or more hormones into the bloodstream.

These hormones are the body's chemical messengers, which speed to target organs and act to control or influence many bodily functions. The pituitary gland, for example, regulates the growth of the body and at the same time influences the

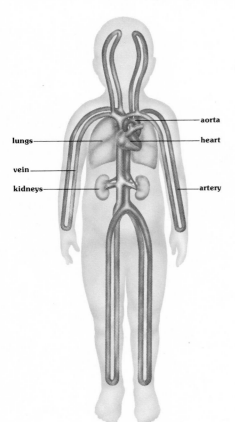

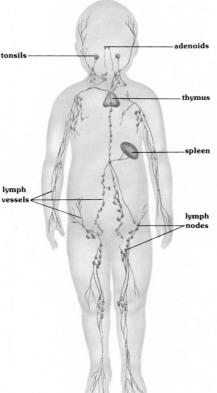

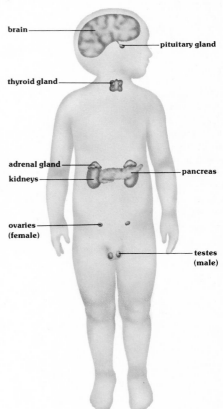

The circulatory system centers around the heart, which pumps blood through the aorta and its branching arteries, sending oxygen and nutrients to the tissues and organs. Blood flows back to the heart through veins, carrying fresh nutrients from the digestive tract. The heart shunts the blood through the lungs to take on oxygen before the cycle begins again. The kidneys filter out wastes picked up by the circulating blood.

The lymphatic system is composed of lymph vessels, circulating fluid, tissues and related organs that fight infection. Bacteria-destroying tissues called lymph nodes filter fluids draining through the lymph vessels; the tonsils and adenoids screen impurities entering through the mouth and nose. The spleen filters impurities from the blood and, along with the thymus, helps manage the child's resistance to infection.

The endocrine system includes several hormone-producing glands that help regulate bodily processes. The pituitary influences growth and kidney function. The thyroid controls metabolism. Adrenal glands produce adrenaline and help regulate blood pressure. Blood sugar is controlled by insulin and glucagon, secreted by the pancreas. The ovaries and testes produce hormones that affect reproduction and sex characteristics.

hormonal production of other glands. The pancreas produces insulin to control blood sugar levels, while the testes or ovaries govern male or female sexual characteristics. An imbalance in the hormonal levels of these glands can result in delayed growth or diabetes, among many other conditions.

As the child grows and matures, body systems adjust to the changing needs. Rapidly growing cells require a faster heart rate to meet their greater demand for nutrients and oxygen. The infant's heart beats 120 to 150 times per minute and may increase to 170 per minute when the baby is crying. Even when the infant is asleep, the heart works at 80 to 90 beats a minute. By the age of three, a child's normal heart rate range is down to 90 to 120 beats a minute, and by five years old to 85 to 110 per minute. By contrast, a normal adult heart rate is from 50 to 95 beats per minute.

A baby's lymphatic system also differs from an adult's: The thymus gland, which produces specialized white blood cells (T-cell lymphocytes) to combat infection, is larger in proportion to body size in an infant than in an adult, reflecting the youngster's greater need for protection against a constant onslaught of new infections. By puberty, the thymus gland has begun to shrink, and by adulthood, it has withered to little more than a bit of fat and connective tissue.

Anemia
Anemia is a disorder in which a deficiency of red blood cells results in a reduction of the blood's ability to ferry oxygen and waste products.

There are many kinds of anemia. Some types, including sickle cell anemia *(page 96)* are hereditary. Other types result from blood loss, long-term use of certain medicines (such as aspirin), poor nutrition or from an underlying disease or disorder that is destroying red blood cells or

producing malformed cells. One fairly common form of anemia among young children is iron-deficiency anemia. It occurs, as its name implies, when a child's diet lacks adequate amounts of iron, which is a necessary building block of hemoglobin, the chemical compound that actually carries the oxygen molecules in the blood.

All full-term babies are born with a four- to six-month supply of iron. After that time, a baby must obtain iron from her diet. For the baby who is still nursing on breast milk or on iron-fortified formula, this is no problem. However, cow's milk is a poor source of iron, and a baby relying on it for complete nourishment is likely to become anemic. You can prevent this by supplementing your baby's diet with such iron-rich foods as egg yolks, meat, green vegetables or iron-fortified cereals. A balanced diet will help keep older children from developing anemia. Any child showing signs of anemia should be taken to a doctor for evaluation. You should not attempt to diagnose or treat anemia yourself, since anemia may be a symptom of other disorders. In the case of iron-deficiency anemia, treatment may be as simple as iron supplements and a change in diet.

Symptoms:
- fatigue, irritability and decreased energy levels at play
- pallor of skin, lips, fingernails and the inside of eyelids
- loss of appetite
- in the more serious cases of anemia, lightheadedness, dizziness, breathlessness and headaches

What to do:
- In iron-deficiency anemia, an ounce of prevention is worth a pound of cure: Be sure that your child's diet provides an adequate amount of iron.
- If iron deficiency is diagnosed by your doctor, you should follow her instructions carefully.

Call the doctor if:
- over a period of several days your child seems pale and less active than usual, or if she loses her appetite.

Congenital heart disease
Congenital heart disease is a common and sometimes serious birth defect found in children. Approximately eight to nine infants of every 1,000 born will show some defect of the heart. Of those, two will face life-threatening difficulties during their first year.

There are about 60 to 70 different abnormalities that can affect the heart, including defects of the organ's pumping chambers or valves, or of the blood vessels that link the heart and lungs. Many of these defects may be identified by the doctor at birth. Others do not become apparent until several weeks or even months later. In minor cases, there may be no outward symptoms, but in general a child will be more prone to infection than his peers and will grow at a slower rate than normal. More serious cases of congenital heart disease cause cyanosis *(below),* which results in a bluish color of the skin. Treatment depends on the kind of defect and the extent of abnormal function. Mild cases of heart disease may require no special treatment or restriction of activities. Even a child with a more serious condition may lead a fairly active life. Today, sophisticated tests make precise diagnosis possible and heart surgery has a high rate of success.

Cyanosis
Caused by a lack of oxygen in the circulating blood, cyanosis is a bluish color of the skin, the mucous membranes and nailbeds. In advanced cases, a child's fingers may become clubbed — that is, the fingertips become enlarged and knobby — and the child may suffer fainting spells. Cyanosis can be caused by a lung disease or an airway obstruction, a cen-

tral nervous system problem, the production of abnormal hemoglobin, or a congenital heart defect or lung defect. Occasionally, otherwise healthy newborns will suffer from a mild degree of cyanosis as their systems become accustomed to life outside the womb. This should pass in a few hours. In any case, cyanosis is a condition that warrants immediate medical attention to identify its cause and prevent complications. Depending on the diagnosis, treatment may include surgery or medication.

Diabetes

Diabetes is a condition in which the body is unable to properly metabolize sugars. One type of the disease most often affects adults. Another type, insulin-dependent diabetes mellitus, also called juvenile-onset diabetes, strikes children. It tends to occur most commonly in children in two age groups: those aged five to seven and those at the age of puberty.

The body breaks down food sugars and starches into a sugar form called glucose, which is then released into the bloodstream. Normally, the pancreas, a gland located behind the stomach, secretes a hormone called insulin that helps the cells use glucose as fuel for energy. In diabetes, the pancreas, for unknown reasons, fails to produce enough insulin, leaving the body unable to utilize the glucose for energy. The glucose remains in the bloodstream at high levels and is filtered out by the kidneys and excreted in the urine. The body, meanwhile, is forced to burn its own fat and muscle to supply its energy needs. The sugar in the bloodstream draws water from body tissues, creating a large volume of urine that must be voided frequently.

In a child, the onset of diabetes is usually sudden and sometimes severe. If early symptoms are ignored, the child could suffer a diabetic coma and even death. Early detection and treatment of diabetes

are therefore essential, and you should contact your physician immediately if your youngster seems to have any symptoms of the disease.

Often urinalysis or a simple blood sugar test is all that is necessary to confirm the diagnosis, although the doctor will probably want to do more precise tests of glucose tolerance and insulin levels as well. Treatment of most cases involves daily injections of insulin, which you can administer at home, as well as regular urine testing and blood monitoring to control dosages and prevent excess sugar in the blood (hyperglycemia) or low blood sugar (hypoglycemia). Hypoglycemia, which can be caused by an overdose of insulin, causes headache, hunger and sweating in mild cases and can lead to convulsions and coma in more severe instances. Long-term care for diabetics includes frequent checkups to help prevent complications affecting the eyes, kidneys and other organs, as well as close attention to infections, which can have grave effects on diabetic children. Although diabetes is a serious disease, with treatment, diabetic children today can lead healthy, normal lives.

Symptoms:
- excessive thirst
- frequent urination, or possibly bed-wetting in a child who has been previously toilet-trained.
- excessive hunger
- weight loss
- dry skin
- weakness and fatigue
- tingling in the hands and feet
- blurred vision
- in more serious cases, difficulty in breathing, abdominal pain, vomiting, nausea, a sweet, fruity odor to the breath and a dry tongue.

What to do:
- If diabetes is diagnosed, follow your physician's instructions regarding insulin injections, urine testing, blood monitoring and dietary changes.

Call the doctor if:
- your child shows any sign of diabetes.
- a diabetic emergency occurs. An emergency could be the result of too much glucose in the blood, which would be signaled by nausea; vomiting; a sweet, fruity odor to the breath; or other symptoms listed above. Or it could be caused by too little glucose, leading to headache; cold, clammy skin; convulsions or even a coma.

Heart murmur

A heart murmur is an abnormal heart sound, which the doctor hears through a stethoscope. The sound — usually described as a hum, buzz or whistle — distorts the steady "lub-dub" sounds the heart normally makes as its valves open and close. As many as 50 percent of all children have what is called a functional, or innocent, murmur at one time or another. Such a murmur, often caused by turbulence in the blood vessels outside the heart and easily heard in children because of their thin chest walls, often presents no other symptoms and is usually first noticed by a doctor during a routine physical examination. In nearly every case, these murmurs disappear by the age of 14. Only a small percentage of heart murmurs are of the organic or acquired types. The organic type is usually caused by congenital heart disease. An acquired murmur might be the result of an infection. In those cases, a doctor will probably order X-rays, an electrocardiogram and blood tests to pinpoint the type and cause of the murmur. Treatment depends on the cause. Surgery is occasionally necessary to correct a structural defect.

Hodgkin's disease

Hodgkin's disease is a form of lymphoma, a cancer of the lymph system. It rarely affects children under the age of five. Swollen glands in the neck, armpits and groin are usually the first signs of the disease. Fever, weight loss, night sweats and persistent itching of the skin are also symptoms. Later, the liver and spleen become involved, and there may be bone pain as the disease invades the skeleton. While early diagnosis is essential, Hodgkin's disease is today one of the most treatable of all childhood cancers, with a cure rate of more than 90 percent. Treatment for the disease includes chemotherapy and radiation therapy.

Hypoglycemia

Hypoglycemia is a condition in which an abnormally low level of glucose is circulating in the bloodstream. It has many causes, including liver-enzyme deficiencies, overproduction of insulin by the pancreas, pituitary- and adrenal-gland deficiencies, and drug and alcohol reactions. Hypoglycemia can also occur in diabetics who are being treated with insulin. In these cases, too great a dosage causes an insulin reaction — a rapid decrease in blood glucose that deprives

muscles and cells of the fuel they need for energy. A glass of orange juice, a candy bar, a piece of fruit or another source of sugar quickly counters the attack *(see Diabetes, page 55)*.

Hypoglycemia is fairly common in newborns and even more so in premature babies because they quickly use up the glucose the mother provided while they were in the womb. This condition passes with the proper treatment. Children from 18 months to five years may also develop hypoglycemia, although doctors do not know the exact cause. Hypoglycemic attacks often occur in the morning after a long night without food. Or you may notice symptoms after the child has had strenuous exercise. Since glucose is necessary for brain metabolism, the first symptoms of a problem are those affecting the nervous system. Emergency treatment for a hypoglycemic attack is the same as that for a diabetic insulin reaction — the immediate ingestion of sugar, in the form of candy, fruit or juice. Afterward, you should consult your doctor, who will probably recommend an overnight stay in the hospital for a thorough blood sugar test. Long-term treatment includes more frequent meals to maintain an adequate intake of carbohydrates. Fortunately, intermittent hypoglycemia of childhood tends to disappear by the age of 10.

Symptoms:
- pale skin color
- hunger, nervousness and irritability, trembling, excessive sweating
- headaches
- fatigue, drowsiness and sometimes slurred speech
- fainting
- vomiting
- in more serious cases, bizarre behavior, seizures, coma

What to do:
- In case of a hypoglycemic attack or an insulin reaction, give sugar, orange

juice, fruit or candy immediately.
- If hypoglycemia is diagnosed, follow your doctor's advice.

Call the doctor if:
- your child exhibits some combination of the symptoms listed above.

Leukemia

Leukemia is the most common form of childhood cancer, with the period of greatest incidence occurring at around the age of four. Its cause is unknown, although previous exposure to radiation, chemicals or certain drugs may be a factor. Research has also implicated a virus as one possible cause. Dramatic improvements have been made in the treatment of childhood leukemia, and today 90 percent of young patients will experience periods of significant remission, and more than half will survive for five years or more, by which time the disease can be considered cured.

Under normal circumstances, the bone marrow manufactures red blood cells, white blood cells and platelets, which respectively transport oxygen, fight infection and help clot blood. Leukemia, however, causes an abnormal multiplication of white blood cells. In the most common form of childhood leukemia, acute lymphocytic leukemia, these abnormal white blood cells crowd out normal bone marrow elements, which causes anemia, infection and bleeding. The onset is often sudden, and a child will show such symptoms as fatigue, headaches, swollen glands, repeated infections, weight loss and easy bruising. Early detection is often difficult, since many less serious diseases share the same symptoms, so prompt medical evaluation is necessary. If the results of blood tests and a biopsy of the bone marrow confirm a diagnosis of leukemia, the child will usually be hospitalized and immediately started on a regimen of drugs to combat the disease. Fortunately, leukemia is rare, and the out-

Clustered in the neck, armpits and groin, lymph glands enlarge as they trap and destroy harmful bacteria and viruses. This swelling, often lasting for weeks after the infection is gone, is a normal reaction caused by a concentration in the glands of infection-fighting cells.

look is continually improving with such new techniques as bone marrow transplantation, in which a portion of a leukemia victim's bone marrow is replaced by healthy donor tissue.

Swollen glands

The lymphatic system is part of the body's intricate line of defenses against disease. Comprised of a network of lymph vessels, the system is strung with knots of tissue called lymph nodes, or glands. These are located throughout the body — with concentrations in the neck, armpits, groin and abdomen — and include the tonsils and adenoids. These nodes serve as tiny manufacturing centers for antibodies against disease, and they also filter out dead bacteria, viruses and white blood cells from the lymph fluid. In the presence of infection, the lymph nodes produce more antibodies and become enlarged, hence the term "swollen glands."

Swollen glands are very common in children. Illnesses such as measles, chicken pox, strep throat, infectious mononucleosis and most other childhood maladies will cause enlarged lymph nodes, as will an infected tooth or an earache. *(See Infection, page 97; Colds, page 75; Sore Throat, page 83.)* These will often persist for weeks and even months after the infection has cleared up. In fact, some youngster's may seem always to have swollen glands or tonsils. In the absence of other symptoms, such swelling is nothing to worry about.

Allergies *(page 46),* too, may produce swollen glands. Even more rarely, such serious disorders as Hodgkin's disease *(page 56)* and leukemia *(page 56)* may cause glands to swell. Since swollen glands are a sign that the body's defenses are working properly, no therapy is necessary other than to ascertain and treat the underlying problem. However, you should contact your physician if you notice red streaks on your youngster's neck, armpits or groin, which are an indication that the lymph nodes themselves have become infected or abscessed.

Thyroid problems

The thyroid gland is located in the front of the neck, below the larynx. It regulates the body's metabolism through the secretion of a hormone called thyroxine, which is necessary for growth and development. Underproduction of this hormone (hypothyroidism) or overproduction of it (hyperthyroidism) can create systemic problems and require a doctor's attention. But it is important to note that both of these disorders are rare, and both are easily treated.

Hypothyroidism can be either congenital or acquired and afflicts both babies and older children. Left untreated, it can cause cretinism, a stunting of physical and mental growth. A child or baby with hypothyroidism will exhibit such symptoms as thick, dry skin; slow growth; enlarged tongue; puffy face and sluggishness. Treatment involves daily doses of thyroxine replacements.

Hyperthyroidism, on the other hand, speeds up the metabolism and mainly tends to affect teenagers, especially teenage girls. Early symptoms include restlessness, sweating, increased appetite and rapid pulse. Later, the eyes may bulge, muscle tremors develop and the youngster loses weight despite her increase in appetite. Some children will have a goiter or enlarged thyroid gland. If hyperthyroidism is diagnosed, the doctor will prescribe antithyroid medication. Surgery may also be necessary. ∵

Common Infectious Diseases

The seemingly endless succession of serious infectious diseases that for centuries were the bane of childhood has largely been eliminated by vaccines. The dread killer smallpox, for instance, has been officially declared nonexistent; the last known case on the face of the earth was reported in 1978, and that was caused by a laboratory accident. Polio, once the crippler of hundreds of thousands of children, has been nearly wiped out. But the battle is not finished. Some serious diseases are still not preventable by vaccines and others threaten to reestablish themselves because too many children are not being vaccinated.

Infectious diseases are caused by bacteria and viruses. In most cases these are spread by sneezing, coughing, kissing or hand contact from an infected person. After the harmful bacterium or virus enters the body of the new host, it multiplies and spreads but does not cause symptoms for days or, occasionally, weeks. During this so-called incubation period before symptoms appear, the ill person may transmit the disease to others. Most

bacteria can be overcome by antibiotics, but for most viral diseases, there is no cure once the incubation period begins: The illness must then run its course.

Even though cures are rare in viral infections, the body can learn to resist invading organisms by producing antibodies to combat them. This resistence is called immunity. It is acquired naturally when a person contracts and recovers from a disease. A vaccination artificially creates the threat of disease in the body so that the immune system produces the specific antibodies needed to fight off the disease, should it ever actually attack a vaccinated child. The immunization is accomplished with agents that cause the body's defensive system to react as if the real disease were at hand. There are three types of these agents: killed disease-

causing bacteria or viruses; weakened live ones; and modified versions of the toxins, or poisons, that are released by certain types of bacteria.

Some vaccinations confer immunity in a single dose. With others, one dose does not produce enough antibodies to guarantee lifelong immunity. Those types must either be taken in stages or reinforced at intervals with boosters.

Newborn babies are temporarily immune to many diseases because antibodies have passed into their bloodstreams from the blood of their mothers. However, these antibodies last only six to 12 months and, since the mother's antibodies are incapable of regenerating, babies have to be vaccinated to stay immune. Vaccines are administered when a baby's inherited antibodies are diminishing and his own defensive system is mature enough to produce new antibodies. Some vaccines are given in combination with others *(chart, below)*. It is essential to keep a record of vaccinations.

All vaccinations carry a small risk of side effects. Normally, these are mild and

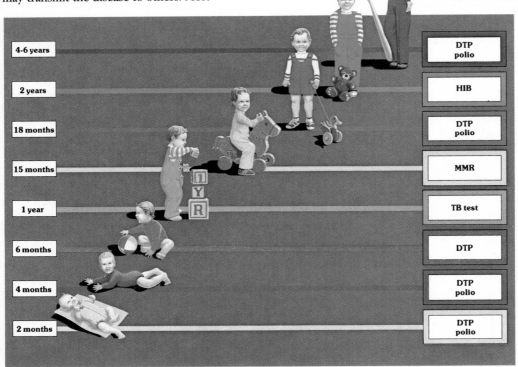

4-6 years	DTP polio
2 years	HIB
18 months	DTP polio
15 months	MMR
1 year	TB test
6 months	DTP
4 months	DTP polio
2 months	DTP polio

A Timetable for Inoculations
To protect children against certain serious illnesses, the American Academy of Pediatrics recommends immunization against eight diseases — polio, measles, mumps, rubella, diphtheria, tetanus, whooping cough (pertussis) and Hemophilus (HIB) infections. The chart at left shows the suggested sequence of the inoculations. Testing for tuberculosis is also recommended.

The shot for measles, mumps and rubella (MMR) and the shot for HIB infections produce protective levels of antibodies with one inoculation. The vaccinations for diphtheria, tetanus and pertussis — combined in the DTP shot — and for polio must be repeated several times.

of little concern. However, the side effects of the whooping-cough vaccine have made it a long-standing source of controversy *(box, page 61)*.

To fight certain diseases, doctors call upon a defense that is similar to but slightly different from the one produced by vaccines. Instead of administering agents that stimulate antibody production, the doctor injects the antibodies directly into the body in what is called immune serum globulin, or gamma globulin. This serum is obtained from the blood of donors who already have the antibodies. Administered after a child has been exposed to disease, these antibodies offer partial or full protection for a while, but they eventually diminish, leaving the body no more immune than before. These shots are essentially stopgap measures and should not be confused with vaccinations.

Chicken pox

Chicken pox is a highly contagious viral disease that is widespread among children, usually striking youngsters between the ages of five and nine. A vaccine was developed in 1974, but as late as the mid-1980s it was still being tested and was not yet approved for general use.

The characteristic symptom of chicken pox — after the appearance of a low fever — is a rash that begins as flat red spots, first appearing on the back, chest and abdomen. The spots rapidly rise to form fragile, watery blisters that are red at the base and easily rubbed open. Within hours, the blisters break and scab over. In the next day or two, the rash spreads to the face, scalp and upper parts of the arms and legs. Two to four crops of the spots may appear in the ensuing two to six days. They may also spread to the mouth, palms, soles of the feet and the genitals. Severe itching accompanies the phase when the blisters are breaking.

Children with chicken pox are contagious from the day before the rash appears until all the blisters have formed scabs — usually a period of seven days. The virus is spread both by droplets sprayed from the mouth or nose and by fluid from the blisters. Once infected, a child will not show symptoms for 14 to 17 days. If you suspect chicken pox, call your doctor and have the diagnosis confirmed. Be sure to tell the physician if your child has another illness as well or if he takes any special medication.

The youngster does not have to be confined to bed or even kept indoors. Just make sure that his activity is quiet and that he stays cool, since perspiration will increase the itching. The child can maintain a normal diet.

Itching will be the main problem. To counter this, use calamine lotion and give the child baths of tepid water mixed with baking soda or cornstarch. Drugs are usually unnecessary and should be used only on the advice of your doctor. Try to keep the child from scratching, which can lead to bacterial infection of the open blisters and can cause scars that last for years. White cotton gloves can help control nighttime scratching.

Count on the child staying home for about one week. When all the blisters have scabbed, the fever will wane and he can return to his day-care center or school if he feels well enough. The scabs may last for another week and leave behind light scars that will gradually fade.
Symptoms:
- low fever (less than 102° F.), loss of appetite, and fatigue during the 24 hours before the rash appears
- a rash that progresses from red spots to blisters and eventually scabs
What to do:
- Clip the child's fingernails and wash his hands frequently during the day, preferably with an antibacterial soap.
- Relieve the itching with calamine lotion or by bathing the child two or three times a day in tepid water mixed with ½ cup of baking soda or ¼ cup of cornstarch.
- Keep the child's skin clean with normal soap-and-water baths. Use tepid, not hot, water. Change his clothing and bedclothes frequently.
- Relieve the child's fever with acetaminophen. DO NOT give the child aspirin, which has been linked to a very dangerous illness called Reye syndrome *(page 105)*.
- If lesions appear in the mouth, have the child gargle with ½ teaspoon of salt mixed with eight ounces of water. Cease this treatment if it pains him. Feed a youngster with mouth lesions soft, bland food.
Call the doctor if:
- you suspect that your youngster has come down with chicken pox.
- the blisters become infected; that is, if they are inflamed and pus-filled.
- you suspect pneumonia *(page 81)*, which can strike up to 10 days after the rash appears.
- the youngster is overly drowsy or suffers severe headaches or a stiff neck. These are symptoms of encephalitis *(page 103)*, a rare complication of chicken pox.
- the youngster vomits profusely or shows any abnormal behavior.

Diphtheria

Diphtheria is an extremely serious disease, which can be fatal if not treated early. It is caused by bacteria that lodge in the nose and throat, then release a powerful toxin that attacks nerves and the muscles of the heart.

A vaccine has made diphtheria a very rare malady in industrialized countries. The vaccine consists of a form of the toxin that is altered in a laboratory to render it safe but still capable of producing immunity. The protection, however, is neither complete nor permanent and the vaccine must be given five times before a child is six years old. After that time, booster shots will be needed every 10 years for life.

The diphtheria vaccine is given in conjunction with vaccines for tetanus and whooping cough in an injection called the DTP shot. (Whooping cough is formally known as pertussis; thus, DTP for diphtheria-tetanus-pertussis.) Your child could suffer an undesirable reaction to this shot (box, page 61).

HIB disease

HIB is an acronym for the name of a bacterium, *Hemophilus influenzae* type B. Oddly, it has nothing to do with what we call influenza, or flu. In the 19th century, when the HIB bacterium was discovered and named, it was thought to cause flu, but in fact it does not: Influenza is caused by viruses.

In the past, HIB infections have affected one child in 200 under the age of five. The infection can lead to several very serious afflictions. One of these is meningitis, an inflammation of the membranes surrounding the brain and spinal cord, a condition that can lead to deafness, mental retardation or death: More than half of childhood meningitis cases in the United States are caused by the bacterium. Another HIB manifestation is called epiglottitis, a severe form of croup in which the windpipe becomes partially or totally blocked. Epiglottitis usually affects children three to six years old. HIB infections also sometimes lead to a potentially crippling form of arthritis. Ear infections, pneumonia and blood poisoning are other potential complications.

A vaccine, first approved for widespread use in 1985, is now available to immunize children against the worst types of HIB infections. It will not protect children from HIB-induced ear infections or from meningitis that develops from other types of bacteria. Nevertheless, it is a powerful deterrent against some dire and all-too-common complications.

The HIB vaccine is given in a single shot. It produces few and minor side effects. Your child should be vaccinated within one month of her second birthday. If she attends a day-care center or nursery school, the risk of infection is higher and your doctor may want to give the injection as early as 18 months. However, if your youngster is vaccinated that young, the inoculation may have to be repeated later. Children up to five years old are vaccinated. It is not necessary to vaccinate older children and adults because there is little risk of HIB disease after the age of five.

Measles

Once, almost no child was spared this highly contagious viral disease, which is sometimes called seven-day or red measles to distinguish it from its milder cousin, three-day or German measles, also known as rubella. But since the early 1960s, when a vaccine became available, the number of cases has plummeted. Some parents, considering measles to be a childhood rite of passage, have wondered whether a vaccine is necessary. But measles makes a child very sick for up to a week and can lead to serious complications, including pneumonia, meningitis and encephalitis. Before the vaccine, measles was responsible for 400 deaths a year in the United States.

Measles is accompanied by a red rash, a bad cough and a high fever. It has an incubation period of about 10 days. The vaccine stimulates antibodies in seven days, so measles is one of the few illnesses that can be successfully countered by a vaccination if it is given within a day or two after exposure. Immune serum globulin, which contains ready-made antibodies from blood donors, is also effective if administered during the incubation period.

The measles vaccine is a weakened virus that is given in combination with vaccines for mumps and rubella. Together they make up the MMR (measles-mumps-rubella) shot. A single injection at 15 months produces lifelong immunity.

Although the MMR shot is cultured in part in the cells of chick embryos, it can be administered to children who are allergic to eggs — except those youngsters whose allergies are so severe that they have suffered anaphylactic shock from eating eggs.

A very small percentage of children suffer a mild reaction six to 11 days after the MMR shot. Normally, the reaction is nothing more than a slight fever and malaise. Let the child rest and treat the fever with acetaminophen. Rarely, a child may develop a rash. An even smaller number will experience aching or swelling of the joints two to eight weeks after the inoculation. This will pass without treatment in a few days' time.

Mumps

Mumps is a formerly common childhood illness caused by a virus that sometimes makes the salivary glands near the back of the jaw swell up. However, almost half the cases of mumps are so mild that the victims are unaware they have the disease, although the infection is sufficient to make them immune for life. Consequently, many adults are immune to mumps but do not know it. In adults, the disease can inflame the ovaries or testes, and in rare instances, mumps has been known to cause sterility.

The mumps vaccine is a weakened virus. It is given when a child reaches 15 months of age as part of a combined shot with the vaccines for measles and rubella — the MMR shot. A single injection gives a youngster lifelong immunity. For more information on the MMR shot, possible reactions to it and measures for dealing with the reactions, see the preceding entry, Measles.

The DTP Shot: Weighing the Pros and Cons

The DTP shot is extremely effective in immunizing children against three very grave diseases — diphtheria, tetanus and pertussis (or whooping cough). It is normally administered to a child five times between the ages of two months and six years. While the shot long ago proved its usefulness, it has also been a source of nagging worry to parents because of doubts about the safety of the pertussis vaccine. In continuing to recommend the DTP shot, doctors weigh the risks of the vaccine against the risks of the disease. You can do the same.

The main agent in the whooping-cough vaccine is dead pertussis bacteria. Unpleasant reactions to this are common, but in the vast majority of cases they are very mild: typically, a low fever, irritability, drowsiness, or soreness and minor swelling where the shot was given. Unfortunately, the vaccine occasionally causes more serious reactions and, very rarely, results in brain damage.

Doctors believe the damage that could be done by the disease if there were no widespread vaccination program far outweighs the risks involved in using the vaccine. Researchers estimate that of 3.5 million children, roughly the number born in the United States in a typical year, more than 350,000 would get whooping cough without a vaccination program — 10 times as many as with vaccinations. It is true that about 51 of the 3.5 million children can be expected to suffer brain damage from the vaccine. But with no vaccinations, 29 would be expected to suffer brain damage from the disease itself. And most telling, almost 460 children would die from whooping cough without widespread vaccinations, more than 10 times as many as are thought to die of the disease now, either because they were not vaccinated or because the vaccinations were not effective.

The disease has staged a comeback in recent years, apparently because of parental reluctance to let their children take the vaccine. Whooping cough is still deadly to small children. It cannot be treated with antibiotics once the telltale cough has developed.

Doctors are now very cautious in their use of the DTP shot. They will not give the pertussis vaccine to a child who is ill or who has had a serious reaction to an earlier DTP injection. They will sometimes administer just the diphtheria and tetanus portions.

If your child does not have a bad reaction to the first DTP shot, it is unlikely that he will react to the later injections. If he does have a reaction, it is very unlikely that he will be in any danger. However, you should call your doctor if the child shows any of these signs within 48 hours after an inoculation: persistent crying for longer than three hours, extreme sleepiness, limpness, paleness, fever over 103° F., undue irritability or a convulsion.

Polio

Polio, known clinically as poliomyelitis and informally as infantile paralysis, is the dread warm-weather disease that as late as the early 1950s crippled many thousands of children. Now, thanks to two types of vaccines, polio is almost eradicated in the United States and other industrialized countries.

Polio is a viral disease that has no cure. It can take a mild course or one that cripples and kills. Early symptoms, after an incubation period of seven to 14 days, are fever, headache, sore throat and sometimes loss of appetite and vomiting. In the harsher version, a stiff neck will develop. If you suspect polio because your child has not been vaccinated and shows some symptoms, put the child to bed at once and call emergency medical help. If the victim is not kept still in this early stage, paralysis is more likely to occur.

Dr. Jonas Salk introduced an inactivated polio virus vaccine (IPV) in 1955. It was given by injection and greatly reduced the number of polio cases. Six years later, Dr. Albert Sabin developed an oral polio virus vaccine (OPV). This contains a live virus and is considered to be more surely effective. It is given four times before a child is six years old, by drops in the mouth. Once the series is complete, immunity should last a lifetime. The vaccine produces no side effects, and your child may eat, drink or play normally after taking a dose.

Very rarely, a parent who has never been immunized against polio may get the disease from a child who has received the live vaccine. An unimmunized parent should be injected with the inactivated vaccine before his youngster receives the first OPV dose.

Rubella

Rubella, also called German measles and three-day measles, is less severe than its cousin, seven-day measles. In fact, rubella is so mild that it would not merit a vaccine at all except for a single disastrous consequence: In the unborn babies of pregnant women who catch it, rubella can cause blindness, heart disease and deafness. Embryos in their first three months are at greatest risk. Thus the main goal of vaccination is to protect not the children receiving the shots, but the unborn. All children should be vaccinated.

Rubella is prevented with a live-virus vaccine given at 15 months as part of the MMR (measles-mumps-rubella) shot (see Measles, page 60). Complications are few and dealt with easily. If you are pregnant, discuss with your doctor whether it is safe to have your child vaccinated.

Symptoms of rubella are often difficult to detect because they are so mild — a light rash, aches, a sore throat, low fever, and enlarged, tender lymph nodes in the back of the neck. If you suspect that your child has rubella, call your doctor. Warn any women of childbearing age with whom your child has had contact in the previous 21 days and keep him away from anyone without immunity until five days after a rash appears.

Tetanus

Tetanus is not infectious in the sense that an ill person can pass it to another person by coughing or through body contact. The disease afflicts its victims when tetanus bacteria and their spores infest tissue under the skin, shut off from exposure to oxygen. Tetanus most often develops in puncture wounds, burns or scrapes, where a lot of dead tissue is present.

Contrary to folklore, rust has nothing specifically to do with tetanus. The bacteria and spores that cause the disease thrive in common dirt and dust, usually in rural areas, where animal feces are often infected. The proverbial rusty nail can be any puncturing object covered with dirt, but a rusty nail in a barn is far more likely to give tetanus than one in a city basement. Once introduced into a body, the bacteria release a powerful toxin, or poison, that attacks the nerves, affecting muscle control and sometimes causing severe spasms of the jaw muscles. This explains the common name, lockjaw, which is often applied to tetanus. The disease can be fatal.

A vaccine can prevent tetanus. It is denoted by the "T" in the DTP (diphtheria-tetanus-pertussis) shot (box, page 62). In addition to the three shots given in the first year of life, shots are needed at the age of 18 months and at four to six years. Tetanus boosters should be given every 10 years thereafter. If a child has been getting his shots on time, he is protected, but will probably be given a booster if he is injured and five years have lapsed since his last shot. If a child is not protected by vaccination, tetanus immune serum globulin, made from human blood that contains antibodies to the disease, may help. If the child develops tetanus, antibiotics can help relieve the disease but will not cure it. As with all inoculations, it is important to keep a record of your youngster's tetanus shots.

Whooping Cough

Whooping cough is a bacterial disease whose course is often vicious and lengthy. The first symptoms appear one to two weeks following exposure. Although some cases are mild and clear up within a week or two, an acute case can cause severe coughing and complications that last up to six weeks. In the worst cases, whooping cough results in brain damage and death. Most of its victims are less than seven years old. A vaccine is available, but the disease has by no means been eliminated. Even in countries where vaccination has been widespread, whooping cough started making a comeback in the 1970s, because some parents began to fear that possible side effects from the vaccine were more dangerous than the disease (box, page 61).

Whooping cough's medical name is pertussis, represented by the "P" in the DTP (diphtheria-tetanus-pertussis) inoculation. Its common name derives from the whooplike sound that a victim makes as he struggles for breath between severe bouts of coughing, which can occur dozens of times per day. Eating and sleeping become very difficult and vomiting often follows the coughing. Other serious consequences of whooping cough are dehydration, weight loss, exhaustion and pneumonia. This disease requires extraordinarily intensive nursing care and, frequently, hospitalization.

Whooping cough is particularly dangerous to babies. A newborn baby has very little immunity because a mother's antibodies for the disease do not pass through her placenta into the baby's bloodstream as easily as do antibodies for other diseases, such as measles. Babies who contract this illness may be so exhausted after a coughing spell that they cannot muster the power to whoop for breath as older children do. The result is that they are deprived of their usual flow of oxygen and may turn blue, have convulsions and lose consciousness. More than half of the fatalities caused by whooping cough occur among children less than one year old.

In order to protect infants, the first DTP shot is administered when the child is two months old. To ensure lifelong immunity, four more injections are needed before the child is six (chart, page 58). Antibiotics may stop the disease if administered before the acute, whooping stage. So if you know your unvaccinated child has been exposed to whooping cough, see the doctor immediately.

Symptoms:
- in mild cases, a coldlike runny nose, slight cough and low fever that lasts for one to two weeks
- in serious cases, coughing in violent spasms, followed by a whoop as the child struggles to breathe in again
- sometimes, vomiting following coughing bouts

What to do:
- Be prepared to hospitalize your child if your doctor feels that is necessary.
- Stay with your child through each bout of coughing to ease his fear if he becomes panicky and to wipe away mucus that is coughed up or vomited. You may need to thump the child on the back to help him bring up mucus from his throat.
- Counter dehydration and weight loss with clear fluids and small amounts of food when the coughing subsides.
- On the advice of your physician, use a sedative to help the child sleep.
- Keep your child isolated from the public until he is no longer contagious — a period of five weeks, the first two of which are the most dangerous. In particular, keep him away from newborn babies and any other nonimmune children.
- Arrange for regular help to come: You will need relief.

Call the doctor if:
- you know your unvaccinated youngster has been exposed to whooping cough, or if your child has symptoms of the disease.
- you suspect pneumonia (page 81).
- your youngster suffers a seizure or if he collapses. ❖

Digestive System

The digestive system breaks down complex foods into basic substances such as proteins, sugars and fats that the body can use for growth or fuel. It also eliminates the solid wastes left over after the food has been digested.

A baby's digestive system is immature and cannot immediately handle adult foods. That is why easy-to-digest mother's milk or an equivalent formula is the baby's first diet. Later, carbohydrate-rich cereals are introduced; later still, foods high in protein; and finally, fats, the most difficult to digest.

The body gets water, too, through the digestive tract. The ratio of water to body weight in infants and toddlers is much higher than it is in adults. And children's small bodies need to renew their water much more often. A quarter to a third of the water in a child's body is replaced every day, compared to only one tenth of the water in an adult's. Because of this, any sudden loss of a child's water, such as that caused by diarrhea or vomiting, can lead rapidly to serious dehydration *(page 65),* and immediate measures must be taken to replace the fluid.

Your youngster's nutritional needs and tastes in food change frequently as he grows and develops. You may occasionally worry that his appetite or eating pattern is somehow abnormal. Be assured that as long as a child is growing and gaining weight at a reasonable rate, sporadic eating binges or finicky periods that last a few days are nothing to be overly concerned about.

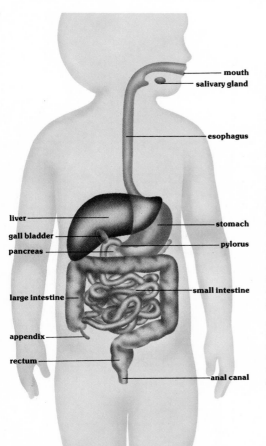

The digestive tract begins at the mouth, where saliva and teeth break up food into small, partially digested bits. The food then passes down a long tube called the esophagus into the stomach. There, gastric juices liquefy and partially digest the food before it is gradually admitted, through a valve that is called the pylorus, into the small intestine. The major portion of digestion occurs in this long, convoluted tube as enzymes secreted by the intestine and pancreas, aided by bile from the liver and gall bladder, reduce the food to chemical components that can be used by the body. These are absorbed through the intestinal walls and enter the blood and lymphatic systems for distribution throughout the body. Undigested food then passes through the large intestine, where water is extracted and absorbed before the residue reaches the rectum for elimination via the anal canal. The appendix, which is a tiny cul de sac on the lower right of the large intestine, serves no apparent purpose in the digestive process.

mouth
salivary gland
esophagus
liver
stomach
gall bladder
pylorus
pancreas
large intestine
small intestine
appendix
rectum
anal canal

Abdominal pain

Abdominal distress — usually called stomachache — is a very common childhood complaint. Depending on the underlying cause, the child may experience anything from mild, intermittent cramps to steady, acute pain. In children too young to describe their symptoms, behavior that indicates pain includes crying, irritability, grasping the belly or pointing to it and, in infants especially, curling the body and tensing the legs. If the child eats, walks, plays and sleeps normally despite her complaints, there is nothing seriously wrong: Something like indigestion or gas may be the problem. You should become concerned, however, if she refuses to eat or move, or cannot sleep. Any constant, unremitting pain that lasts longer than three hours should be reported to your doctor.

Knowing the type of pain and accompanying symptoms will help pinpoint the cause. One common cause, constipation *(page 65),* results from hardened stools in the lower bowel and is characterized by a dull, steady pain. Bacterial and viral infections of the stomach or intestines usually produce cramps, along with vomiting or diarrhea or both. In cases of intussusception *(page 70)* — when a section of the intestine telescopes into itself, causing a blockage — the child usually vomits and has severe cramps. After the pain subsides she is likely to remain very still. Appendicitis *(page 64)* is also signaled by pain in the abdomen.

Abdominal pain may also be a symptom of a disease outside the digestive system, such as pneumonia, urinary-tract infection or sore throat. Emotional upsets, even in a very young child, can also trigger belly pain *(see Stress-related illness, page 107).* Though the pain does not originate in a physical problem, it is still real and must be taken seriously. The best treatment for this kind of pain is parental sensitivity and attention.

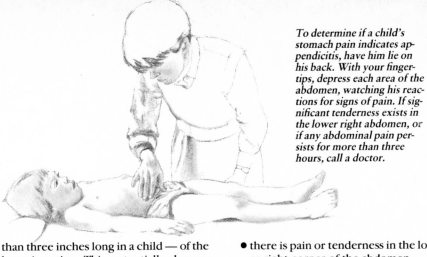

To determine if a child's stomach pain indicates appendicitis, have him lie on his back. With your fingertips, depress each area of the abdomen, watching his reactions for signs of pain. If significant tenderness exists in the lower right abdomen, or if any abdominal pain persists for more than three hours, call a doctor.

Whatever its cause, DO NOT give aspirin or paregoric for abdominal pain. DO NOT give a laxative or an enema unless your doctor specifically recommends it. Such treatments may mask a problem or make it worse. Applying a hot-water bottle — wrapped in a towel and not hot enough to burn the youngster — provides safe and, in most cases, substantial relief. Temporarily eliminating all dairy products — which are difficult to digest — from the diet may also help curb discomfort. Instead of milk, the child should drink such clear liquids as water, apple juice, flat soda, sweetened gelatin solution or weak tea.

Anal fissure

A small crack in the tissue at the open end of the rectum is often signaled by streaks or spots of bright red blood on the surface of the stool or on toilet paper. The condition is more common in infants than in older children. It is usually associated with constipation, which can either cause it or result from it. Hard, constipated stools irritate the anal opening and widen tiny cracks in the tissue. But when a crack is present for some other reason, a child may try to avoid pain by withholding bowel movements and so become constipated. The result is a worsening cycle of constipation and tissue injury. To break this cycle, take action to soften the stool, thus lessening the irritation so that the crack can heal. One way you can help soften the stool is by increasing dietary fiber. For example, feed your child fruits, whole-grain cereals and bran breads.

If a change in food does not help, your physician may recommend a medicinal stool softener. Laxatives are seldom a useful treatment for anal fissure because they provide only temporary relief.

Appendicitis

Appendicitis is an inflammation of the appendix, a worm-shaped protrusion — less than three inches long in a child — of the large intestine. This potentially dangerous ailment, which rarely strikes a child younger than two, produces constant pain that usually begins around the navel and then shifts to the lower right area of the abdomen. However, in about 20 percent of cases, the pain is more widespread. When your child complains of abdominal pain, try to determine if it is localized by gently pressing his belly with your hand *(above)*. Marked tenderness in the lower right abdomen should be reported to your doctor promptly. Early diagnosis is crucial, since a diseased appendix can rupture and spread infection to the abdominal cavity. If the child is diagnosed as having appendicitis, he will probably be admitted to the hospital to have the appendix removed surgically. When he goes under general anesthesia, it is important that the stomach be empty; so make sure your child has only clear liquids to drink if there is a possibility he has appendicitis.

Symptoms:
- pain beginning near the child's navel and moving to the lower right section of the abdomen
- temperature of 100° F. or more
- loss of appetite
- nausea and vomiting

What to do:
- Determine whether one area is noticeably tender.
- Take the youngster's temperature every two hours.
- Give the child clear liquids in small quantities only.
- DO NOT give the youngster a laxative or any other medicine unless approved by a physician.

Call the doctor if:

- there is pain or tenderness in the lower right corner of the abdomen.
- any abdominal pain lasts for more than three hours, whatever the location of the pain.
- the pain stops suddenly. This could mean the appendix has ruptured.

Celiac disease

This is an intestinal disorder caused by an intolerance of gluten, a protein found in wheat and rye. Symptoms include greasy, foul-smelling, runny stools, a distended belly, weight loss and even a failure to grow. Once a physician has made the diagnosis, treatment is simple: All wheat and rye products — breads, cakes, most pastas — are omitted from the child's diet for the rest of his life. A nutritionist can help choose replacement foods and vitamin and mineral supplements.

Cleft lip and cleft palate

These fairly rare birth defects — a notch in the upper lip, called cleft lip or harelip, and a gap in the roof of the mouth, called cleft palate — can impede sucking and severely interfere with the feeding of the child. They arise from incomplete development of the embryo within the mother's womb. The embryo's lower head develops first as separate parts that normally later join to form palate, lips and nose; sometimes this fusion is incomplete, leaving a gap that may extend from the teeth all the way back to the throat.

Their causes are not known, but cleft lip and cleft palate sometimes run in families. A child may be born with one or both of the defects. They can make it impossible for the child to speak intelligibly. Surgery can repair both defects, but it should be undertaken at an early age.

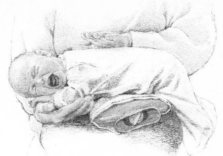

Resting your infant on his stomach on top of a warm hot-water bottle may help ease colic. For increased relief, try rubbing the baby's back as well. Check the water bottle's temperature before use by holding it against the inside of your wrist; you should feel no discomfort. Then wrap the bottle in a towel or diaper to prevent it from burning or irritating the child's skin.

Colic

Prolonged, recurring bouts of hard crying — sometimes lasting hours despite every effort of parental solace — usually indicate colic, abdominal pain that is probably caused by feeding problems or gas. It rarely occurs before the baby is two weeks old and almost always wanes by the age of three months.

Although colic appears to be painful to the baby and certainly is very stressful to parents, it is not dangerous unless there are symptoms other than crying and abdominal pain. If prolonged crying is accompanied by fever, vomiting or diarrhea, or if the baby seems listless or uncomfortable before or after the crying bouts, then illness, not common colic, is the problem. Colic should not be treated with medicines unless your physician recommends doing so.

Symptoms:
- loud, hard crying with few or no interruptions
- sudden onset of crying in the late afternoon or evening
- rejection of bottle or breast after eager acceptance
- tense position with legs drawn up, hands clenched and feet cold
- tight, distended abdomen
- bowel movement or passage of gas near the end of an attack

What to do:
- Burp the baby.
- Avoid frequent feedings.
- If you are nursing the baby, abstain from drinking cow's milk for a brief period to see if the colic stops.
- Try cuddling, soothing talk, soft music, rocking and walking.
- Swaddle the baby snugly.
- Lay the baby stomach down on your lap or on a hot-water bottle wrapped in a towel, and rub the child's back gently *(above).*
- Give the baby a pacifier.
- Check bottle nipples and the position of the bottle during feeding to make sure the baby does not suck in air.

Call the doctor if:
- the youngster continues to cry for longer than four hours.
- the child exhibits other symptoms of illness, such as fever, runny nose, coughing or vomiting.
- such long bouts of crying still occur after four months of age.

Constipation

Infrequency of bowel movements alone does not constitute constipation. Whereas one child has one or more bowel movements every day, another child's normal pattern may be one bowel movement every three or four days. DO NOT attempt to use medicines, enemas or changes in diet to force the child into a pattern you consider desirable. Instead, familiarize yourself with your child's pattern of regularity so that you will be able to recognize an abnormal absence of bowel movements.

The constipated child has stools so hard that they can be passed only with difficulty and, sometimes, pain. Occasional constipation in a child who is otherwise healthy can be corrected by adding fiber to the diet and limiting milk products. However, check with your doctor before making changes in the diet.

During toilet training, a child may become constipated simply because he resists his parents' directions by withholding bowel movements. If so, stop toilet training for a while, and start again later when the child seems ready.

Breast-fed infants, who are rarely constipated, usually have regular, yellowish, loose stools: Bottle-fed infants have firmer, brown stools. Any infant who ceases to have regular bowel movements may have an intestinal obstruction *(page 69)* and should be seen by a doctor immediately. Constipation may accompany other conditions that call for a doctor's attention *(see Encopresis, page 66; Abdominal pain, page 63; Anal fissure, page 64; Intussusception, page 70).*

Symptoms:
- hard stool that may be large
- straining and pain during defecation

What to do:
- With your doctor's approval, change the child's diet in any of several ways. For babies, give one half to one ounce of prune juice daily, or add a tablespoon of dark corn syrup to a four-ounce bottle of water or milk, or add one teaspoon of Maltsupex® to the child's bottle twice daily. For toddlers and preschool children, increase the intake of fruit (except bananas), fruit juices, raw vegetables and liquids. You can also give additional fiber in the form of bran or whole-wheat cereals to children of six months or older. Limit dairy products. Call the doctor again if home treatment does not relieve the constipation.

Call the doctor if:
- the child passes infrequent but very large, dry stools.
- hard stools recur frequently.
- the child cannot pass a movement though obviously trying hard.
- there is involuntary soiling of the youngster's underwear between hard bowel movements.
- there is blood in the stool.

Dehydration

An abnormal loss of fluids — usually as a result of prolonged vomiting or diarrhea — is a highly dangerous, even life-threatening condition. The best treatment is prevention: When an infant or child is losing fluids rapidly, try to maintain recommended levels of fluid intake *(see Diarrhea, page 66); Vomiting, page 72).* Mixtures known as oral rehydration fluids can be purchased at pharmacies. They are recommended for infants in danger of dehydrating, whereas older

To prevent dehydration during a fever, diarrhea or other illness, make sure your child consumes every hour at least the amount of fluids indicated for her age in the chart at right.

Fluid Intake per Hour

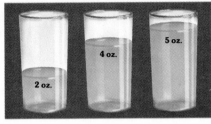

infants   1-5 years   older

children can be offered flat soda, flavored gelatin water or weakened tea.

If, despite your efforts to get liquid into the youngster, you notice serious indications of dehydration — sharply decreased urine output; a lack of tears; a dry mouth and tongue; sunken eyes; inelastic, doughy-textured skin; or lethargy and drowsiness — call the doctor at once. Dehydration demands immediate professional attention.

Diarrhea

The typical case of diarrhea — unusually loose or watery stools — is a symptom of a viral infection and usually clears up within four days. Other common causes of diarrhea are overfeeding, bacteria *(see Food poisoning, right),* parasites *(see Giardiasis, page 68),* a change in diet, antibiotic medicines, difficulty in digesting milk or dairy products, or a formula that is too concentrated or too sugary. When diarrhea is the result of an infection, the condition may be accompanied by other symptoms, such as abdominal cramps, fever, runny nose, fatigue, sore throat or vomiting.

Diarrhea rarely afflicts breast-fed infants, although their normal bowel habits often are mistaken for the condition. Breast-fed babies have softer, more frequent stools than bottle-fed babies — more than a dozen a day are not unusual. Bottle-fed babies generally pass fewer stools a day. However, if diarrhea is present in any child, prompt treatment is necessary: The ailment drains liquids from the body and can lead to dehydration. For symptoms of dehydration, see the previous entry.

Symptoms:

- a sudden increase in the number, volume and fluidity of stools in children of any age
- liquid, runny stools in infants
- more than two runny stools a day in children older than a year

- abdominal cramps before the child has a bowel movement

What to do:

- Stop all solid foods and milk — except breast milk — for 24 hours. For bottle-fed babies, provide oral rehydration fluids, which can be bought at pharmacies. In a pinch, you can give infants water or apple juice. Older children can drink those beverages or flat soda, weak tea or sweetened gelatin solution. (Avoid using red-colored gelatin, which may be mistaken for blood in the stools.) To prevent dehydration, keep fluid intake high: two ounces of liquid an hour for infants, four ounces an hour for children between one and five years of age, and five ounces an hour for older children. Offer this to the youngster in small sips — one or two teaspoonfuls every 10 to 15 minutes.
- After 24 hours — provided there is no vomiting — begin to give the child soft foods such as bananas, rice, applesauce, oatmeal, crackers, gelatin, sherbet and toast. For bottle-fed infants, resume formula at half-strength.
- If, after two to three days, stools are returning to normal, put the youngster back on a regular diet, but withhold milk, other dairy products and fatty foods for a day or two longer.
- Spread petroleum jelly over the buttocks or diaper area to prevent irritation. But if sores are already present, do not use petroleum jelly or other ointments, and keep the child as clean and dry as possible.
- DO NOT use any antidiarrheal medicines unless your doctor tells you to.

Call the doctor if:

- the child with diarrhea is less than six months old.
- the child is taking an antibiotic.
- watery stools continue after three days of home treatment.
- loose stools occur as often as once

an hour for four hours, or more than once an hour for two to three hours.
- there is fever of 102.5° F. for more than four hours.
- abdominal pain lasts for longer than half an hour.
- there is blood or mucus in the stools.
- the youngster exhibits signs of dehydration *(page 65).*
- the child is unable to consume or keep down the liquids that are suggested at left.

Encopresis

When a toilet-trained child withholds stools long enough for them to harden, liquid stool may still leak around the partial plug to soil underpants. The child is most likely to soil himself in the late afternoon, sometimes after complaining of abdominal pain.

This condition, encopresis, or soiling, has several causes. One is chronic constipation *(page 65).* Other cases may involve an emotional factor, such as fear of the toilet or of the painful bowel movements associated with anal fissure *(page 64).* A child unable to cope with family stresses may withhold bowel movements. Discuss the condition with your doctor; do not attempt to treat it with enemas or laxatives.

Food poisoning

Any illness brought on by eating food contaminated with bacteria is called food poisoning. Under certain conditions, bacteria that are normally or accidentally present in food can multiply and release harmful chemicals. Although most cases of food poisoning cure themselves within a few days, they can be serious in children younger than four because they can lead to dehydration *(page 65).*

One type of food poisoning — botulism — is exceedingly dangerous, though

How to Keep Foods from Spoiling

Bacteria that can lead to food poisoning are almost everywhere — in soil that clings to raw vegetables, in raw meat or fish, on human hands. Not all bacteria can be washed away, but they can be killed by cooking and their harmful growth can be limited by storing food properly. The following rules are merely simple kitchen routine:

- Keep hot foods hot and cold foods cold. High heat kills most bacteria and low temperatures inhibit their growth. Food temperatures between 60° F. and 120° F. provide ideal growing conditions for dangerous bacteria. After just two hours within that temperature range, a food may be highly contaminated and unfit to eat. To allow a margin of safety, you should store food at 40° F. or less. If you are keeping a dish hot to eat later, it should stay at 140° F. or higher until you let it cool down sufficiently for serving.
- If you are not serving food soon after it is cooked, then you should cool it quickly, either in the refrigerator or on ice. Do not leave the food sitting out at room temperature to cool gradually.

- When you reheat leftovers, be sure that they are hot all the way through — 140° F. or more. If the food contains liquid, heat it to the boiling point to kill any bacteria that might have grown since the dish was first prepared. Of course, allow food to cool to about body temperature before feeding it to children. You can test how hot it is with your own tongue first.
- Be attentive to hygiene when you handle food. Wash your hands carefully and keep utensils, containers and work surfaces scrupulously clean to avoid contamination.
- Keep raw fish, meats and poultry and anything they have touched away from foods that are already cooked and from salads, breads and other foods that require no cooking. Do not, for instance, slice salad ingredients with a knife you have just used for cutting up a raw chicken, since the knife will almost certainly harbor bacteria.
- Try to avoid handling food others will eat when you are suffering from a bacterial infection. Bacteria in or on your body can be transferred to

food when you touch it.
- Store canned goods and dry-packaged goods in a cool, dry location. Most perishable items should be stored in the refrigerator; the few exceptions to this rule include potatoes, bananas, hard-rind squash and unripened fruits.
- Be particularly careful with foods that provide especially good growing mediums for bacteria. Chief among these are dishes that combine eggs with milk and sugar, but all foods containing eggs — and uncooked eggs themselves, once they are out of their shells — spoil very readily. Eggs that have cracked shells should be used only in foods requiring a lot of heating, such as casseroles or baked goods. Do not use them for poached, boiled, scrambled or fried eggs, and you should certainly not use them in mayonnaise or other foods that will not be cooked. Other foods in which bacteria grow quickly include all dairy products, meat (especially pork, chicken and ground or chopped meat), fish, shellfish, leftovers, gravies and stuffings.

fortunately very rare. Avoiding botulism calls for a special precaution in feeding infants in the first year of life. The digestive tracts of a few infants, unlike those of older people, cannot destroy the spores of botulism bacteria that are normally present in honey. Although only a handful of babies who eat honey will come down with botulism, such an attack — however rare it may be — is so dangerous that honey should not be fed to young children until they are at least one year of age.

If you prepare, store and serve food properly, the chances of bacterial contamination are slim *(box, above)*.

Symptoms:
- abdominal cramps, fever, diarrhea and vomiting
- in the event of botulism — general feeling of weakness, double vision, impaired speech, and difficulty chewing and swallowing 12 to 36 hours after eating contaminated food

What to do:
- Alleviate vomiting *(page 72)* and diarrhea *(page 66)*.
- Give acetaminophen for fever higher than 102° F.

Call the doctor if:
- you notice any of the symptoms of botulism in your child.
- your child is younger than four years old and you suspect food poisoning of any kind.
- vomiting and diarrhea in a youngster become severe.
- symptoms persist for longer than two to three days.
- the youngster exhibits signs of dehydration *(65)*.

Gas

Crampy discomfort results when bubbles of gas form in a youngster's digestive tract. The pain can be severe and cause long bouts of crying *(see Colic, page 65)*. Infants who suck vigorously at

the bottle or breast are prone to gas problems since they swallow large quantities of air along with the milk.

To relieve or prevent a baby's gassiness, burp him frequently during feedings — after every one or two ounces of a bottle or after every five to 10 minutes when breast-feeding. If you suspect that gas is making a baby uncomfortable and if burping does not help, try laying the baby on his stomach across a hot-water bottle. Make sure it is at a comfortable temperature by touching it with your wrist, then spread a towel across it before laying the baby down.

In older babies and children, gas pains are most often caused by diet. Cabbage, beans and other foods high in nitrogen are the principal offenders. Gassiness may also be a symptom of an allergy *(page 46)*. If gas pains or excessive flatulence continues or is accompanied by cramping or bloody diarrhea, you should call your doctor.

Gastroenteritis

Inflammation of the lining of the stomach and intestines, known as gastroenteritis, is usually caused by a bacterial or viral infection. The symptoms are nausea, vomiting, diarrhea, and occasionally fever. See those entries, as well as the entry on intestinal infection, *(page 69),* for advice about treatment.

Giardiasis

Giardiasis is an intestinal illness caused by *Giardia lamblia,* a one-celled parasite that enters the body through contaminated food or water. Symptoms occur one to three weeks after ingestion of the parasite and usually include diarrhea, severe abdominal cramps and weight loss. If you suspect giardiasis, take stool samples to your physician. Several samples may be needed to verify the presence of the parasite. Once diagnosed, the illness can be treated with any of a number of effective drugs. To prevent giardiasis, avoid drinking water from untreated sources, such as mountain streams or lakes, unless the water has been boiled or otherwise disinfected.

Hepatitis

The term "hepatitis" is sometimes used for any liver inflammation, which can arise from a variety of causes. Most often, however, hepatitis means liver inflammation that has been brought on by one of several viruses, identified simply as Type A, Type B and non-A/non-B.

Early symptoms of the illness are similar to those of flu: fever, headache, muscle ache, nausea, diarrhea and loss of appetite. Later symptoms may include abdominal pain, dark urine, foul breath and jaundice — a yellowing of the eyes and skin. Your child may also cry or complain of tenderness when touched in the upper right area of the abdomen, where the liver is located.

All three types of viral hepatitis are infectious in one way or another, although only Type A is commonly termed infectious hepatitis. Type A, which is more common in children, can be contracted by direct contact with an infected person or by ingesting contaminated food or water. Symptoms of Type A hepatitis appear four to six weeks after exposure to the virus. Type B hepatitis, also known as serum hepatitis, enters the body through the bloodstream, usually on unsterile needles or syringes, or through contaminated blood transfusions. Its incubation period ranges from two to five months. The third type of viral hepatitis, the kind called non-A/non-B, is caused by viruses that scientists have not yet identified. However, these unknown viruses are believed to find their way into the body through the bloodstream.

There is no cure for hepatitis, but in children it is usually mild and runs its course within four weeks without complications. Only rarely is the liver permanently damaged. Treatment involves rest and a low-fat, high-carbohydrate diet. If your child's appetite is low, increase the frequency of feedings to make sure he gets enough nourishment. Also, encourage your child to drink plenty of fluids high in calories, such as milk shakes. Because viral hepatitis is contagious after symptoms appear as well as beforehand, the patient should be kept quarantined for at least one week after the first indication of hepatitis to reduce the chances of infecting others. For further protection, have all family members wash their hands before and after meals; also, clean all toilets and potty chairs with a disinfectant several times a day.

Your doctor may prescribe that your entire family receive injections of immune serum globulin, blood protein that contains antibodies to fight the infection. Although it does not prevent the onset of viral hepatitis, it can make the illness milder. Immune serum globulin is also often prescribed for people who are planning on making a trip to an area where viral hepatitis is common.

Hernia

If the wall of a muscle in the abdomen or groin is weak, an internal organ may poke through the weakened tissue to produce a bump in the skin. This protrusion is a hernia. In children, two types, each affecting a different muscle and part of the digestive system, are common.

An umbilical hernia occurs when the opening in the abdominal muscle under a baby's navel does not close completely after birth. Part of the baby's small intestine then pushes up under the navel, causing a lump at the navel that becomes larger when the child cries or tenses her body. This type of hernia, which is not painful to the child, is often diagnosed at birth and will usually disappear without treatment by a child's third birthday, because the separation in the muscle wall closes naturally. If an umbilical hernia persists beyond the age of five, your doctor may recommend surgical correction. Do not attempt the old-fashioned remedy of tying a belt around the child's stomach. The belt will have no effect on the hernia, but it can make the baby's skin sore and cause considerable discomfort.

The second type of hernia, called inguinal, is much more serious. It occurs when the intestines protrude into the inguinal canal, a small, muscle-lined passageway that extends from the abdomen down into the groin area near the juncture with the thigh. An inguinal hernia can create a small lump in the groin that becomes larger when the child is crying. It is more common among boys than girls and may appear in the scrotum, the sac that contains the testes.

If you detect any lump in your child's groin, report it immediately to your doctor. The intestines can become strangulated, or trapped, by the muscles that

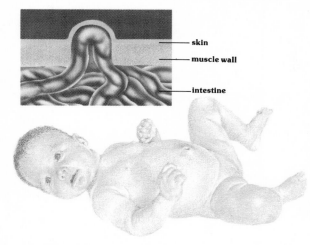

skin

muscle wall

intestine

Hernias form when part of an internal organ bulges through an opening in a muscle wall. When a part of an infant's small intestine pushes through the abdominal wall under the navel (top), the result is an umbilical hernia. The hernia can appear as a small bump at the navel (bottom) or as a protuberance up to several inches in length.

line the inguinal canal. Blood may stop circulating to the trapped part of the organ, causing the tissue to die and become gangrenous. This is an extremely critical situation that requires immediate medical attention.

If a nonstrangulated inguinal hernia is diagnosed, your youngster will probably be admitted to the hospital — often on an outpatient basis — to have it surgically corrected. A strangulated hernia requires emergency surgery.

Symptoms:
- a lump in the abdomen or groin
- in the severe case of strangulated hernia — constipation, severe abdominal pain or vomiting.

What to do:
- In the case of inguinal hernia, elevate your youngster's hips. Umbilical hernia usually requires no treatment.
- DO NOT push on the lump with your fingers or hand.
- DO NOT give any medicine unless approved by a physician.
- DO NOT give any food if inguinal hernia is suspected.

Call the doctor if:
- you detect a lump in the abdomen or groin. If the lump is accompanied by abdominal pain and lack of bowel movements, take your child immediately to a hospital emergency room.

Indigestion
Eating fried, fatty or undercooked foods or eating too much or too fast can cause indigestion, the discomfort felt when the stomach and intestines are unable to digest foods properly. Emotional tension is another common cause. Symptoms include gas, abdominal pain and heartburn — a burning sensation in the chest caused by stomach acids rising into the esophagus. Babies may also spit up small amounts of milk. To prevent indigestion, avoid overfeeding your baby and teach your older child to chew food slowly and thoroughly. Also, try to keep mealtimes quiet and unrushed.

For treatment of indigestion, see the entries on gas *(page 67),* abdominal pain *(page 63),* and colic *(page 65).*

Intestinal infection
Intestinal infection is a general term used to describe a variety of attacks on the stomach and intestines by viruses or bacteria *(see Gastroenteritis, page 68),* or intestinal parasites *(see Giardiasis, page 68, and Pinworms, page 71).* Symptoms often include diarrhea, abdominal cramps, fever, nausea and vomiting.

These infections, sometimes misnamed "stomach flus," usually last a day or two and then go away without special treatment. However, if diarrhea or vomiting persists, call your physician. Special drugs will be prescribed for infections that are caused by parasites.

Give your child plenty of fluids during an intestinal infection to protect against dehydration *(page 65).* If the child is having trouble holding down food, you may wish to withhold solid food until the infection runs its course.

To prevent an intestinal infection from spreading to other family members, you should take extra care to wash your hands after changing diapers or helping the child use the potty or toilet. Also, set aside special eating utensils and dishes for exclusive use of the ill child until the infection has gone.

Intestinal obstruction
A child's intestines may become blocked, creating a potentially dangerous problem, for a variety of reasons, including an intestinal inflammation *(see Gastroenteritis, page 68),* an inguinal hernia *(see Hernia, page 68),* a sudden telescoping of one section of the intestine into another *(see Intussusception, page 70),* and the swallowing of a small toy or other object. In some newborns, the obstruction is caused by the failure of meconium — the dark, sticky substance that accumulates in the intestine before birth — to pass out of the body after birth. Some babies are also born with a malformation of the intestine that can block the passage of food — either a narrowing of the intestinal walls, called stenosis, or a separation of the small intestine into one or more sections, called atresia.

Symptoms of an intestinal obstruction usually include abdominal cramps, vomiting and a swollen abdomen caused by a build-up of gases. The child's vomit may resemble a bowel movement or contain green bile, the liquid produced by the liver to aid digestion. The child may also be constipated or may alternate between diarrhea and constipation.

Intestinal blockage, whether complete or partial, is very serious. Because it keeps food and water from being absorbed into the body, the blockage can lead to severe dehydration *(page 65).* Blood may be cut off from the blocked section of the intestine, causing that section to die and become gangrenous. The section may then rupture and infect the

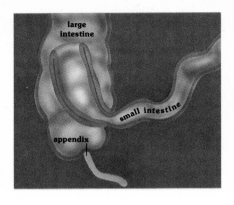

Intussusception occurs when a section of intestine telescopes into an adjacent section. The obstructed area swells painfully and the intestinal lining becomes inflamed, producing a bloody mucus the child may pass in a stool. This condition usually develops at the junction of the small and large intestines, as seen here.

lining of the abdominal cavity, a dangerous condition called peritonitis.

The treatment of a blocked intestine varies, depending on its cause, but corrective surgery is often required.

Symptoms:
- abdominal cramps
- distended abdomen
- persistent vomiting or projectile vomiting, in which vomit is spewed a foot or more from the child's mouth
- chronic constipation or no bowel movements for several days
- constipation that alternates with diarrhea
- bloody or pellet-like stools

What to do:
- Give the child clear liquids in small quantities, at frequent intervals if dehydration appears possible.
- DO NOT give an enema or laxative or apply any other medicines unless approved by a doctor.

Call the doctor if:
- any abdominal pain lasts for more than three hours.
- the youngster's abdomen appears to be bloated or distended.
- the vomit resembles a bowel movement or contains green bile.
- signs of dehydration appear.

Intussusception

If a section of the intestine telescopes into itself, a process called intussusception, the result is a dangerous blockage. Intussusception is most common in children six months to three years old and usually involves a portion of the small intestine telescoping into the large intestine. The cause of most intussusceptions is unknown, although noncancerous growths called polyps within the lining of the intestines are sometimes blamed for the condition.

Symptoms occur suddenly. The child will turn pale, cry and pull his legs up sharply to ease the pain in his abdomen. The pain and crying often come in short spurts, with intervening periods of quiet. The most telltale sign of intussusception, however, is a bloody, mucous, jelly-like bowel movement. It is produced when pressure from the blockage causes blood and mucus to be squeezed from the intestinal lining.

Because the obstructed segment of the intestine can rupture and infect the abdominal cavity, intussusception must be treated immediately *(see Intestinal obstruction, previous entry)*. In cases where the intestine has not yet ruptured, your physician may give your child an enema containing barium sulfate, a phosphorescent substance that can be seen on a fluoroscope. Besides being needed to diagnose the intussusception, the enema may push the bowel back into its correct configuration. If the intestine has been perforated or become gangrenous, however, the enema will not be given and emergency surgery will be required.

Symptoms:
- bloody, mucous, jelly-like stools
- short spurts of severe abdominal pain followed by periods when the child lies very still

What to do:
- Give clear liquids in small quantities.
- DO NOT give an enema or laxative or any other medicines unless approved by a physician.

Call the doctor if:
- any blood or mucus appears in the youngster's stool.
- any abdominal pain lasts for more than three hours.

Jaundice

Jaundice, a yellowing of the skin and eyes, is not an illness itself, but a symptom of a variety of afflictions, including hepatitis and some types of anemia. In newborn babies, it may also be the result of a reaction between the blood types of mother and infant, or of a rare defect — the absence of a duct that normally carries the digestive chemical bile away from the liver.

The yellow color of jaundice is caused by bilirubin, a pigment produced as the liver processes red blood cells. Ordinarily, the liver disposes of the bilirubin. But when it does not, and bilirubin levels in the blood become too high, jaundice results. Very high levels in a newborn can damage the infant's brain.

Mild jaundice, sometimes called physiological jaundice, is common in more than half of all newborn babies. Their livers are simply not yet mature enough to process bilirubin quickly. Mild jaundice usually appears two or three days after birth and disappears by the end of the child's first week. If the jaundice persists or worsens, call your doctor at once, for the condition may be a symptom of a more serious illness.

In older children, jaundice is usually a symptom of viral hepatitis or anemia; both of these ailments require treatment by a physician.

Because of a hormone found in breast milk, breast-feeding can sometimes prolong jaundice in newborn infants. Treatment, therefore, may include a halt in breast-feeding until the jaundice disappears. More serious cases of jaundice are treated with blood transfusions or with an ultraviolet-light treatment that helps the liver form the chemicals needed to process bilirubin.

Motion sickness

Motion sickness is nausea that is caused by the movement of a car, boat, airplane or amusement ride. It stems from disruption of the body's balancing mechanism in the inner ear and often leads to vomiting. See page 81 for a discussion of motion sickness and suggested treatment.

Nausea

This unpleasant queasiness is one of the body's basic signals of trouble. It can be triggered by anything from an emotional upset, an unpleasant odor or motion sickness to poisoning, influenza or heart failure. Sucking on crushed ice or drinking a mildly flavored soft drink can sometimes relieve nausea. If the nausea persists, or if it is accompanied by high fever, pain or diarrhea, consult your physician.

Pica

The compulsion to eat substances normally considered inedible, such as dirt, ashes, wool or paint, is called pica. It should not be confused with the normal childhood practice of licking or sucking an object as a form of exploration. Pica, which is most common among children one to three years old, is a dangerous habit and must be stopped immediately, for it can lead to poisoning and infections. If your child shows signs of pica, keep the substances she is eating out of her reach and consult your physician promptly.

Pinworms

These small, white, threadlike worms infest the intestines of many small children, causing itching around the anus. The microscopic eggs of the pinworm collect on fingernails, clothing, bedding — even on dust in the air — and are then easily swallowed. They hatch in the small intestine and then the larvae travel to the large intestine, where they mature. Adult female pinworms crawl out of the intestines, usually at night, to lay their eggs around the anus. The egg-laying causes severe itching. As the child scratches, more eggs are picked up on his fingernails and the cycle is repeated when the child puts his fingers in his mouth.

To confirm that your child has pinworms, look for adult worms around his anus at night *(below),* or press a piece of easily-removable cellophane tape onto the area near the anus in the early morning before the child has had a bowel movement. The pinworms' eggs should stick to the tape. Save the tape and take it to your physician.

Pinworms are usually harmless, although in rare cases they can migrate to the appendix and trigger appendicitis. They can be eliminated with drugs, but usually the entire household must be treated to stop the infestation. Pinworms frequently recur because their eggs are easily picked up through contact with other children.

Symptoms:
- itching of the skin around the anus, particularly at night
- difficulty sleeping

What to do:
- Apply petroleum jelly or zinc oxide ointment to the affected area to relieve itching.
- Keep the child's fingernails clean and cut short.
- Make sure that the child's hands are washed often throughout the day.
- Change the youngster's sheets, pajamas and underwear daily and wash them in very hot water to kill the pinworms and eggs.

Call the doctor if:
- your youngster complains of itching near the anus.

- you find thin white worms on your child's bed sheets or clothes.

Pyloric stenosis

The pylorus, the muscular valve that connects the stomach and the small intestine, sometimes thickens and then obstructs the flow of food from the stomach. This pyloric stenosis, or constriction of the passageway, usually occurs in infants two to 10 weeks old. Its cause is unknown, but the condition is more common among boys than girls.

An early sign of pyloric stenosis is persistent vomiting after a feeding. The vomiting becomes more forceful as the condition worsens. Because the obstruction keeps food and water from being absorbed into the body, it can lead to severe dehydration and malnutrition and must be treated immediately. Surgery is required to correct the problem; babies recover fully within two to three weeks after the operation.

Symptoms:
- projectile vomiting, which causes material to spew over a distance of one foot or farther
- visible stomach spasms
- weight loss or failure to gain weight
- small, infrequent stools
- dehydration *(page 65).*

What to do:
- Give the youngster small, frequent feedings throughout the day.
- Keep the baby in a semiupright position for one hour after feeding.

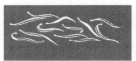

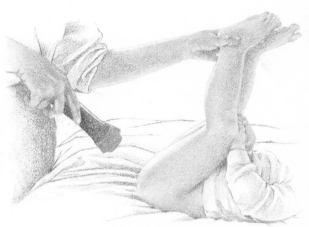

White, threadlike, and about ⅛ to ½ of an inch long (above), pinworms live in the intestines, but emerge from the anus at night to lay eggs on the surrounding skin. If your child complains of intense anal itching, or if you observe her scratching her bottom frequently, lift her legs at night and shine a flashlight onto the rectal opening (left). If pinworms are present, consult a doctor.

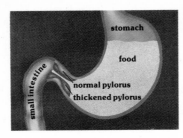

The muscular walls of the pylorus, the valve connecting the stomach to the small intestine, sometimes thicken, obstructing the flow of partly digested food to the intestines. This condition, pyloric stenosis, usually affects infants two to 10 weeks old. It is signaled by forceful vomiting soon after feeding.

Call the doctor if:

- your baby projects vomit a distance of a foot or more.
- your youngster continues to vomit his food soon after feeding for a period of two to three days.
- your baby either loses weight or fails to gain weight.

Stomach flu

Stomach flu is a general term that is used to describe a variety of infections affecting the stomach or intestines. More often than not, the infection is not a true influenza and may not have anything at all to do with the stomach *(see Intestinal infection, page 69).*

Vomiting

The forceful ejection of the contents of the stomach is a symptom of many illnesses, including intestinal infection, appendicitis, intestinal obstruction, pyloric stenosis and Reye syndrome. Or it may be related to spoiled or allergy-causing foods or other toxic substances.

In some children, vomiting may result from a congenital defect: a weak muscle between the stomach and the esophagus, the pipe that connects it to the throat. If the muscle is too weak to close off the stomach, food and gastric juices rise into the esophagus and are vomited. This so-called gastroesophageal reflux usually corrects itself by the time a child is two years old. Until then, a youngster may require propping up into a near-vertical position for an hour after meals, or in severe cases, for longer periods. Your pediatrician may prescribe drugs that can lessen vomiting.

In infants and babies, it is important to differentiate between ordinary regurgitation, or spitting up, and more serious vomiting. When a baby brings up small amounts of milk during or after a feeding but otherwise appears well, she is probably regurgitating rather than vomiting.

Regurgitation in an infant is normal and nothing for a parent to worry about; it usually stops by the time the youngster begins to walk.

Overfeeding, swallowing air during a feeding or feeding too fast can all cause a baby to regurgitate food. Try feeding your baby more slowly and stop often to burp the child. Avoid giving the youngster too much food and make sure that your baby does not take in air when being fed from a bottle.

True vomiting is visibly different from regurgitation, bringing food forcibly out of the stomach. Sometimes it involves projectile vomiting, in which food shoots with great force out of the mouth over a distance of a foot or more. A single episode of vomiting in an infant or young child is not a cause for concern. But if your child vomits all feedings within a six-hour period or if he shows other symptoms of pain or distress along with vomiting, call your doctor immediately. Besides being an indicator of a variety of serious illnesses, vomiting can result in an excessive loss of body fluid, a dangerous condition in young children *(see Dehydration, page 65).*

When you call your doctor, be prepared to answer the following questions about your child's vomiting:

- When did the vomiting occur?
- What type of food was vomited?
- How frequent is the vomiting?
- What is the color, consistency and amount of the vomit?
- Is the child showing other symptoms of discomfort?

What to do:

- Avoid feeding your child for several hours after vomiting. Then offer clear fluids in small amounts, as little as one to two teaspoons, every 10 to 15 minutes to avoid dehydration.
- If the youngster is older than one year, offer small portions of bland solid foods — such as bananas, apple-

sauce, diluted skim milk or refined cereal (rice or Cream of Wheat®) — after about 24 hours.

- If vomiting occurs in an infant, temporarily stop feeding the baby breast milk or formula. As a substitute, offer the youngster oral rehydration fluids, which can be purchased at pharmacies. If one is not immediately available, provide the child with clear fluids such as flavored gelatin water or fruit-flavored syrup drinks that have been diluted with extra water. (Note that red-colored gelatin can stain the baby's stool red, so use gelatin of another color that cannot be mistaken for blood in the stool.) Feed this to the infant in teaspoon amounts until the baby can keep down an ounce or more at a time. Gradually reintroduce milk or formula.
- Watch the youngster for additional symptoms of an illness.
- DO NOT give your child any food or water if he vomits after an accident or injury.
- DO NOT give your youngster an antiemetic to stop the vomiting without consulting your doctor.

Call the doctor if:

- the child's vomiting is accompanied by drowsiness, headache, sharp or constant abdominal pain, high fever, difficult breathing, a bloated belly or painful urination.
- an infant vomits repeatedly and forcibly, with or without exhibiting other symptoms of illness.
- your infant's vomiting is accompanied by bowel movements that are watery and frequent.
- an older child vomits all feedings within a six-hour period.
- your youngster vomits after an accident or injury.
- your child vomits after seeming to recover from chicken pox, influenza or another viral illness. ❖

Ear, Nose, Throat and Respiratory System

Coughs, colds and infections of the interconnected passageways of the ears, nose, throat and lungs are the most common illnesses of childhood. In part, this is because the immature physical structure of a child's ears and respiratory tract renders them more susceptible to disease. In a young child's breathing system, the airways are still comparatively short, which allows infection in one part of the system to spread easily to other parts. A youngster's air passages are also very narrow, so that swelling caused by infections will quickly block the passages and thus hamper the breathing.

The smallness of a child's body parts sometimes makes diagnosis a challenge. Narrow nasal passages coupled with normal amounts of mucus turn even healthy babies into noisy breathers. If the passages are further obstructed by the added mucus of a cold, the breathing can begin to sound disturbingly labored. And because the nose, throat and lungs are all so close together, the rattly sound of simple nasal congestion may sound like congestion in the chest.

Because the ears and respiratory tract continue to develop throughout childhood, many problems in this area clear up as the child grows older. Ear infections, for example, are a problem in the early years because of the shape of the Eustachian tubes, which form wide and nearly horizontal corridors connecting the nasal cavity with the inner portions of the ear. With time, these tubes become narrower and shift to a steeper angle, thereby restricting the movement and spread of infection.

On the positive side, there is at least one disorder that seldom troubles younger children because their respiratory systems are still developing: The sinus infections that plague many adults are not as common during childhood because the major sinus cavities do not finish forming until adolescence.

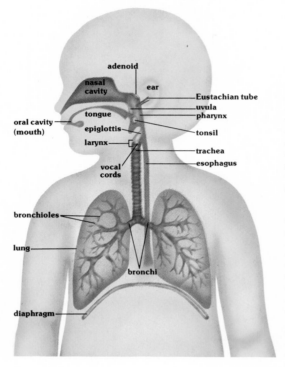

The respiratory and digestive systems share some common passageways. In breathing, the contraction of the diaphragm allows the lungs to inflate, pulling air in through the mouth and nose and down through the pharynx, or throat. Bypassing the entrance to the esophagus, incoming air moves through the larynx, which contains the vocal cords, and into the trachea. This windpipe branches into a pair of bronchi, which enter the lungs and there divide into smaller airways called bronchioles. Food from the mouth and fluid from the nose and middle ear — which drains via the Eustachian tubes — also pass through the pharynx en route to the esophagus, which leads to the stomach. The epiglottis, a flap of cartilage, covers the trachea during swallowing.

Apnea

A pause in breathing that lasts longer than 15 seconds is referred to by doctors as apnea. It is a symptom of various other medical conditions, rather than a disorder in itself. Apnea is most common in premature babies. Its usual causes are infections, anemia, seizures, metabolic disturbances and certain types of heart conditions. Apnea is believed to be related to sudden infant death syndrome *(page 85)*, but that connection has yet to be substantiated and medical research is still being conducted on the subject.

The length of time that breathing stops is important in distinguishing apnea, because it is not unusual for small babies — particularly premature ones — to breathe irregularly or even to stop taking in air for a few seconds at a time. With apnea, however, the interruption of the oxygen flow lasts long enough to pose a danger to health. In a severe episode, you will be able to observe that the child's chest stops moving, he becomes pale and may start to turn blue. Oxygen deprivation can damage the brain within as little time as four minutes. For instructions on how to assist a child who is not breathing, see Breathing Difficulties *(page 16)*.

If your youngster has more than one episode of apnea, your physician will attempt to determine the cause by compiling a detailed medical history and performing a physical examination. Since the causes of apnea are often difficult to pinpoint, it is sometimes necessary to test the child at a center that specializes in the disorder. A common precaution in situations where the cause cannot be determined and thus cannot be treated is the use of a monitor that sounds an alarm when the child's breathing stops for longer than 15 seconds.

Asthma

Asthma is a chronic condition, usually allergy-related, which is characterized by attacks of wheezing, tightness in the chest and shortness of breath. During an asthma attack, the air passages leading out of a child's lungs are constricted by swelling and muscle spasms. The airways also become clogged with thick mucus, making both inhaling and exhaling difficult. Some bouts of asthma are mild and end naturally without treatment, while others are serious enough to require hospitalization.

It is estimated that asthma affects 5 to 10 percent of all children, though in most cases the condition is not severe. Most youngsters who get asthma show the first symptoms before they reach five years of age. Asthma commonly occurs in families that have a history of the illness or a history of other allergic conditions such as hay fever or eczema.

Asthma is rarely fatal to children, but unless it is controlled, it can be very disruptive. If your child is asthmatic, he may miss more school than other youngsters and his activities may have to be restricted. Even a mild asthmatic condition demands good communication with your pediatrician, so that you can keep informed on up-to-date treatment methods. And because some of the most effective treatments for a bad bout of asthma can be performed only in the hospital, you will need to be familiar with emergency facilities in your area. You should also take extra care in selecting and training baby-sitters.

Many asthma attacks are caused by allergic reactions. The source of the allergy may be anything from pollen and household dust to tobacco smoke and certain kinds of food and drink. The best way to control asthma, therefore, is to identify the allergens that affect your child and try to limit his exposure (see Allergies, pages 46-48). Unfortunately, asthma attacks also seem to be aggravated by infections, stress and even physical exercise, especially in cold weather.

Though there is no actual cure for asthma, several medicines are effective in controlling the illness. These medications, which are usually taken as aerosol inhalants by older patients, are available in pills and drops for administering to small children.

The medication falls into two categories: prophylactics and bronchodilators. Prophylactics, designed to prevent asthma attacks by relaxing the bronchial muscles and thus keeping the airways open, are most often prescribed for frequent sufferers. In some cases, they are used on a daily basis; for the most part, however, they are used only when the child is about to exercise or when you know that he will be particularly susceptible to his allergies. Bronchodilators, on the other hand, are used to relieve the symptoms once an attack has begun, by opening up the constricted air passages.

Fortunately, more than half of all asthmatic children outgrow the condition completely by their middle teens. And for many of the rest, the attacks become milder and occur much less frequently as the child approaches adulthood.

Symptoms:
- labored breathing
- wheezing when exhaling, ranging from loud to barely audible
- tightness in the chest
- in severe attacks, anxiety, sweating, lips turning blue

What to do:
- If the symptoms of an asthma attack are appearing in your child for the first time, seek medical help.
- If asthma medication has previously been prescribed for the child, administer it according to instructions. Note the time the dose is given, so that you can keep track of the medicine's working time.
- Remain calm, to avoid contributing to your child's anxiety.
- Help the child find a comfortable position; sitting up is usually best. Prop him up in bed with pillows supporting his back or have him straddle an upright chair with the backrest supporting his arms.
- Offer sips of a warm liquid to loosen congestion in the chest, but stop if the child seems nauseated.
- If the attack becomes severe and you cannot contact your physician by phone, quickly and calmly take the child to an emergency room.

Call the doctor if:
- your child displays symptoms of an asthma attack and has not been previously diagnosed as asthmatic.
- you are not able to provide the child rapid relief by following your doctor's most recent instructions.

Bronchitis

In the aftermath of a cold or sore throat, a child may develop bronchitis — an inflammation of the windpipe and the large bronchial tubes branching off from the windpipe into the lungs. In the usual pattern, the youngster's previous fever has just abated and recovery seems to be in sight, when a low fever reappears and she starts coughing, apparently feeling even worse than before.

Bronchitis is usually caused by a viral infection and sometimes is complicated by secondary bacterial infections. Children generally recover from it without specific treatment of the infection, although antibiotics may be given to minimize complications when a child suffers recurrent episodes of the illness. Drugs will not speed up the child's recovery, however. Bronchitis normally lasts from seven to 10 days.

Coughing is the most bothersome symptom of the illness, but you should consult your doctor before giving the child any cough medicine. Most often, in the course of bronchitis, the cough progresses from a dry, hacking cough to a productive one that brings up mucus, so you need to take care that you are using the right type of cough medicine at the right time *(see Cough, page 76)*.

Symptoms:
- dry, hacking cough that gradually turns into a wet cough
- low fever
- loss of appetite
- a burning feeling in the chest when the child breathes deeply
- raspy breathing, similar to the wheezing of asthma, but noisier during inhalation
- greenish yellow sputum in the airways, which may cause vomiting in children too young to cough it up

What to do:
- If your youngster is still an infant, shift her position frequently in the crib to facilitate quick drainage of the respiratory tract.
- Use a cool-mist humidifier or vaporizer to loosen secretions by making them more liquid.
- Have the child rest quietly, and minimize her contact with other people.
- Use acetaminophen to relieve fever.
- Make sure that the youngster takes in plenty of liquids.
- Give cough medicines, but only under a doctor's instructions. DO NOT give antihistamines.

Call the doctor if:
- an infant develops a persistent cough, or if an older child is prevented from sleeping by the cough.
- the child's fever rises above 101° F. more than once.
- your child suffers repeated episodes of bronchitis.

Bronchiolitis
Like bronchitis, bronchiolitis is a chest infection that usually starts as a cold. It is less common than bronchitis but potentially more serious, since it can sharply restrict a child's breathing. Bronchiolitis is a contagious viral infection that makes its way into the bronchioles — tiny air passages that spread throughout the lungs — and causes inflammation. In a severe case, the bronchioles also fill up with mucus, further reducing the flow of air. The child breathes quickly and shallowly, with considerable coughing and wheezing as he struggles for breath. At this point, the youngster needs immediate medical attention.

Bronchiolitis occurs during the first and second years of life, most often when a child is about six months old, and it usually strikes during the flu season — in winter or early spring. The body normally fights off the infection fairly quickly — generally in one to three days. In the meantime, however, bottle-feeding is very difficult, and because the breathing problems may be quite severe, your doctor may suggest that the child be cared for in a hospital until the infection is brought under control.

Symptoms:
- very shallow, rapid breathing, accompanied by wheezing and coughing
- low fever
- loss of appetite

What to do:
- Notify the child's physician immediately, then follow the treatment that the doctor recommends.
- Use a cool-mist humidifier or vaporizer, or sit with the youngster in a steamy bathroom.

Call the doctor if:
- a child shows any of the symptoms of bronchiolitis.
- while you are following the physician's suggested treatment, the infant's lips or fingernails begin to turn blue, or he refuses to take any fluids for a full day or he vomits the fluids that he does accept.

Common cold
Frequent colds seem to be an inescapable fact of life in early childhood: Preschoolers suffer an average of six to nine colds a year. Despite its classic discomforts, a cold is a relatively harmless viral infection of the upper respiratory passages that generally runs its course in a week or two. Because colds occur so often, you will probably become an expert at nursing your achy, runny-nosed child back to health without your doctor's assistance. You really only need to seek medical advice if a cold deviates dramatically from the usual pattern or if your child is younger than two months old.

Most colds develop very quickly: If the child shows a fever or begins sneezing at bedtime, the full force of the cold will probably be upon her by morning. The most acute phase lasts from three to four days, but it may be several more days before the swollen mucous membranes in the nose and sinuses return to normal

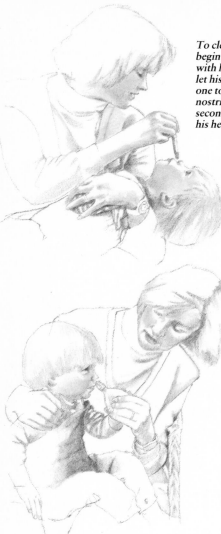

To clear mucus from a child's nose, begin by laying the child across your lap with his neck supported by your arm; let his head drop backward slightly. Place one to two saline drops (left) in each nostril. Keep the child's head still for 30 seconds, then seat him upright and tilt his head slightly forward.

Compress the bulb of a nasal aspirator and insert the nozzle into one nostril. Slowly release bulb to collect mucus. Repeat for other nostril. Apply saline drops and resuction in five to 10 minutes, if needed.

and the child feels fit again. A runny nose or cough may last for an additional week. The cold is contagious from a day or two before the symptoms appear until a day or two after their appearance.

Infants under three months old are particularly susceptible to cold viruses and other infections, though they do not develop a fever as a barometer of their illnesses as readily as older children do. Small babies also suffer extra hardship with ordinary colds because the excess

mucus produced by the illness stops up their tiny airways and makes it difficult for them to breathe while they are sucking from the breast or bottle. Therefore, if your baby is younger than three months old, you should call your doctor at the first signs of a cold.

It is probably impossible to protect your baby from all exposure to cold viruses, but you should try to limit her exposure, within reason, by keeping her away from anyone whom you know to be suffering from a fresh cold.

A child with a cold should drink plenty of fluids, including orange juice and other fruit juices. However, dosing a child with massive amounts of vitamin C — or any other vitamin, for that matter — is a highly questionable practice. And you should use cold medication only under a doctor's guidance.

The youngster's main complaint will be a stuffed-up nose, and for that a batch of homemade nose drops of plain salt and tap water *(page 75)* gives the simplest and best relief. Suctioning out a child's nostrils can be difficult but is effective if done correctly *(left)*. Sometimes it is the only way to clear a baby's nose sufficiently to enable her to nurse.

Symptoms:
- dryness and itchiness in the nose, followed within a few hours by sneezing
- stuffed-up nasal passages accompanied by clear discharge, which later becomes thick and greenish yellow
- low fever
- chills and aching muscles
- loss of appetite; sometimes, temporary constipation
- in some cases, coughing

What to do:
- Use nose drops to relieve nasal congestion *(page 75)*. For a baby, use a nasal aspirator to clear the nostrils prior to feedings.
- Offer fruit juices or water frequently throughout the day.

- Use a cool-mist humidifier or vaporizer to ease breathing.
- Prop up the child's head with an extra pillow when she sleeps. Elevate an infant's head by placing books or pillows under the mattress; lay the baby down on her stomach, rather than on her back.
- Use acetaminophen to relieve fever.

Call the doctor if:
- a baby under three months old shows cold symptoms.
- an infant of any age with a cold refuses to nurse.
- your youngster's fever lasts longer than three days, stays above 101° F. for more than five hours or suddenly surges much higher.
- the child complains about throat pain.
- the youngster has a cough that brings up heavy mucus.
- the youngster has enlarged, tender glands in her neck.
- the child develops any of these additional symptoms: excessive listlessness, chest pain, shortness of breath, rapid breathing, headache or earache, extreme irritability, blueness around the lips or under the fingernails. These symptoms can be signs of a secondary infection.

Cough

Coughing is essentially a reflex action that prevents the lungs from taking in foreign matter such as dust or crumbs or mucus from an illness. All coughs are symptoms of some irritation in the respiratory tract, but their sources are so varied that the cause can often be difficult to pin down.

In newborns, a cough is very unusual because the chest muscles are so weak: Coughing during the early weeks of life can be a warning sign of problems in the lungs. In toddlers, who have a tendency to inhale crumbs or other small objects, coughing may signal breathing distress

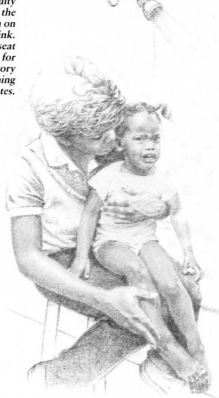

To relieve the breathing difficulty caused by croup, take your child into the bathroom, close the door, and turn on the hot water in both the shower and sink. Since steam rises, hold her up or seat her as high as you comfortably can for faster relief. Calm her by telling a story or speaking in a soothing tone; breathing should ease within 20 to 30 minutes.

(page 16). Most of the time, however, coughing is triggered by colds and other infections that irritate the breathing passages by producing excess mucus. The tickling irritation of a post-nasal drip — mucus draining from the nasal cavity down the back of the throat — is the most common problem, although mucus may also aggravate the bronchial tubes and lungs enough to cause coughing.

The sensible course in treating a child's cough is fairly simple. If the cough is productive — if it is bringing up mucus that might otherwise congest or infect the lungs, as is the case with such illnesses as bronchitis and asthma — do not try to stop the coughing. On the contrary, give the child fluids and add moisture to the air with a cool-mist humidifier or vaporizer to further loosen the mucus. There are cough medicines called expectorants that are designed to promote this process, but they are often ineffective.

If, on the other hand, the cough is dry and unproductive — as are those caused by postnasal drip or the flu — talk to your physician about using a decongestant or a cough suppressant, particularly if the cough is keeping your child awake at night. Cough suppressants contain drugs that block the coughing reflex.

Both suppressant and expectorant formulas may also contain a decongestant, which acts to reduce inflammation. Decongestants are most effective in the case of unproductive coughs caused by simple throat irritation — for example, the soreness that results from postnasal drip.

If you are not certain what is causing a cough or if coughing persists for more than a few days, consult your doctor. Using the wrong cough remedy may produce an effect that is precisely the opposite of the treatment your child needs. Some parents find that home remedies such as lemon juice thickened with honey or warm apple cider are effective in quieting a dry, hacking cough. However, a child younger than 12 months should not be given honey, because it contains botulism spores that can cause food poisoning in some infants.

Croup

The term "croup" is applied to a severe form of laryngitis and to a number of other infections of the larynx and the windpipe, among them a very dangerous illness called epiglottitis *(page 78)*. Croup primarily affects children three months to four years old. It usually strikes at night during the winter, often in the wake of a bad cold or cough.

Croup infections cause inflammation that drastically obstructs a youngster's already-narrow breathing passages. The common forms of croup are characterized by a peculiar, hacking cough that sounds like the barking of a dog or seal. A child with severe croup may also develop stridor, which is a harsh, shrill sound emitted when the child breathes.

While it can be frightening to watch your youngster struggle for breath, it is important for you to remain calm — and to keep the child from panicking — so that you can take the necessary steps to ease the child's breathing. At the first signs of croup you should place an emergency call to your doctor or, better still, have someone else call while you assist the child. During later episodes, you may be able to help the youngster without the doctor's advice.

The immediate remedy for breathing distress caused by croup is inhalation of either warm, steamy air *(left)* or cool, moist air from a cool-mist humidifier or vaporizer, whichever you can produce most quickly. Croup rarely cuts off the oxygen supply altogether, and getting moist air into the child's airways should deliver rapid relief. It is a good idea to use this remedy even if the coughing seems mild; a bout of croup can worsen rapidly and should be treated at the onset.

Attacks of croup often come in cycles: One moment the child is struggling noisily for each breath, and an hour later he is resting peacefully. A few hours later he may have yet another attack. Croup may go on for five or six nights in a row. It is a good idea to sleep in the child's room while the attacks continue, so that you can respond quickly. The youngster may lose his appetite for a few days. Make sure that he drinks enough liquids so that he does not become dehydrated.

The mildest and most common croup infection is laryngitis, which affects the vocal cords and their surrounding structure. In older children and adults, laryngitis is an uneventful illness marked by hoarseness, sore throat and sometimes, temporary voice loss. In small children, however, the swelling in the larynx is often enough to obstruct the breathing passages. The inflammation sometimes spreads to the windpipe as well.

Symptoms:
- a distinctive barking cough
- difficulty in breathing that intermit-

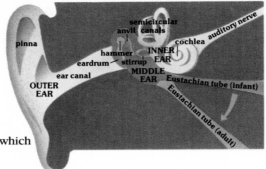

The ear has three parts: the outer, middle and inner ear. The outer ear includes the ear flap, or pinna, and the ear canal. The middle ear starts with the eardrum stretching across the canal's end. The Eustachian tube regulates pressure in the middle ear and drains fluid into the nasal cavity. Almost horizontal at birth, this duct slopes downward by the age of eight. Bones in the middle ear — the hammer, anvil and stirrup — carry sound vibrations to the cochlea in the inner ear. In this chamber, vibrations are transformed into nerve impulses and sent to the brain along the auditory nerve. The semicircular canals of the inner ear sense movement and help maintain balance.

tently produces a shrill sound, which is called stridor
- low fever
- hoarseness

What to do:
- If it is the child's first attack of croup, notify his physician immediately.
- Treat the breathing distress with steam or cool, moist air.
- If steam or moistened air does not provide relief within 20 minutes, hold the child by an open door or window to breathe the cool night air.
- Stay with and comfort the youngster throughout the attack.
- DO NOT give cough medicines.

Call the doctor if:
- it is the child's first attack of croup.
- the breathing difficulty does not lessen within 30 minutes.
- the fever rises above 103° F.
- there is blueness in the youngster's lips or fingernails.
- the child starts to drool or seems reluctant to swallow.

Dizziness

A child who feels dizzy has the sensation that her surroundings are spinning wildly around. Also referred to as vertigo, this condition occurs when the balance mechanism in the inner ear has been disturbed. Except when it can be explained by the child's play — too many somersaults, too much running in circles — or by the motion of riding in a car or boat, dizziness is usually attributable to an ear infection, which will require prompt medical attention.

Dizziness will usually pass in a few moments if the child lies still. If it persists, try giving the child some nose drops *(page 75)*, which will relieve congestion in the nose and thus open up the Eustachian tubes and equalize the pressure in the youngster's middle ear.

You should consult your doctor any time that dizziness goes on for more than

an hour, occurs following a head injury or seems to be caused by a medication.

Earache

Earache is one of the most frequent complaints in infants and small children. It can be caused by such diverse problems as a foreign object in the ear, a sore throat or uneven pressure inside and outside the ear during air travel *(page 85)*. But earache is usually associated with an ear infection — either otitis externa, infection of the outer ear *(page 81)*, or otitis media, middle-ear infection *(page 80)*. Learn to recognize the symptoms of both so that treatment can be promptly begun.

All complaints about ear pain must be taken seriously. Even mild ear infections should receive medical attention, for without proper treatment, an infection can lead to permanent hearing loss.

Epiglottitis

Epiglottitis is a relatively rare but potentially life-threatening infection of the epiglottis, which is a lidlike protuberance in the throat that stops food from entering the windpipe. This infection is the most

severe form of croup — one that threatens total obstruction of the airway. For a more extensive discussion of the treatment, see the entry for Croup *(page 77)*.

Signs of epiglottitis usually appear several hours before it becomes a breathing emergency. If you see the symptoms, call your doctor immediately. If you cannot reach the physician, move your child quickly and calmly to the nearest hospital emergency room.

Symptoms:
- fever, usually reaching 102° F., sometimes higher
- muffled voice
- sore throat and reluctance to swallow
- labored breathing; child often sits up with his chin jutting forward as he struggles to breathe
- blueness in the lips or fingernails
- drooling

What to do:
- If you suspect epiglottitis, get medical help immediately.
- Have the child breathe steam from a hot running shower *(page 77)*.
- Do your best to keep the child calm; panic will make matters worse.

Call the doctor if:
- your child displays any symptoms of epiglottitis.

Hay fever

Hay fever, or allergic rhinitis, which affects the nose, throat and upper respiratory tract, is caused by an allergy. *(See Hay fever, page 48)*.

Hearing problems

Good hearing is essential to a child's ability to learn to talk. Any hearing problem — even one that is temporary — can hinder that learning process and should be investigated with your doctor's assistance. Aided by computers that measure changes in a child's brain waves, hearing specialists, or audiologists, can test the hearing of even very young infants. For

Signals of a Hearing Problem

As you observe your child's behavior at the ages noted here, ask yourself the following questions. If the answer is no to one or more of them, talk to your pediatrician about a hearing test.

Birth to six months:
- Is your baby startled by loud sounds?
- When spoken to, does your three- to six-month-old infant turn his head to look for the person who spoke to him?
- Does he recognize your voice?
- Does he frequently repeat sounds?

Six months to one year:
- Does the baby respond to his own name when called?
- Does he understand words such as "no" and "bye-bye"?
- Does he use his voice to attract your attention?

One to two years:
- By 15 months, is the child speaking his first words?
- Can he follow a simple sequence of directions such as, "Pick up the toy and come here"?
- By the age of two, does he have command of 10 to 15 words?

- Does he sometimes try to repeat the words you speak?

Two to five years:
- At two and a half years of age, can he point to pictures of objects in a book when you say their names?
- By three years of age, does he understand conversation easily?
- Does he hear you when you call from another room?
- Does he hear whispered speech?
- Is his voice as clear as other children's voices?
- Can he make all speech sounds correctly, except the "s" and "th"?

signs that indicate whether your youngster should have her hearing tested, see the box above.

Hearing problems can be divided into two broad categories: conductive hearing loss and sensorineural hearing loss. Conductive problems are often temporary. They are caused by some form of blockage — either in the canal that leads to the eardrum or in the middle ear, beyond the eardrum. Blockage on the inner side of the eardrum occurs when infection creates a build-up of fluid there (see Middle-ear infection, page 80). Such infections must be treated with antibiotics to prevent the eardrum from rupturing, possibly resulting in permanent damage.

Blockage in the canal outside the eardrum can also be caused by infection and, again, will need professional treatment (see Outer-ear infection, page 81). Other sources of outer-ear problems are accumulated wax, insects lodged in the ear canal, or small objects such as beads or peanuts that the child has pressed into her ear. Do not try to remove such an object yourself. You may damage the child's ear or push the object farther in. Let a doctor remove the foreign item.

If the cause of hearing loss is a build-up of wax, you may be able to help the child at home, but even here you need to exercise caution. You can try to flush out the wax with a stream of warm water from an ear syringe. If the wax is very hard or packed into the ear, you may have to soften it first. Wax softeners are available in drugstores; simply follow the instructions on the label. Always use water that

is close to body temperature for flushing out the ear; cold water can cause dizziness or even vomiting. Never employ this procedure unless you are certain the eardrum is intact. Therefore, never flush out the ear of a youngster who has had a recent ear infection.

Sensorineural hearing problems, which are permanent, result from damage in the inner ear, in the nerves that connect the ear to the brain or in the brain itself. These varieties of hearing loss can be identified by tests but cannot be cured. The question becomes one of how you can best help your child cope with the hearing impairment.

The degree of impairment can range from mild, in which the child has difficulty hearing distant speech or faint sounds, to profound, in which the child may hear very loud sounds but cannot rely upon hearing for communication. In between, there are several gradations of hearing loss, each of which calls for some remedial measure, such as a hearing aid, preferential seating in classrooms, speech therapy or special schools. It is important that any hearing impairment be identified early, so that, with the help of a doctor and an audiologist, you can give the child the greatest possible support and help.

Herpangina

Herpangina is an infection of the throat caused by a virus. It is a contagious disease that usually strikes children who are between the ages of one and seven years, most often in the summer or early fall, and lasts about a week.

An early sign of herpangina is a sudden high fever — generally 102° F. to 103° F., but sometimes as high as 106° F. Once herpangina develops, the most prominent symptom is the appearance of tiny blisters or sores inside the throat and at the back of the palate. Other symptoms include backaches, stomachaches and, in some cases, vomiting.

There is no specific medication given for herpangina, but you may have to take measures to reduce the high fever (page 94), and you should keep the child isolated to prevent the spread of the disease.

Hiccups

Hiccups are caused by an involuntary spasm of the diaphragm, a large muscle that separates the chest from the abdomen. Frequent bouts of hiccups are common in young children — they can even occur before birth — and often continue into early childhood.

Sooner or later an attack of hiccups will cease on its own, but to hasten that moment there are several strategies that sometimes provide relief. Try having your child hold her breath for as long as she can while exerting pressure with her abdominal muscles, as though she were having a bowel movement. Other home remedies that may be worth a try are drinking a glass of water without taking a breath, swallowing crushed ice and eating a teaspoonful of dry sugar.

Hoarseness

Hoarseness is a raspy-sounding quality in the voice or in breathing. In many cases, it is caused by nothing more serious than prolonged crying or some other strenuous use of the vocal cords, and it will disappear in a day if the youngster rests his voice. In a child younger than three months, however, hoarseness can sometimes indicate a more serious problem, such as a thyroid disorder or a birth defect. And if it lasts longer than a day in older children, the cause is most probably a virus.

If the hoarseness is accompanied by labored breathing and a distinctive cough that sounds like a barking dog, the child may have croup (page 77). Hoarseness accompanied by drooling, severe pain in swallowing or gasping for air may be a symptom of epiglotittis, which is a medical emergency. You should have the child examined by your doctor if hoarseness persists for more than a week with no obvious explanation.

Influenza

Influenza — flu — is an infection of the respiratory tract, spread by highly contagious viruses and characterized by chills, fever, coughing and body aches. Flu usually lasts from three days to a week, with a cough sometimes persisting for an additional week. Like the common cold, it is difficult to avoid and has no cure. And while it is usually not serious in itself, it does make a child more susceptible to other diseases and thus must be watched very carefully. One possible complication is pneumonia, signaled by chest pain and a prolonged high fever that appear after the initial flu symptoms have abated.

Flu is most prevalent in children older than five years. About half of these children will catch every new strain of flu virus that comes along. Influenza vaccines are not recommended for most children, but they are recommended for youngsters who run a high risk of complications, such as: children with congenital heart conditions, cystic fibrosis, severe asthma, emphysema, chronic bronchitis or tuberculosis.

Symptoms:
- sudden fever of up to 106° F.
- a dry, hacking cough and sore throat
- chills
- headaches, muscle aches and fatigue
- in some cases, diarrhea

What to do:
- Encourage the child to rest in bed.
- Take her temperature at the same time each day and give acetaminophen to reduce fever and relieve muscle aches. DO NOT give aspirin (see Reye Syndrome, page 105).
- Use a cool-mist humidifier or vaporizer. Moisture in the air makes breathing much easier.
- Ask your doctor about giving a cough suppressant if the child is losing sleep because of a cough.
- Isolate the sick child to prevent the spread of the illness.

Call the doctor if:
- the fever rises to a significant level for a child of that age (page 93) or diminishes and returns several times.
- the cough worsens or the child experiences breathing difficulty, chest pain or blood-tinged sputum.
- vomiting or diarrhea occurs.
- there is thick yellow or green discharge from the nose or ears.
- the child has ear or sinus pain.
- the lips or fingernails start turning dusky blue or purple.
- your child has any chronic disease and catches the flu.

Laryngitis

Laryngitis is an infection of the larynx — the vocal cords and the portion of the throat around them. In older children the symptoms are hoarseness, sore throat and voice loss, but in children under three, laryngitis can also cause the breathing difficulties that are associated with croup (page 77).

To instill medicated drops in a child's ear, have her lie down with the infected ear facing up. Hold her head steady while depositing the prescribed number of eardrops into the ear canal and for a full minute afterward.

Middle-ear infection

Known by the medical term "otitis media," middle-ear infection usually arises from a cold or other upper respiratory infection. In fact, mild inflammation of the middle ear — often unrecognized — accompanies most colds suffered by children under four years of age. One reason that a child's middle ear is peculiarly susceptible to infections is a quirk of childhood anatomy: Until a child is eight or so, the Eustachian tubes — ducts that drain fluid secretions from the middle ear into the back of the nose — are shorter than those of older children and adults. This makes it easier for infectious organisms to reach the middle ear. The tubes are also more nearly horizontal than those of older people, which makes it more difficult for them to drain and easier for them to be flooded with milk or formula if an infant is fed while lying flat. If the tubes or surrounding tissue become irritated and swell shut, bacteria and viruses can thrive in the closed space, causing fluid to build up in the middle ear.

As the fluid pressure increases, the eardrum bulges outward painfully. In some cases, particularly if the infection is left untreated, the pressure may rupture the eardrum, releasing pus or a watery discharge into the ear canal and simultaneously relieving the pain. Although the eardrum will heal itself in time, your doctor should be notified immediately to begin proper treatment and to prevent the possibility of further injury.

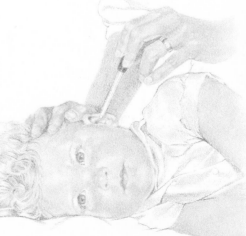

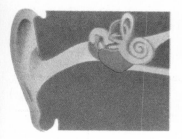

Middle-ear infections occur when the Eustachian tubes have become blocked and prevent normal drainage of fluid from the ear into the back of the throat. The trapped fluid (red) provides a fertile breeding ground for bacteria. If the ear is left untreated, increasing pressure from the fluid may cause the eardrum to burst.

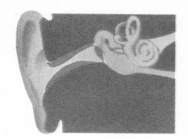

Often the first indication of an outer-ear infection appears when the entire ear becomes extremely tender. There may also be a white cheesy discharge, consisting of wax and sloughed skin. The reason for the pain is an infection — usually hidden from view — that has caused the ear canal to become swollen and inflamed (red).

Even mild ear infections should be treated promptly. If the doctor believes an eardrum rupture is imminent, he may choose to make a tiny incision, called a myringotomy, in the eardrum to drain the infected fluid from the middle ear. This is a simple procedure done in the doctor's office, often requiring only local anesthesia. The incision heals within a week to 10 days.

To prevent middle-ear infections, keep an infant's head raised during feedings, so that milk or formula cannot run into the Eustachian tubes. For an older child, sleeping with a pillow helps keep fluid draining from the middle ear.

Mild hearing loss is common during an ear infection and for a few days afterward, but rarely is there permanent damage. On the other hand, a child's ability to hear may be diminished or may fluctuate if middle-ear infections become chronic. This can impair the acquisition of complex social and language skills during critical periods of development. If a child with chronic ear infections does not respond to antibiotic therapy over a period of months, doctors sometimes recommend surgery to implant tiny drainage tubes in the youngster's ear to prevent the build-up of fluids.

Symptoms:
- ear pain or stuffiness, shown by the child's rubbing or pulling at the ears
- high fever in babies, low-grade fever in older children
- crying, irritability
- loss of appetite

What to do:
- Call the doctor immediately.
- While waiting to see the doctor, give acetaminophen and hold a hot-water bottle filled with warm water or a heating pad set on low against the ear to ease the pain.
- Complete the full course of medication that the doctor prescribes even if the symptoms improve.

Call the doctor if:
- your child displays any symptoms of middle-ear infection.

Motion sickness

Many children are subject to motion sickness in just about anything that moves — cars, boats, buses, airplanes or rides at the amusement park. The symptoms are dizziness, nausea and vomiting, which come on suddenly during or just after the trip. The cause of the problem is overstimulation of the semicircular canals in the inner ear, which help the body maintain balance, but why this upsets the stomach remains a mystery. Sometimes the smell of engine fumes or other strong odors, such as cigarette smoke, will aggravate the problem. A heavy meal just before beginning the ride also seems to make matters worse.

When traveling in a car, keep a window open. If a child is large enough to be properly secured by a safety belt, let him sit in the front seat, where he can focus on the horizon ahead rather than being dizzied by the quickly passing sights to the sides. Discourage reading or playing with small toys: The constant refocusing of vision from close-up objects to the world outside the car seems to increase motion sickness. If you know that your child is prone to this problem, plan for the worst and bring along a resealable plastic bag and some tissues.

On boats, keep the youngster above deck, toward the bow if possible, and away from the engine exhaust. On airplanes, the ride is a little smoother if you are seated above the wings. But more important, choose seats that are as far as possible from the smoking section. Focus a stream of cool air on the child's face and if he starts to look queasy, ask the flight attendant for a cold cloth. Flat sodas and mildly salty foods such as soda crackers or pretzels will sometimes help to stabilize the stomach.

Over-the-counter medication based on meclizine or dimenhydrinate is effective in reducing nausea, although drowsiness is a frequent side effect. These medicines are available in tablets or drops. Fortunately, most children outgrow their sensitivity to motion in time.

Outer-ear infection

Formally called otitis externa, outer-ear infection is also known as swimmer's ear because it occurs often in children who swim frequently. The infection develops when bacteria invade the constantly moist skin lining the external ear flap, or pinna, and the ear canal. Occasionally an external infection is caused by bacteria that find their way into a scratch or other opening in the skin. Unlike a middle-ear infection, otitis externa will make the child's ear flap tender to the touch.

To help your child avoid outer-ear infections, caution him against scratching or attempting to clean the ears himself. If the child gets these infections often, sterilize each ear canal after swimming with two or three drops of isopropyl alcohol. Keep the drops in the ear for about five seconds, then let the alcohol drain out.

Symptoms:
- ear pain, indicated by scratching or pulling at the ear while crying
- red, swollen ear canal
- appearance of a white, cheesy substance consisting of wax and sloughed-off skin

What to do:
- Contact your child's physician. You can usually wait until regular office hours, although if the pain is increasing, call the doctor immediately.
- Give the child antibacterial eardrops if the doctor prescribes them.
- Keep ear dry until infection clears.

Pneumonia

Pneumonia is not always caused by the same organism. It can result from any of several different causes — ranging from viruses, bacteria and fungi to foreign objects inhaled into the lungs — and it varies greatly in its severity. Any case of pneumonia requires a doctor's care, but nowadays, because of the medicines that are available, the illness is rarely life-threatening, as it used to be. Pneumonia is most dangerous for babies under a year old and for youngsters with asthma or cystic fibrosis. Such children may have to be hospitalized with the illness. Except for a rare type caused by tuberculosis, pneumonia is not a highly contagious disease, but it is caused by organisms passed from person to person.

In children, pneumonia often spreads downward from upper respiratory infections, usually as a complication of influenza or bronchitis rather than of a common cold. The course of the illness and the necessary treatment will vary depending upon the cause, but you can expect the youngster's recovery to be rather slow. It is common for fatigue and feelings of weakness to last for as long as one month to six weeks.

Symptoms:
- coughing — either a dry, hacking cough or a wet cough that produces rust-colored or pink-tinged sputum
- fever
- shortness of breath or breathing that is labored and noisy
- chest pain, especially with cough

What to do:
- Follow your physician's instructions with regard to all medication.
- Offer plenty of fluids to prevent dehydration and to thin the mucus.
- Use a cool-mist vaporizer or humidifier to ease breathing.
- To relieve chest pain, use a hot-water bottle filled with warm water or a heating pad set on low.
- Keep the youngster in bed until the fever and shortness of breath have been gone for 48 hours.

Call the doctor if:
- the child has pneumonia symptoms.
- the fever suddenly worsens.
- chest pain is not reduced by heat or the prescribed medication.
- any blueness appears in the child's lips or under his nails.
- there is blood in the sputum.
- the youngster is nauseated, vomits or has diarrhea.

Rheumatic fever

Rheumatic fever is a rare but dangerous disease that is a complication of untreated strep infections *(see Strep throat, page 84)*; it rarely affects children younger than five years. Rheumatic fever can be life-threatening: The disease carries a 50 percent chance of permanent damage to the heart. Or it can be a mild episode with little residual damage. In any case, professional medical care is indispensable and should begin as soon as possible.

A prompt diagnosis and treatment of strep throat will prevent the occurrence of this illness. If a child does develop rheumatic fever, it is likely to appear 10 days to three weeks after the sore throat subsides. The disease will also have a tendency to reappear if the child contracts subsequent strep infections. This can be prevented by keeping a child on penicillin for an extended period of time.

The most prominent symptom is a painful swelling of joints, most often the elbows, wrists, knees and ankles. Typically, the swelling shifts from one joint to another before the illness subsides. These symptoms should not be confused with common growing pains behind the knees or in the calf or shin muscles, which sometimes awaken a child at night. Rheumatic fever, unlike growing pains, makes joints tender to the touch and painful when moved. It sometimes leads to chorea *(page 102)*.

Symptoms:
- red, swollen, tender joints

- generally low fever, but sometimes as high as 104° F.
- chest pain and shortness of breath
- in some cases, a lattice-like red rash on the torso or limbs

What to do:
- Call the child's doctor immediately.
- If antibiotics are prescribed, carry out the full treatment even if the symptoms seem to disappear.
- Your doctor may also suggest using aspirin to reduce the swelling, but DO NOT give aspirin if there is any possibility that your youngster has been infected by chicken pox, flu or any other viral infection *(see Reye syndrome, page 105)*.

Call the doctor if:
- your child shows the symptoms of strep throat *(page 84)*.
- she has sore, swollen joints.

Scarlet fever

Also known as scarlatina, scarlet fever is a highly contagious streptococcal infection marked by a rough, red rash on the chest and abdomen or sometimes over the entire body *(right)*. It is a variant of strep throat, caused by a particular streptococcal bacterium that manufactures a toxin that causes the rash. In itself, scarlet fever is not serious. But like strep throat, it carries the risk of dangerous complications: rheumatic fever, hearing impairment, meningitis and pneumonia.

A throat culture is necessary to confirm the strep infection; the rash alone is not sufficient evidence because it closely resembles measles, heat rash or sunburn. Once identified, scarlet fever is treated with antibiotics — preferably penicillin, but erythromycin if the child is allergic to penicillin. The youngster is contagious until 24 hours after the antibiotics are begun. The rash usually fades after about a week, and then the skin flakes or peels.

Symptoms:
- high fever, up to 104° F.

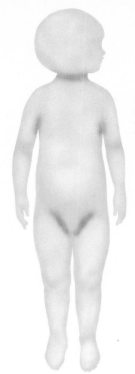

The red, sandpaper-like rash that accompanies scarlet fever appears first, and remains most intense, around the skin folds of the neck, groin and armpits. After a week the rash usually disappears and the skin flakes or peels.

- chills
- often, vomiting early in the illness
- swollen glands in the neck
- sore throat
- after one day, a rough, red rash
- tongue coated white with bright red showing through

What to do:

- Call the doctor immediately; antibiotics will be necessary. Continue giving the full course of medication even if the child seems better.
- To soothe a sore throat, have the youngster gargle a salt-water solution: one teaspoon of salt mixed in eight ounces of warm water.
- Give acetaminophen to relieve fever.
- Isolate the child until he is no longer contagious. The whole family may need to have throat cultures tested.

Call the doctor if:

- you suspect scarlet fever, even if the symptoms are mild.

Sinusitis

When bacterial or viral infections invade the membranes lining the sinuses — air-filled cavities tucked among the bones of the face *(right)* — the resulting condition is called sinusitis. Connected with the nasal passages through small openings, the sinuses have the same kind of mucous-membrane lining as the nose and often develop secondary infections in the aftermath of colds. Excess mucus trickling from the sinuses into the throat causes coughing, particularly at night when the child is lying down in sleep. Sinus infections are usually short in duration, but they can make a youngster extremely uncomfortable, and in some cases the infections become chronic.

Until they are at least 10 years old, children usually do not get the full-fledged sinusitis attacks marked by severe headaches that afflict some adults. This is because the sinuses form gradually over the course of childhood. Before the age of two, only the sinuses behind the bridge of the nose and inside the cheekbones are large enough to become infected. If your toddler develops a fever or swelling around the eyes in the wake of a cold or upper respiratory infection, have her examined by a doctor right away. Though sinusitis at this age is relatively rare, the infection can spread to the eyes or the brain. Between the ages of three and five, the sinuses behind the eyes also mature and become susceptible to infection. At 10 years of age, the cavities in the forehead are fully formed.

Symptoms:

- opaque, yellow or milky discharge from the nostrils
- coughing, sometimes severe; may be followed by gagging or even vomiting if it occurs while the child is sleeping
- a headache or pressure behind the eyes, especially when bending over

What to do:

- Give the child nose drops; do not exceed the recommended dosages.
- Use a cool-mist vaporizer or humidifier to ease breathing.
- Encourage the child to drink plenty of fluids to keep secretions thin.
- Apply a warm, wet cloth to the affected area of the face.
- Consult your physician about the use of decongestants.

Call the doctor if:

- the sinusitis becomes severe or recurs frequently.
- there is swelling around the forehead, eyes, nose or cheeks.
- the youngster suffers a severe or persistent headache.
- vision becomes blurred.

Sore throat

The throat — or technically, the pharynx — is a high-traffic passageway con-

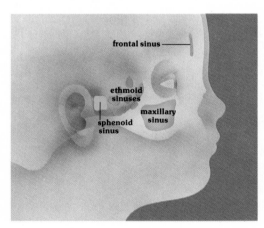

frontal sinus

ethmoid sinuses

maxillary sinus

sphenoid sinus

The sinuses, which are air-filled cavities situated among the bones of the face, lend resonance to the voice and lighten the weight of the skull. Lined with mucous membranes, the sinuses drain excess mucus directly into the nasal cavity. Until the age of two, only the maxillary sinuses, which are located in the cheekbones, and the ethmoid sinuses, which are located behind the bridge of the nose, are fully formed. The sphenoid sinuses, situated deeper behind the nose, develop between the ages of three and five, while the frontal sinuses, which are positioned above the eyebrows, develop when the child is between the ages of six and 10.

necting the mouth with the nasal cavity above and the larynx, windpipe and esophagus below. It also houses the adenoids and the tonsils. Inflammation in this part of the body, referred to as a sore throat or by the medical term "pharyngitis," is quite common in childhood. The cause of a child's sore throat can be as simple as the postnasal drip of a cold or the breathing in of dry air from forced-air heating and cooling systems. If soreness persists for more than a day, however, it may be due to an infection caused by viruses or bacteria.

The source of the problem may be ascertained by a painless procedure called a throat culture, which involves swabbing out a sampling of throat mucus for laboratory analysis. In many labs, test results can be obtained in a matter of minutes. When bacteria are at fault, they are usually of the streptococcal type, which produces the illness known as strep throat *(following entry)*, and which can be eliminated by antibiotics.

Unlike bacterial throat infections, sore throats caused by viruses cannot be treated with drugs. Once begun, they must run their course. The duration can be as brief as 24 hours or as long as five days. Viral sore throats normally develop more gradually than strep infections do: The beginning of the illness is marked by fever and feelings of tiredness; soreness of the throat sets in after two or three days.

An overall sore throat may encompass infections of the tonsils and adenoids — specifically termed "tonsillitis" and "adenoiditis." These glands are lumps of lymphoid tissue that are most useful in infancy and early childhood: They act as filters to prevent disease from entering the body by way of the throat. As the baby grows older, the glands gradually lose their function and diminish in size; eventually, both all but disappear.

Until fairly recently, doctors thought the tonsils and adenoids were the starting point for many throat infections and, because the glands can obstruct breathing when they become swollen, they were routinely taken out if a child had frequent sore throats. Doctors now know that tonsils and adenoids have nothing to do with the frequency of throat infections. Operations to remove them have become much less common and are never performed simply to avert sore throats.

Symptoms of viral sore throat:
- general fatigue
- fever of 101° F. to 103° F.
- throat pain
- sometimes, coughing, hoarseness, and congestion of the nose

What to do:
- Have your doctor arrange a throat culture if there is a likelihood of strep throat *(following entry)*.
- Use a cool-mist vaporizer or humidifier to ease breathing.
- If the youngster is old enough, have her gargle as often as necessary with a solution of one teaspoon of salt dissolved in eight ounces of warm water to relieve pain. (Gargling will not shorten the course of the illness.)
- Use acetaminophen to relieve pain and fever. DO NOT give aspirin *(see Reye syndrome, page 105)*.

Call the doctor if:
- your child gets a sore throat.
- the soreness persists for more than seven days.

Strep throat

The most serious type of sore throat is an infection named strep throat, after streptococcus, the bacterium that causes it. Although its symptoms are similar to those of viral sore throats — chiefly, throat pain, fever and malaise — the strep infection must be handled more cautiously because it can lead to grave complications. A small percentage of children who are left untreated will develop a kidney inflammation called nephritis, or, more seriously, rheumatic fever. Another variation of strep infection that will sometimes accompany the sore throat is scarlet fever.

There is an incubation period of one to three days from the time of exposure to the appearance of symptoms, when they are present. However, many people infected by strep throat suffer only mild symptoms or do not develop symptoms at all. In the winter, some 25 percent of school-age children with no symptoms of the disease carry the streptococcal bacteria. Strep throat can be diagnosed only by means of a throat culture. Once identified, the infection is treated with antibiotics, which usually provide very rapid relief. As with any prescribed course of medication, it is important to complete the entire drug treatment even if your child starts to feel better right away. To be sure the infection is gone, your child's doctor may want to repeat the throat culture five days after the antibiotic treatment has ended.

Strep infections are sometimes passed from one family member to the next; when a child comes down with strep throat, doctors sometimes suggest that the whole family come in for throat cultures. The sick youngster ceases to be contagious 24 hours after beginning the course of antibiotics.

Symptoms:
- fever as high as 104° F.
- throat pain
- headache, loss of appetite and general feeling of being ill
- swollen lymph nodes in the neck
- abdominal pain
- bad breath
- sometimes, pain in the ears
- sometimes, a red rash under the armpits or elsewhere on the body

What to do:
- Arrange for a throat culture to identify the illness. If strep is diagnosed, follow your doctor's instructions.

- Have a child older than three or four gargle a solution of one teaspoon of salt in eight ounces of warm water.
- Give acetaminophen to relieve fever.
- Provide a diet of soft foods such as ice cream, milk shakes, flavored gelatin or applesauce, until the child can swallow more easily.
- Make sure that the youngster drinks plenty of liquids, despite the discomfort from throat pain.

Call the doctor if:
- your child gets a sore throat.
- the child's fever suddenly returns after a few days of treatment.
- your youngster has any of these symptoms: vomiting, earache, skin rash, chest pain, shortness of breath or a severe headache.
- the child develops a cough, especially if the sputum is green, yellow-brown or blood-streaked.

Sudden infant death syndrome

The sudden, unexplained death of an infant who showed no previous signs of illness is known as sudden infant death syndrome (SIDS). Sometimes called crib death, this alarming phenomenon is undoubtedly the greatest unsolved mystery of pediatric medicine. It claims the lives of about 10,000 babies each year in the United States — roughly three out of every 1,000 children born.

SIDS occurs worldwide and has been recorded as far back as biblical times. It usually strikes babies who are two to four months old and rarely occurs after six months of age. The greatest number of deaths occur in the winter, the smallest number in summer. And the SIDS victim is more often a boy than a girl. It is not yet certain what role genetics plays in predisposing babies to SIDS, but some studies have revealed a tendency for the calamity to recur in families. Low birth weight and a mother with a history of smoking ap-

pear to be predisposing factors as well.

Doctors are also investigating possible links between SIDS and other medical conditions — a breathing disturbance called apnea, a combination of neurological and biochemical abnormalities, and failure of the cardiorespiratory controls — but so far none of these suspected causes have been proved. At the same time, recent research has disproved earlier theories that SIDS is often caused by suffocation from bedding in the crib, spinal-cord damage, pneumonia or bacterial infections.

The sudden loss of an infant is, of course, the most grievous shock that any parent can suffer. There are a number of local and national support groups — and in many areas, SIDS hotlines — available to help a family cope with this tragedy.

Swimmer's ear

Swimmer's ear is an outer-ear infection that often afflicts frequent swimmers *(see Outer-ear infection, page 81).*

Thrush

Thrush, the informal name for a form of the fungal condition candidiasis, is a common yeast infection of the mouth. A newborn may acquire the infection while passing through the birth canal if the mother has a vaginal yeast infection at the time of delivery. In this case, the problem usually does not show itself for a week or more after birth. Older children also sometimes get thrush when they have been taking antibiotics, which promote the growth of the offending organisms by killing the friendly bacteria that normally keep them in check.

The signs of the infection are white patches, which look like curds of milk, appearing on the tongue and the insides of the child's cheeks. The white patches will not wipe off.

Thrush does not cause any pain and often clears up on its own with no treat-

ment. Your doctor can speed recovery, however, by prescribing medication that is applied directly to the white patches.

Tonsillitis

Tonsillitis is an infection of the tonsils — small lumps of lymphoid tissue located in the folds at the back of the throat. Marked by fever and localized pain, the illness is usually part of an overall throat infection *(see Sore throat, page 83).*

Traveler's ear

Small children often experience pain in their ears while traveling on airplanes, which has lent the condition the popular name "traveler's ear." Problems typically occur during ascents and when planes begin to descend for landing.

The pain, which is caused by a difference between the internal and external pressure on the eardrums, can also occur on fast-moving elevators or while traveling in automobiles at mountain elevations or through tunnels that descend below ground level.

The body normally adjusts for changes in air pressure by means of the Eustachian tubes: They act as valves for air moving back and forth between the inner ears and the nose, thus equalizing the pressure inside and out. Young children, however, often do not act to facilitate the process by swallowing or yawning, as adults learn to do. And because children's Eustachian tubes are very small, they are more susceptible to blockages that prevent the movement of air.

Whenever possible, it is advisable to avoid air travel if your child has a bad cold or an ear infection: There is a risk of temporarily muffled hearing or bleeding inside the ear in addition to the pain. If you must travel, give the child a decongestant or use a decongestant nasal spray prior to boarding and again just before the plane descends. Decongestants work by shrinking swollen tissues, thus widen-

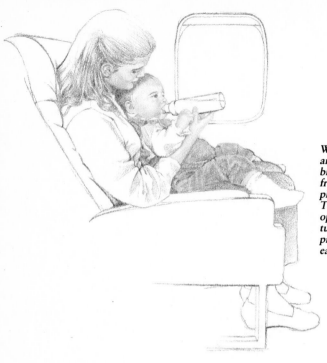

When traveling by air, allow an infant or small child to breast-feed or take liquid from a bottle during the airplane's ascent and descent. The swallowing motion will open the child's Eustachian tubes, equalizing the air pressure on either side of the eardrum and relieving pain.

ing the Eustachian tubes of a child with a cold. If you are traveling with a baby, breast-feed the child or give him a bottle or pacifier during take-offs and landings. The swallowing action will enhance the movement of air to equalize the pressure. A baby's crying, too, will help equalize air pressure — however disturbing it may be to parents and other passengers.

Give an older child gum or hard candy to promote swallowing. As a last resort, instruct the child to take in a mouthful of air, hold his nose and, with his mouth closed, gently try to blow the air out through his blocked nose. This will force air into the Eustachian tubes.

Wheezing

Wheezing is a high-pitched sound that a child makes when he breathes through obstructed air passages. The sound is similar to the harsh, whistling sound known as stridor, but it emerges from deeper in the chest. Wheezing is usually most pronounced when the child exhales, but it can sometimes be heard when he inhales as well. It is an important signal that your child is having trouble breathing. Any time you detect wheezing you should be watchful for more serious signs of shortness of breath: very shallow, rapid breathing or blueness in the lips or the fingernails.

The usual causes of wheezing are asthma and lower respiratory infections such as bronchitis and bronchiolitis. Pneumonia can also cause wheezing. Less frequently, wheezing results from foreign objects that are lodged in the airways and from allergic reactions caused by insect bites or medication.

The remedy for wheezing will depend on the specific cause. If you do not know the cause, get in touch with the child's doctor. Aside from prescribed medication, the most effective measures you can take are to make sure that the youngster drinks plenty of water and to add moisture to the air with a cool-mist vaporizer or humidifer. ❖

Eyes

The eyes of a newborn baby are always beautiful, yet they look different from those of older people. The whites of the eyes may appear bluish or grayish, a tint that disappears within a few months as the whites thicken. Or they may be yellowish, a sign of a form of jaundice *(page 70)* that soon passes. The iris (the colored part of the eye surrounding the pupil) is usually blue at birth in a white baby, while irises in the newborn of dark-skinned peoples are brown. By six months, the iris often changes to a different, permanent color. The eyes may appear crossed, a condition that probably will soon correct itself. They should be the same size and shape, however, and the pupils should widen equally as the room is darkened and contract equally as the light increases.

Newborns can respond to facial expressions, and by the age of four months your child should be able to focus his eyes well enough to follow an object moving in an arc across his field of vision. Between four and six months, a baby's eyes should be moving smoothly and in a coordinated fashion, much like an adult's.

From this point on, you should watch for changes in the appearance of the eyes, lids or surrounding tissue, as well as for signs in your child's visual behavior that might indicate any of the problems described in this section. The common diffi-

culties in seeing clearly — nearsightedness, farsightedness and astigmatism — may appear when children are very young, but can be recognized only after the age of three, when development of the shape of the eyeball is complete and visual acuity can be accurately assessed. Therefore, every child should have an eye examination at the age of three and another before beginning school.

Blocked tear duct
Tears, which continually flow over the eye to wash dust off, normally drain away through a small duct that runs from the inside corner of each eye to the nasal passage. If this duct is blocked, tears spill onto the cheek and dry to a yellowish-white residue that sometimes cakes the eyelids together while a baby sleeps.

In some infants younger than nine months, the duct has not yet matured and is not completely open. Mucus and skin can obstruct the movement of tears in such a narrow passage. This blockage is harmless and will cure itself, but it can be eased by a massaging technique that your doctor can demonstrate.

A nose injury or, occasionally, allergies may cause a blocked duct in older children. Blocked ducts can lead to infection in a child of any age. You should watch for redness, pus-filled discharge, itchiness or swelling in the corner of the

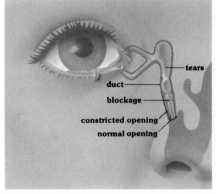

Lubricating tears wash over the eye continually, draining through a duct into the nose. If the duct is not completely developed at the time of birth or if it becomes blocked by small particles, tears back up and spill onto the cheek.

child's eye, and tell the doctor, who may prescribe antibiotics.
Symptoms:
- continuous overflow of tears
- yellowish-white mucus at the inside corner of the eye and edges of the lids
- redness and pus-filled discharge in the inside corner of the eye — an indication of infection

What to do:
- If an infant's duct is blocked but not infected, massage the area according to your doctor's instructions.
- Wash residue of tears away with a moistened washcloth.

Call the doctor if:
- the cause is an injury.
- tears are continually present and the child is older than nine months.
- puslike discharge, redness and itchiness indicate infection.

Conjunctivitis
An inflammation of the membrane lining the inner eyelids and the whites of the

The wall of the eyeball is composed of three layers covered by a clear membrane, the conjunctiva. The outer layer consists of the sclera, visible as the white of the eye, and the cornea, which is clear to admit and focus light. Beneath the sclera is the choroid, the pigmented layer that forms the iris at the front of the eye. An opening at the iris's center, the pupil, controls how much light enters the eye. Behind the iris, the lens focuses light on the retina, the eye's innermost lining. From there, the optic nerve carries messages to the brain. The eyeball is filled with clear, jelly-like vitreous humor.

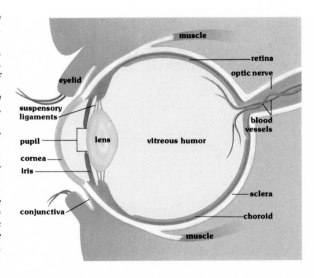

eyes, conjunctivitis can be caused by bacteria, viruses, allergies, chemicals or foreign objects. The bacterial type is often called pinkeye. Symptoms vary slightly for each type but include itching, burning, discharge of tears or mucus, and whites that turn pink or red. Treatment depends on the cause.

Advice on removing foreign objects is on page 30; redness and burning may linger for as much as 48 hours after the object is removed. Allergic reactions may be somewhat relieved with home treatment but are best prevented as other allergies *(page 46)* are.

Mild chemical irritations, such as those caused by soap or cosmetics, usually clear up quickly. One form of chemical conjunctivitis often affects newborns after their eyes have been treated with infection-fighting silver nitrate. Their eyelids may swell, but this is harmless and goes away in two or three days.

Viral conjuctivitis, which sometimes accompanies a cold, is not really treatable at all. Bacterial conjunctivitis can be relieved by eyewashes, eyedrops or ointments prescribed by your doctor. Do not attempt to use the commercial eyedrops that adults use for pinkened eyes. Both viral and bacterial conjunctivitis are highly contagious, spreading from eye to hand to hand to eye unless careful sanitation measures are taken.

Symptoms:
- of bacterial conjunctivitis — redness, swelling of the eyelids, itching and a yellow-green pus that seems to clear by day but cakes eyelids shut overnight, usually affecting both eyes
- of viral conjunctivitis — watering and slight redness, often affecting only one of the eyes
- of allergic conjunctivitis — watering, slight redness and itching, equally affecting both eyes
- of conjunctivitis in a newborn that is caused by silver nitrate — puffy lids

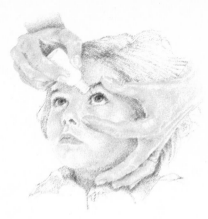

To give eyedrops, stand behind your child and tilt her head back slightly. Gently push downward on the cheek skin to depress the lower eyelid; place the drops in the channel between the eyeball and lid.

and sticky discharge from the eyes
- of conjunctivitis caused by chemical irritation or foreign objects *(page 30)* — redness, burning, running tears

What to do:
- For bacterial conjunctivitis, apply warm compresses to the eye. Several times a day, at bedtime and when the child wakens, hold cotton balls soaked in boiled water and cooled to a bit warmer than body temperature against his closed eyes for 10 minutes.
- Apply antibiotic drops or ointment according to your physician's instructions. Use the medication for the indicated number of days, even if the symptoms have abated. DO NOT use over-the-counter eye preparations unless the doctor recommends them.
- Prevent the spread of viral or bacterial conjunctivitis by insisting on frequent hand-washing by all members of the family; using disposable paper towels; and keeping washcloths, towels and bedding of affected children separate from those of others. Although his eyes itch terribly, try to keep your child from rubbing them. Do not let him swim until 24 hours after the redness has gone.
- For allergy-caused conjunctivitis, keep your child away from the irritant and apply cool compresses to closed eyes. Eyedrops or antihistamines prescribed by a doctor may help.

Call the doctor if:

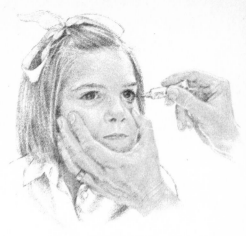

To give eye ointment, gently pull down the lower lid. Starting at the inner corner, squeeze a thin line of ointment into the channel between the lid and eyeball. Take care not to touch the eye with the applicator.

- you suspect bacterial conjunctivitis.
- puffy eyelids in an infant last longer than about three days.
- conjunctivitis that appears to be caused by chemicals or a virus lasts longer than three days.

Cross-eye

When a child's eyes do not coordinate to provide a single image of an object to the brain, the symptom is called strabismus. If one or both eyes seem to look toward the nose, the child is said to be cross-eyed. If one or both eyes wander outward, she is wall-eyed. Strabismus is serious — threatening blindness in one eye — and it must be treated promptly.

Strabismus may be caused by one of several underlying conditions. The two most common are vision defects, such as farsightedness in one eye or weakness in the muscles that control eye movement. In rare instances the cause is retinoblastoma, a curable cancer of the eye.

The misalignment of the eyes causes one eye to send the brain a view so different that it cannot fuse them into a single image, as it normally does with the views from both eyes. Instead the brain chooses the view from one eye over the other. This condition is called amblyopia, or lazy eye. Eventually, the signals from the second eye are totally ignored by the brain; the sight in that eye is seriously diminished and may be lost permanently.

Although parents should watch for

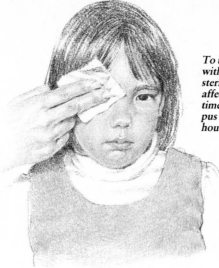

To treat a sty, moisten a piece of gauze with warm water that has been boiled for sterilization. Hold the compress to the affected area for about 15 minutes, three times a day. The warmth will bring the pus closer to the skin's surface; within 48 hours the sty should drain.

cross-eye in their children, apparent signs of the condition are not always cause for worry. The muscles controlling the movement of the eye do not develop fully until the child is three to six months old, so you may observe a lack of coordinated movement during this part of infancy. In addition, some babies have a flat, broad-bridged nose or a wider fold of skin at the inside corner of the eye. Since this hides part of the white of the eye, the eyes can appear to be crossed when, in fact, they are normal — a condition known as pseudostrabismus, or false strabismus. False strabismus normally disappears by the age of six months as the eyes grow larger in relation to the surrounding skin and more of the whites comes into view. If the eyes still appear to be crossed beyond this age, the condition should be evaluated by a doctor.

In children older than six months, there are varying degrees of strabismus. Sometimes the signs are obvious: The eyes seem to look in two directions at once, or they do not always move together, or one eye wanders, taking longer than the other to focus on an object. Strabismus is always serious, however mild a case it may appear to be. It may be indicated by such clues as the frequent rubbing of one eye (the weaker one), tilting of the head to see, the frequent covering of one eye (the weaker one), a dislike for games that require estimating distances or catching a ball or, in babies, a cry of displeasure when one eye (the stronger one) is covered.

If you are concerned about your child, you can perform a quick test for strabismus at home. Hold a penlight several feet from your child's face, aimed at her nose. When she looks straight at the light, its reflection should appear at the identical location on each pupil. In misaligned eyes, the points of light will not be symmetrical; one reflection will rest on the pupil while one may appear on the iris.

If you believe your six-month-old's eyes are not coordinating properly, or you begin to notice symptoms in your toddler or preschooler, you should take the child for an eye examination. An ophthalmologist will be able to determine if strabismus exists and by what it is caused. Cross-eye can generally be cured and the vision of both eyes preserved if treatment begins soon after the condition is first noticed. Treatment usually involves special exercises that strengthen the muscles of the weaker eye; a patch over the stronger eye, which helps force the weaker one to work; special glasses that equalize the focusing ability of the two eyes; or surgery that tightens and strengthens the weak muscles.

Ptosis

Ptosis is a drooping of the upper eyelid over a portion of the eye. Caused by weakness in the muscle controlling the lid, it should be corrected because the affected eye can become a so-called lazy eye *(see Cross-eye, page 88)* and eventually lose its ability to see. In rare cases, ptosis may be an indication of an even more serious underlying problem, so a child should see a doctor promptly if the condition appears. If ptosis is present at birth, it usually affects only one eye and does not worsen with age. Ptosis of this sort tends to run in families and is readily cured when a child is three or four years old by surgery that shortens and strengthens the eyelid muscle.

Ptosis may also be caused at any age by

damage to the muscle that operates the lid or to the nerve that works the muscle. A physical injury, diabetes, muscle disease, infections, or a brain tumor may all lead to ptosis. In such cases, the underlying cause must be treated.

Sties and chalazions

A sty is a pimple-like bacterial infection in a hair follicle along the margin of the upper or lower eyelid. It grows red and painful in one or two days and subsides in about five more, usually after bursting and releasing pus.

A sty should not be confused with a chalazion, a painless swelling on the inside of either the upper or lower lid caused by plugged tear glands. Small chalazions may disappear in a month or two; large ones require surgery.

For a sty, home treatment is usually sufficient. The goal is to thin the skin at the top of the swelling with warm wet compresses, so that the sty eventually opens. If this fails, a doctor may pierce the sty or prescribe antibiotic eyedrops.

Symptom:
- a painful, pimple-like bump at an eyelash base on an upper or lower eyelid

What to do:
- Hold a compress, soaked in boiled water that has cooled to warm, over the sty for 15 minutes three times a day.
- DO NOT squeeze or puncture the sty.

Call the doctor if:
- the top of the swelling does not open after 48 hours of home treatment.
- the eyelid itself swells or the white of the eye turns reddish.

Vision problems

The three most prevalent vision problems — nearsightedness, farsightedness and astigmatism (blurry vision caused by irregularities in the cornea or lens) — are common indeed. Some 10 to 20 percent of all children wear corrective glasses by the time they enter school. Less com-

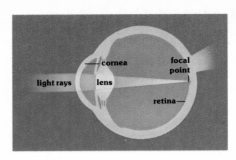

Light rays travel in straight, parallel lines. When they strike the eye the rays are bent, or refracted, first by the cornea and then by the lens. This focuses the light onto a point at the back of the eye on the retina. The nerve cells on the retina transmit visual information to the brain.

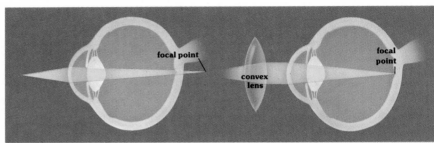

Farsightedness, or hyperopia, occurs when an eyeball is too short for the focusing power of the lens and cornea. In a far-sighted eye, light rays converge on a focal point beyond the retina, which makes close-up objects appear blurred. A convex corrective lens begins bending the light rays before they enter the eye, so that they converge earlier and focus on the retina.

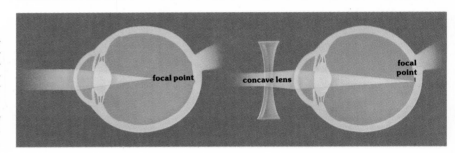

Nearsightedness, or myopia, is the result of an eyeball that is too long for the focusing power of the lens and cornea. In a myopic eye, light rays reach a focal point short of the retina and diverge again, creating a blurry image of faraway objects. A concave corrective lens spreads the light rays slightly before they hit the eye. This moves the focal point of the rays farther back inside the eye, to the nerve cells of the retina.

mon, and much more worrying, are three other problems: Blurred vision, double vision and cloudiness of the cornea are all symptoms of damage to the nervous system or the eyes, or symptoms of conditions that can lead to such damage.

Sudden blurred or double vision can be caused by a blow to the eye, injury to the brain, a brain tumor, poisons or drugs. Double vision may also arise during early stages of strabismus *(see Cross-eye, page 88).* Cloudiness of the cornea and an inability to tolerate light may suggest glaucoma, an increase in pressure inside the eye that can destroy vision. Cloudiness may also be a sign of cataracts — opaque spots in the lens that can interfere with vision. If your child exhibits any of these symptoms, call your doctor right away.

The more common vision defects are not dangerous. They are easily remedied with eyeglasses. But if not corrected, they may handicap a child at play and can seriously interfere with schoolwork.

Nearsightedness, or myopia, often runs in families. Only objects held close can be seen clearly. If your child squints, holds books close to her eyes or insists on sitting very close to the television screen, you should suspect myopia if she is older than five — many younger children just prefer to look at things close up, even though their vision is perfect. For a home test of your child, try to find out if she can distinguish an approaching object at the same time that you can. Your child should recognize you as you walk toward her at the same moment you recognize her. Since you know her vocabulary and language skills better than anyone else does, take note if she mistakes distant objects with which she is already familiar — such as referring to pears as oranges.

Farsightedness, or hyperopia, is the opposite of myopia — close objects are not seen clearly. All newborn babies are born somewhat farsighted, but this nearly always corrects itself within a few months. If it persists past infancy, the child may

back away from objects being examined, lose things that are close, lack interest in such sit-down play as reading or stringing small beads, rub the eyes often or complain of tired eyes.

Astigmatism produces a blurry view somewhat like that seen through a wavy pane of glass. The symptoms of astigmatism are similar to those of myopia, but may also be accompanied by headaches and complaints of eyestrain.

The most difficult part of remedying these vision problems may not be in detecting them but in persuading your child to wear the corrective glasses. Letting her select the frames may help. Also, your child probably will not have to wear glasses at all times, and you can help ease her into the habit of using them by not insisting that she put them on except when they are truly necessary. Shatterproof plastic lenses, which are safer and lighter in weight than glass and therefore a less noticeable burden, also help make glasses more acceptable to children. ❖

Fever

Fever is one of the most common symptoms of childhood illness and probably the most misunderstood. Many parents view this elevation in body temperature as an illness in itself. In fact, the existence of fever is a healthy sign that the body is actively fighting off some form of disease.

A fever usually arises in response to obvious viral or bacterial infections, such as those that cause earaches or sore throats, but it may also result from minor illnesses with no other symptoms. If your child has picked up a "bug," she may feel fine but still have a fever. Whether you decide to call the doctor, treat the fever at home or simply keep an eye on it will depend on a number of variables. Remember that fever is only a symptom; reducing a child's temperature does not treat the underlying cause.

To understand how fever is generated, it helps to look at the way the body's heat-regulating system works. Under normal conditions, the body maintains a fairly constant core temperature that is regulated by the hypothalamus, a natural thermostat in the brain. As the environmental temperature increases or decreases, the brain receives signals to readjust the thermostat, and this sets in motion certain coping mechanisms. If the outside temperature is cold, the blood vessels constrict to lessen heat loss through the skin; involuntary shivering may begin, generating heat through the movement of contracting muscles. If it is warm, the blood vessels dilate and the sweat glands are activated to release moisture, which cools the body as it evaporates.

Fever is the result of another complex reaction involving the body's thermostat, this one triggered not by the environment but by an invasion of infectious organisms. As white blood cells fight off the intruders, chemical by-products released into the bloodstream travel to the brain and prod the thermostat to a higher level. As a result, blood vessels near the skin's surface constrict to conserve heat and the body's temperature rises. This excess heat is believed to inhibit the growth and reproduction of the offending organisms and to help stimulate the production of infection-fighting antibodies.

Because of these apparently beneficial aspects of fever, most doctors recommend treatment to reduce a temperature only if the child is feeling discomfort or if the fever exceeds 102° F. *(For guidelines on treating fever, see page 94.)* It is more important to observe a feverish child for other symptoms, such as coughing, diarrhea, ear pain, lethargy, stupor or a rash — clues that will help the doctor diagnose the underlying illness.

The standard normal temperature —

How Ill Is Your Feverish Child?

The chart below will help you judge how ill your feverish child is, regardless of his temperature level, which is not always an accurate gauge of a patient's condition. Note the child's behavior or appearance in each of the categories at left and rate your observations as follows: Assign one point to mild symptoms, three points to moderate symptoms and five points to serious symptoms, then add the six scores. A total of 10 or fewer points indicates a child is only mildly ill in most cases; a score of 11 or more means there is greater likelihood of serious illness.

	Mild Symptoms	Moderate Symptoms	Serious Symptoms
crying	strong with normal tone or content and not crying	whimpering or sobbing	weak, moaning or high-pitched cry
when patted or held	content or stops crying	cries off and on	cries continually or hardly responds
waking and sleeping	if awake, then stays awake; if stimulated when asleep, awakens quickly	awakens slowly when roused, or awakens only with prolonged stimulation	falls to sleep on and off during play, or will not rouse from deep sleep
skin color	pink body, palms, soles of feet, mouth	pale or blue hands and feet	overall: pale, blue, ashen, gray or mottled
hydration: moisture in skin, eyes, mouth	skin normal, eyes and mouth moist	skin and eyes normal; mouth slightly dry	skin doughy and inelastic, eyes and mouth dry
response to hugs, kisses, warm talk	smiles; if younger than two months, takes notice	brief smile; if younger than two months, is briefly alert	no smile; face anxious or expressionless; if younger than two months, takes no notice

Taking a Young Child's Temperature

To monitor a child's temperature, a reliable thermometer is a necessity. In recent years several new types have become available. Heat-sensitive strips, when pressed to the forehead, indicate fever through a color change or numerical reading. Digital-display thermometers are also easy to read, and some have a heat sensor covered by a throwaway plastic sheath that can be changed after each use.

But despite these conveniences, most physicians still recommend the mercury-filled glass thermometer. This old stand-by is less expensive, more reliable and more precise than newer models — accurate to within .1° F. of the true temperature. There are two distinct kinds of glass thermometers *(below),* and every household should have one of each. You should use the oral type for taking a temperature by mouth and the rectal variety for use in the child's rectum.

For an oral reading, the thermometer is placed under the child's tongue for three to four minutes; the lips must be closed and the youngster cautioned against biting down on the glass. Since these instructions may be difficult to follow for children under the age of five, the rectal method or the underarm method is suggested for infants and young children.

A rectal reading, the most accurate temperature measurement, is usually 1° F. higher than an oral measurement. While taking a rectal temperature *(below),* be prepared to remove the thermometer to prevent breakage if the child moves suddenly. Never leave the child alone with a thermometer in place.

If symptoms such as a stuffy nose or diarrhea preclude taking an oral or rectal temperature, or if the child will not cooperate with these methods, a third alternative is the axillary, or underarm, method. Place an oral or rectal thermometer in the youngster's armpit, hold the arm snugly to his side, and keep it in place for at least five minutes. This external reading is not as true as one taken orally or rectally, however, and it generally falls about 1° F. below that of an oral measurement.

To factor in normal daily fluctuations, you should take the child's temperature at the same time each day. When the youngster has taken anything hot or cold by mouth, wait at least 15 minutes before taking an oral temperature. Wait 20 minutes after a bath to take a rectal reading.

Following each use, wash the thermometer with soap and cool water, and wipe it with rubbing alcohol.

Before using a thermometer, make sure its column of mercury is registering less than 95° F. To force the mercury below that level, grasp the top of the stem firmly between your thumb and index finger, and then shake the thermometer vigorously with quick downward snaps of the wrist.

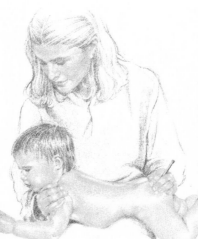

To take a rectal temperature, first coat the bulb of the thermometer with a lubricant such as petroleum jelly. Lay an infant on his stomach across your lap; place a toddler on his side with knees bent. Steady the child with one hand, then gently insert the thermometer's tip no more than one inch into the rectum. Holding the thermometer between your index and middle fingers, press the child's buttocks together with your hand to prevent slippage. After three minutes, remove the thermometer and wipe it clean. To read the temperature, rotate the thermometer slowly in a good light until you see the silvery strip of mercury appear beneath the numbers; record the number where the column of mercury ends.

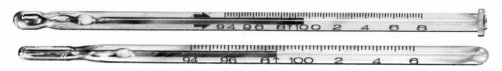

The two types of glass thermometers are recognizable by their design: The rectal thermometer has a short, round bulb at the working end to facilitate entry into the rectum; the oral thermometer has a long, slim tip to afford more heat-sensing contact in the mouth. Both types enclose a thin column of mercury, which expands along the length of the tube when heated. In a pinch, a rectal thermometer can be used orally; it must be left in the mouth for at least three minutes to achieve accuracy. An oral thermometer, however, because of its more pointed tip, should not be used in a child's rectum.

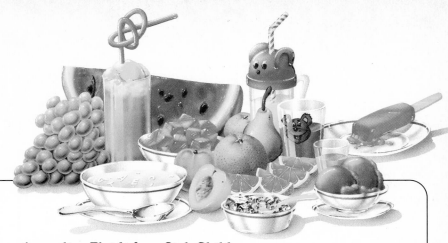

98.6° F. measured orally — is only an average, and to judge when your child is feverish, it first helps to know her usual range. These levels vary from child to child and by age. Temperature also fluctuates a few degrees over a 24-hour period, with its lowest point at about 4 a.m. and its highest at about 6 p.m.

A number of factors other than disease or body rhythms — such as the air temperature, the type or amount of clothing worn, warm food or drink, vigorous activity or even anxiety — may temporarily elevate temperature. A child overdressed for the weather or hard at play could easily raise her temperature to 100° F.

Children also tend to have more rapid temperature fluctuations than adults do. Whereas an adult will probably know he has a fever by the achy feelings that accompany it, a child can develop a fever so quickly and with so few outward signs that parents may not detect it right away. However, your child may very well exhibit the usual signs: She may experience chills or shivering (a clue the temperature is rising), appear flushed (a sign a fever has peaked), feel hot to your touch, seem unusually irritable or complain of an aching, tired feeling.

If any of these symptoms appear, you should take your child's temperature, using the method appropriate to her age or other conditions *(left)*. It is particularly important to watch the temperature of infants under the age of four months. A fever may be the only observable symptom of illness that a young baby exhibits, so any rise in temperature warrants an immediate call to the doctor.

Most doctors have their own guidelines as to what temperature in what situation warrants a call from a child's parent. If you do not know your pediatrician's fever guidelines, here are some widely approved ones. In addition to calling anytime a child under four months has a fever, notify the doctor if:

Appealing Fluids for a Sick Child

To prevent dehydration, offer a feverish child a drink every half hour while he is awake. Water, fruit juices, flat sodas, weak tea, soup and gelatin desserts are all good fluid sources. Here are suggestions for presenting liquids in appealing ways:
- Pour the drink into a favorite mug or cup and add a straw.
- Give the child crushed ice.

- Make ice pops with gelatin water or fruit juice.
- Offer slices of orange, watermelon and other juicy fruits.
- Let a recently weaned child drink from a bottle. He can return to using a cup when he recovers.
- Give clear, low-salt broths with alphabet noodles mixed in.
- Offer water-based fruit ices.

- a child between four months and 12 months old has a rectal temperature of 101° F. or greater.
- a one- to two-year-old has a rectal temperature of 103° F. or more.
- any child has a rectal temperature over 104° F. (103° F. taken orally).
- a child has a fever that lasts for 24 hours without any other symptoms.
- a child has a fever that lasts more than three days, even if other symptoms of the causative illness are present.

A temperature of 100° F. measured orally, or 101° F. rectally, is considered by many physicians to be a low, illness-induced fever. But for a child, behavior and appearance, not the temperature level, are the best measures of the severity of the illness *(box, page 91)*. Children may run a low-grade fever and be very ill, or run an extremely high one — 105° F. to 106° F. — with even a minor ailment.

While a fever of 105° F. or 106° F. can pose danger for adults, this level is not always critical for children under eight. Most childhood illnesses will not cause a fever to exceed 106° F., though a more serious disease such as meningitis can send temperature as high as 107° F.

Parents often worry that even moderately high temperatures of 103 or 104° F. will cause brain damage or other permanent effects. Actually, such results are extremely rare: Each individual has a fever threshold — a point beyond which the body's thermostat usually prevents temperatures from climbing — and fevers seldom cross it. In some young children, however, there is a chance that a fever may induce a convulsion, or febrile seizure. Sometimes the reason seems to be not the level of the temperature, but the speed at which it rises. In fact, most seizures occur at the very start of a fever, before the child has shown any outward signs of elevated temperature.

A febrile seizure *(page 106)* occurs when the brain, overstimulated by the fever, begins transmitting irregular signals that cause involuntary muscle responses. The child's body may stiffen, his limbs may beat rhythmically, his eyes may roll and he may lose control of bowels and bladder. As frightening as it may appear, a seizure usually lasts only a few minutes and rarely causes any damage. Research shows that fewer than half the children who experience a febrile seizure will have a recurrence; fewer than half of those will have a third seizure.

Techniques for Bringing a Fever Down

Although fever is part of the body's defenses against infection, it can make the sick child feel very uncomfortable and it can produce some effects that may require countermeasures.

One of the most potentially serious of these effects is dehydration. The heat generated by a fever causes the body to dissipate fluids more rapidly than normal, and it is important to replace them. If vomiting or diarrhea is also present, the danger of dehydration greatly increases. You should make sure that your youngster consumes plenty of liquids; offer small quantities at frequent intervals throughout the day.

Encourage drinking only clear fluids, as the stomach of a feverish child cannot absorb milk easily and he is likely to vomit it up. For a child who is nauseated or has been vomiting, give carbonated soft drinks that have been allowed to go flat. Your child will also burn calories at a higher rate and should be persuaded to eat, if possible. Taking food, however, is not nearly as vital at this time as drinking fluids.

During a fever, excess body heat may be given off in a number of ways — through dilation of the surface blood vessels, sweating or rapid breathing. To help this heat escape, you should avoid overdressing your child or covering him with blankets, even if he feels chilled; bundling him up will only force his body to retain heat and might even result in heatstroke, which can be fatal. Dress the youngster in a T-shirt and a diaper or underwear, or in thin cotton clothing, and cover him with a light sheet. Keep the child's room at a cool, even temperature, about 70° F.

Although most mild fevers can be allowed to run their course, your doctor may recommend medication to bring the fever down if it climbs over 102° F. or persists for more than two days, if the child is suffering from headaches or body aches and is unable to sleep, or if there is a history of febrile seizures.

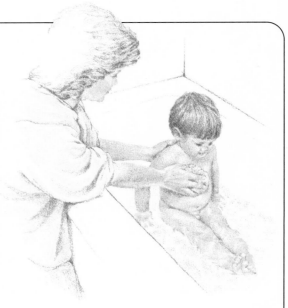

To bring down a fever by sponging, seat a small child in a tub filled with two to three inches of lukewarm water; lay an infant on a towel placed over a waterproof sheet. Wet a sponge or washcloth and rub the child's body briskly, especially over the face, neck, stomach and insides of elbows and knees, where blood vessels are concentrated. Continue for 20 minutes, adding more warm water if the child starts to shiver. Then pat the child dry with a towel and dress him lightly.

The two most commonly used fever-reducing drugs, known as antipyretics, are aspirin and the aspirin substitute acetaminophen. The two are equally effective in reducing fever by lowering the body's thermostat. But increasingly, physicians are recommending acetaminophen over aspirin, because the latter has been linked with Reye syndrome — a rare disease that strikes children who are recovering from viral infections, particularly chicken pox and influenza, especially those who took aspirin during the illness. Reye syndrome *(page 105)* can cause major damage to the liver and the brain, and in some cases the disease proves fatal.

Acetaminophen is free of this danger, and it has several additional advantages. It is less irritating to the stomach than aspirin, and it comes in a liquid form, which is easier to measure precisely and administer to babies and young children. Before giving your child any medication, however, you should check with your pediatrician for guidelines on which product to use and the correct dosage to give.

Occasionally, when a temperature reaches 104° F. or higher, antipyretic drugs are not enough to bring the fever down. Sponging the child with tepid water may be necessary as well *(above)*. Rubbing the skin briskly with a very wet sponge or washcloth brings blood to the surface, and heat is carried away as the water evaporates from the skin. You should not use cold water to bring a fever down: The cold will cause the blood vessels to constrict and make the child shiver, driving the youngster's temperature up even more. And do not use rubbing alcohol for sponging the child; the fumes are dangerous to children if inhaled.

Treating the child's fever will help lower the temperature and make her feel better temporarily, but it may not return the temperature to normal. Remember that aspirin or acetaminophen and sponge baths will not cure the underlying cause of the fever; therefore, it is important to observe your youngster closely for other indications of illness and contact your physician when appropriate *(box, page 91).*

Genetic Disorders

Just as parents' genes can make a child grow up to be short, or give her curly or straight hair, so they may also transmit to a child a medical disorder. There are more than 3,000 diseases that are known to be hereditary, but fortunately, all of them are rare, and most are treatable to at least some extent.

A child's basic physical characteristics are fixed at the moment of conception, when the egg and sperm, each carrying genetic material, combine to form the embryonic beginning of a new individual. Hundreds of thousands of genes — bits of chemical information — are embedded in microscopic, threadlike structures called chromosomes. Each gene carries a piece of information that is essential in the development of the body. At conception, a gene from one parent is usually paired with a gene from the other parent that applies to the same trait.

If one gene in a pair overrides the other in its effect on the child's development, it is called a dominant gene. Its less assertive partner is a recessive gene. The gene for brown eyes is dominant; the gene for blue eyes is recessive. Thus, blue eyes show up in a child when both parents transmit the recessive genes for the trait. If one parent were to hand on a brown-eyed gene instead, it would dominate and the child would have brown eyes.

An adult with a disorder resulting from a dominant gene has at least a one in two chance of passing the disease on to any offspring, since at least one of the two relevant genes that the adult inherited carried the code for the disorder. But many genetic disorders crop up unexpectedly, the result of two faulty recessive genes, one bestowed by each of the two healthy, symptomless parents. Every time parents who carry these hidden traits conceive a child, they run a one in four risk of producing an afflicted offspring. Finally, a genetic disorder can arise spontaneously, from an error during cell division — either during the development of the egg or the sperm, or when the two combine at conception.

While many genetic disorders cannot be diagnosed until a child is born, some can now be detected beforehand. Blood tests can alert parents if they are carriers of some particular traits. And a procedure called amniocentesis can give specific genetic information about an unborn child, including the existence of some disorders. In this process, a hollow needle is inserted into the pregnant woman's abdomen to withdraw from her womb a sample of amniotic fluid containing fetal cells, which are then analyzed.

Cystic fibrosis

Cystic fibrosis, the most common fatal hereditary disease, is passed on through recessive genes and affects the cells that produce mucus and sweat. These faulty cells in the digestive and respiratory tracts then excrete a thick, gummy mucus rather than a clear, free-flowing fluid. The viscous mucus accumulates in the mucous and sweat glands, leading to swelling, cysts and finally plugged ducts in the lungs, pancreas and intestines. The most common symptom is chronic coughing, as the child's lungs attempt to expel the thick mucus. The result is chronic lung infections such as pneumonia — a frequent cause of death among children with cystic fibrosis. They also suffer from runny noses, wheezing and difficulty in breathing. Most of these symptoms show up during infancy.

Other children with cystic fibrosis produce bulky, foul-smelling stools and gain weight slowly; the disease interferes with the flow of their digestive enzymes, preventing the children from extracting sufficient nourishment from what they eat. The first clue to what is wrong, however, may come from a kiss: The sweat of cystic fibrosis children tastes excessively salty.

Although there is no cure, and prenatal diagnosis is not yet generally available, the disease can be treated. The sick child is fed digestive enzymes and kept on a well-balanced, high-calorie diet. Antibiotics are used to battle the recurrent bacterial infections, while a regimen of chest pounding shakes loose the sticky mucus in the lungs. All this is done to make the lungs and digestive system work as normally as possible. If treated early and continuously, a child with cystic fibrosis can expect to live to young adulthood.

Down syndrome

Down syndrome, formerly known as mongolism, causes mental retardation in most who have the disorder, although five to 10 percent have I.Q.s in the normal range. An extra chromosome is usually the culprit. Normal individuals have 46 chromosomes in every cell. Most Down syndrome children have 47, because of an error that occurs during cell division, either in the development of the egg or the sperm or at conception.

There are distinct physical characteristics associated with the disease, including slanted eyes, a protruding tongue and a tendency toward obesity. Down syndrome children often have trouble learning to speak. They may suffer from chronic respiratory infections, and 30 to 40 percent have heart defects. However, the average life expectancy of a Down syndrome child is 50 to 55 years, and with early intervention programs and supportive families, many grow up to hold jobs and lead semi-independent lives.

A woman over forty is more likely than a younger one to give birth to a Down syndrome child. The chromosomal defect can be diagnosed by amniocentesis as early as the 18th week of pregnancy (*see introduction to this section*).

Hemophilia

Hemophilia is a rare genetic disorder characterized by slow-clotting blood, which can lead to excessive bleeding from superficial wounds. With treatment, a child with hemophilia can expect to lead an almost normal life. Most hemophiliacs are male, because the disorder is sex-linked and usually passes from mothers — who may not know they carry the gene — to their sons. Their daughters will not have the disease, but there is a 50 percent chance that they will be carriers.

Parents and doctors often first suspect hemophilia when a minor cut continues to bleed long after it should have stopped or when a large bruise develops following a shot. Or the problem may become evident when a newborn male is circumcised. Hemophiliacs always face the danger of internal bleeding, sometimes undetected, that can cause damage as blood seeps into and around the joints.

But hemophilia can be controlled. Since it is caused by an abnormality in one of the several blood factors responsible for the formation of clots, treatment focuses on providing the deficient factor. The clotting agent comes in a plasma concentrate that can be kept in a home freezer and injected by a parent when the child begins to bleed. Severe blood loss can be made up by transfusions.

Blood tests usually can identify women carrying the trait, so they can decide whether to bear children. Amniocentesis can foretell the sex of an unborn child *(see introduction to this section)*.

Muscular dystrophy

Muscular dystrophy is actually a group of diseases that cause the body's muscles to weaken and waste away. The most common form of this rare but deadly disorder is the sex-linked Duchenne muscular dystrophy, which affects boys. Thus healthy women with brothers or maternal uncles who have had the disease should consider genetic counseling before having children.

The disease will become evident by a boy's third birthday. His gait and movements become awkward, because among the first muscles to weaken are those of the buttocks and abdomen. He has trouble standing up properly and waddles when he walks. He falls frequently and finds it difficult to run or climb stairs.

There is no cure for the disease and profound muscle atrophy eventually sets in. The child usually does not live past the age of 20, because of respiratory or cardiac failure. Treatment focuses on keeping the child mobile and the joints limber for as long as possible.

Phenylketonuria

The ravaging effects of the metabolic disorder called phenylketonuria, or PKU, are now routinely overcome. Left untreated, PKU — which is conveyed by recessive genes — causes mental retardation, but a test of blood drawn by simply pricking the newborn's heel will tell your doctor if your child is affected or carries a gene for the disorder.

Children with PKU are not able to break down an essential amino acid called phenylalanine. When they are fed breast or cow's milk — both rich in phenylalanine — their bodies cannot process it properly. The accumulation in the body of too much phenylalanine leads to brain damage. If the blood test — done routinely in most hospitals in the U.S. — shows that the child has PKU, milk is eliminated from the baby's diet and a special formula is used instead. As the child grows, fruits, vegetables and certain cereals are substituted for foods with a high phenylalanine content. Most PKU children are taken off the special diet around age six and can eat normally thereafter.

Sickle cell anemia

Sickle cell anemia, a recessive-gene blood disorder that primarily affects blacks, causes recurrent bouts of excruciating pain and makes its victims susceptible to deadly blood infections. Most die in early childhood; a few live into young adulthood.

A defect in the hemoglobin — the molecule in red blood cells that carries oxygen to the body's muscles and organs — changes the normally round, flexible cells into misshapen crescent, or sickle-like, forms. Rather than nourishing the body's tissues, the sickle-shaped red cells get stuck in small blood vessels and block them. This prevents oxygen from reaching tissues and organs, resulting in a damaging and painful episode known as a sickle cell crisis. Among the first symptoms, usually appearing between the ages of six months and two years, are pain and swelling in the fingers and toes. Affected children are likely to be chronically tired and may have difficulty breathing.

Treatment involves alleviating the crises through pain killers, trying to prevent damage to major organs and combating infections. While there is no cure, carriers of the trait can be identified through a blood test and should consider genetic counseling before having children.

Tay-Sachs

This lethal disorder, found most often among Jews of Eastern European descent, destroys the nervous system by depositing abnormally large amounts of fat in the brain cells. An affected baby seems normal at birth and for the first few months. By six months, however, physical development halts and the child begins to regress. The baby soon goes blind. Further deterioration follows: deafness, retardation, seizures, paralysis. Children born with Tay-Sachs disease usually die before their fourth birthday. While there is no effective treatment, adults who are carriers can be identified by blood tests, and prenatal diagnosis of the disorder is possible. All adults of Jewish descent who are considering becoming parents should be tested. ❖

Infection

Simply by having your child immunized, you can help protect her against many common childhood diseases *(pages 58-62)*; but short of raising a child in an isolated and absolutely sterile environment, there is little you can do to prevent occasional infectious illnesses. Colds, intestinal upsets, earaches and many other ailments are a normal part of growing up, as your child's body struggles to adapt to a world teeming with minute, unseen, infective agents.

These include bacteria, one-celled microscopic organisms that exist virtually everywhere. Others are viruses, tinier and simpler agents made up of chemical components and not even considered a form of life by many scientists. Then there are fungi, which, like bacteria, are living things, and rickettsiae, microbes that fall midway between most bacteria and viruses in size and complexity.

Among these germs — as all microbes that cause disease are called — are some of earth's simplest life forms. Yet given a chance, they can wreak havoc inside the body. And they are easily spread from one person to another. Germs can be coughed, sneezed or breathed into the air to be inhaled by another person, or they can be transmitted directly by a handshake or a kiss. Germs can also enter the body through a cut or a scrape, or as the result of an animal or insect bite.

Once they are established in the body, germs undergo an incubation period, during which they multiply to disease-producing strength. This incubation period can vary from mere days to several months or longer; then the body signals its distress by displaying a variety of symptoms, which are the result of both the tissue damage caused by the invading microbes and the body's response to the invaders. Fever, inflammation and swollen glands are often the first noticeable signs that the body has mobilized its immune system to fight off an infection.

But not everybody reacts to infection in the same way. In some people, an attack by a particular germ may produce no symptoms at all, even though an analysis of germ-fighting antibodies in the blood of those persons would reveal that they currently have or recently had a mild case of the disease. Such symptom-free infections indicate that an invasion of germs was successfully and quietly thwarted by the body's immune system.

It is important to remember, however, that even though a certain strain of bacteria or virus may not produce symptoms in some people, those persons remain carriers of the disease and can easily pass it on to more susceptible hosts. Likewise, people who are immune to some particular diseases — through either vaccination or previous exposure to the illnesses — can still carry the causative bacteria or viruses and transmit them to others.

Faced, then, by what amounts to a constant onslaught of microbes, how is it that you and your child almost always manage to overcome the threat posed by these invaders and remain in good health?

The answer is in your body, which is protected by an imposing battery of natural defenses. The skin, for example, forms a tough outer barrier — one that most microbes find impenetrable unless a cut or other injury opens a path to the more vulnerable underlying tissues. The eyes, another avenue of microbial invasion, are continually bathed in fluid containing an enzyme called lysozyme that can kill bacteria. Stomach acid is equally destructive to many kinds of microorganisms, protecting the gastrointestinal tract from microbes in swallowed food. The defenses in the respiratory tract, where most infections begin, are especially formidable. They include secretions that kill invaders and a cough mechanism that violently heaves them back into the air.

Inevitably, some microbes do manage to evade the body's defenses or, in the case of an injury, pour in through an open wound. To destroy them, the body employs a sophisticated immune system that, triggered by the presence of invading microorganisms, launches a counterattack. Often, the body's opening salvo is signaled by the dilation of small blood vessels that bring an increased flow of blood to the site of the invasion. The result is the redness and swelling that are associated with a wound, or the sore throat and congestion of an upper respiratory infection. Signals sent out by a part of the brain called the hypothalamus raise the body's temperature, causing the familiar fever that is believed to inhibit the growth of germs and enhance production of germ-fighting antibodies.

At the same time, the lymphatic system and the bone marrow are stimulated to manufacture more white blood cells, the body's scavengers, which are then dispatched to the site to hunt down, engulf and destroy any microbes they encounter. In addition, other specialized cells in the blood and lymphatic system swing into action, producing antibodies that are custom-made to react to the specific kind of attacking microorganism or its chemical by-products. These antibodies coat the cell walls of bacteria and other microbes to make it even easier for white blood cells to identify and destroy the intruders. The same coating action disarms viruses by preventing them from locking onto the surface of body cells — a necessary step for a virus, which can reproduce only by taking over living cells.

The dead or neutralized microorganisms and the white blood cells are then swept along in the blood and lymph fluid, broken down by the liver and spleen, and eventually filtered out of the system by the kidneys. The contest continues round the clock until the body has at last rid itself of the invaders. And after victory, the body carries a helpful memento of the battle: One type of white blood cell can remember each germ it has encountered and stands ready for years afterward to mobilize antibodies in the event of future attacks by the same microbes, thus ensuring immunity to those germs. The concept of immunity is the basis for vaccination, a technique that uses dead or weakened germs to trick the immune system into producing antibodies against a particular disease.

Since the number of types of antibodies for which the body carries patterns reflects the number of illnesses a person has been exposed to, it would seem that a baby would have few or no antibodies in her system and thus be highly susceptible to attack by any microorganism. But in fact, a baby is born with a supply of antibodies donated by her mother. These give the child temporary immunity to those illnesses to which the mother herself has been exposed, until the infant's own immune system starts to develop. Breast-feeding can prolong this immunity for some illnesses, since breast milk — and especially the colostrum, or first milk — is rich in both antibodies and antibody-producing cells. Later, as this natural immunity wears off, your youngster will have to be vaccinated in order to stave off attack by many of the contagious diseases of childhood.

In general, however, younger children do suffer more illnesses than teenagers or adults. The average two-year-old, for example, will come down with at least eight respiratory infections during the year. Children in day-care centers may experience even more bouts of illness because they are being exposed to more germs. Children attending day-care centers, for example, suffer an average of 30 percent more cases of diarrhea than youngsters kept at home. The number of infections declines as the child grows older and the immune system grows stronger, since every bout with a new infection adds to a child's arsenal of antibodies, making her

more resistant to future exposures. And adequate rest, exercise and a proper diet will help keep the body's defenses in good shape, ensuring that your youngster is as resistant to disease as possible.

Any infection serious enough to cause a fever, rash or other inflammation should be brought to your doctor's attention. Sometimes the doctor can make a diagnosis after a brief physical examination. At other times, a germ culture test will be needed to identify the infective agent. In this procedure, a laboratory cultivates and examines microbes taken by means of a throat swab or stool sample.

The treatment, of course, will depend on the kind of invader. With proper care and medication, a child should recover quickly from most infections. Only rarely do serious complications develop.

AIDS
Acquired immune deficiency syndrome — AIDS — is caused by a virus that attacks the immune system itself, destroying one type of white blood cell that normally defends the body against infection. Thus it makes the victim helpless prey for other diseases and generally leads to death within 12 to 18 months

Tips for Preventing the Spread of Infection

- Have all family members use their own washcloths and towels.
- See that all wash their hands thoroughly and frequently: before meals and at bedtime, before preparing food, before handling the baby, after dealing with soiled items or tending to someone who is ill, and after every trip to the toilet. Wash with soap and warm water, lather the wrists and the backs of the hands as well as the palms, and dry with a clean towel. Clean often beneath the fingernails, preferably with a brush.
- Use disposable cups in the bathroom or at least have an individual cup for each member of the household. Get new toothbrushes often, certainly for anyone who has just recovered from an infectious illness.
- Use paper tissues instead of handkerchiefs. Teach your children to cover their mouths and noses with tissues when they cough or sneeze and to promptly dispose of their used tissues in paper or plastic bags.
- If you have a toddler or crawling baby, try to keep the floor scrupulously clean, being especially quick to wipe up bits of food or a pet's urine or feces.
- Keep a pet's food and water dishes away from the child, and make

sure she does not stroke an animal and then put her hands in her mouth. If she is playing outside, watch for animal feces.
- If someone in the family has a communicable disease or other infection, keep his toilet articles, including his soap, separate.
- Use disposable dishes for the patient or wash his dishes immediately after use, rinsing them in near-boiling water and then drying them in a rack.
- If you have a cut, avoid its contact with a patient's infected area or with any of his soiled clothing or bedclothes.
- If your child attends a day-care center, choose one that is staffed by sanitation-conscious people who quickly clean up any spills or toileting accidents, and who wash their hands and the children's hands often, especially after diaper changes. Studies show that the spread of viral disease in day-care centers is 10 times greater in states that permit diapered children to be enrolled than in states where centers are forbidden to accept children in diapers. For this reason, you may want to arrange for at-home or family-based day care until your youngster can attend a day-care center that accepts only toilet-trained children.

after full-blown symptoms develop. In the mid-1980s, researchers identified the virus and began working to develop a vaccine for this fast-spreading but still rare ailment, for which no cure is known.

AIDS is believed to be transmitted only by the passage of bodily fluids from a carrier to a host. Of the fewer than 250 U.S. children under the age of 13 who were diagnosed as AIDS victims by the beginning of 1986, some 70 percent caught the disease from their mothers, either in the uterus or during delivery. In about half of those instances the mothers were intravenous drug abusers who probably acquired AIDS from shared hypodermic needles. Another 20 percent of the afflicted children were believed to have received the virus in blood transfusions or blood products, such as those used in treating children with hemophilia. Comprehensive tests to screen out blood donors who might carry the AIDS virus are likely to reduce or eliminate the chances of getting AIDS in this way.

For parents, the chief worry is likely to be whether their children might catch the disease from an AIDS-carrying child at school. The issue of whether AIDS victims should be allowed to attend school has been widely debated; different states and local jurisdictions may handle the issue in various ways. Researchers have maintained that transmission of the virus in the course of normal contact is virtually impossible.

Among other conditions and illnesses that commonly hit children with AIDS early in the course of the disease — and therefore among the indications that the AIDS virus might be present in a child — are failure to thrive; enlarged lymph nodes, liver and spleen; chronic diarrhea; and bacterial bloodstream infection.

Bacterial infections
Most bacteria are harmless. Billions of these microorganisms live on your skin and inside your body without causing any trouble. Some, including those that inhabit the intestines, are actually beneficial, breaking food down into necessary nutrients and manufacturing such essential chemicals as vitamin K. A small proportion of bacteria are pathogenic, or disease-producing, however, and it is those strains that are responsible for the familiar staphylococcal and streptococcal infections, as well as for such serious illnesses as whooping cough, diphtheria, tetanus and tuberculosis.

A bacterial infection can be localized in one area of the body, or it can be generalized — spread throughout the body. In some cases, the bacteria themselves cause the damage by disrupting the regular functions of normal body cells. In other bacterial infections, the bacteria release potent toxins that do the dirty work. Such poisonous bacterial waste products are responsible for the devastating effects of diphtheria, cholera and tetanus. Many bacteria-killing antibiotics, the first of which was penicillin, have been developed to combat infections.

Follow the doctor's instructions regarding a prescribed antibiotic to the letter, giving your child the specified dosage for the specified length of time. DO NOT stop giving the medicine after a few days just because your child seems better. The infection may not yet be completely eradicated. Without continued doses of the antibiotic, it could erupt again, perhaps in a form that has grown resistant to the prescribed medication. In contrast, doubling the dosage or giving the medication more often than directed, in a vain attempt to speed recovery, may result in dangerous side effects.

Occasionally, a child may suffer an allergic reaction to an antibiotic — hives, perhaps, or a fever or joint swelling. A common offender is penicillin: Some 10 percent of adults in the United States are allergic to it. If a drug reaction occurs, you should contact your doctor. The chance of such a reaction increases with the frequency with which a drug is taken.

Blood poisoning
Septicemia, a dangerous complication commonly known as blood poisoning, occurs when bacteria from a rampant infection spill into the bloodstream, multiply and spread throughout the body. Septicemia can cause high fever, chills, irritability, rash, delirium and, in more serious cases, shock. A child in shock will have a fast but very weak pulse, breathe very slowly, become sweaty and clammy, and might lose consciousness or even fall into a coma. The infection may further spread to attack other parts of the body — such as the membranes covering the brain and spinal cord, where it causes meningitis. Blood poisoning is a true medical emergency and you should contact your doctor at once if you suspect it.

Fungal infections
Most of the childhood diseases that are caused by the microorganisms known as fungi are spread by contact, being picked up from another person or from a surface or water that was in contact with a fungus carrier. Different species of fungi cause such diseases as ringworm and the yeast infections that can affect throat or vaginal tissues. (Ironically, one of the most useful weapons in the war against infection — the antibiotic penicillin — is produced by a type of fungus.) Some fungal infections can be treated with powders and ointments available without prescriptions. It is best, however, to check with your doctor about appropriate treatment.

Rickettsial infections
Rickettsiae are like viruses in that they must parasitize living cells in order to reproduce. But unlike viruses and bacteria, most rickettsiae cannot survive in the atmosphere or in water while waiting to

prey on a susceptible host. Instead, they are carried by such pests as lice and ticks and are transmitted through their bites. Inside the human body, rickettsiae attack the small blood vessels, producing widespread inflammation that often results in a characteristic rash and is accompanied by fever. In more serious cases, rickettsiae can damage the central nervous system and lead to death. A tickborne rickettsia is the cause of Rocky Mountain spotted fever, while lice carry the rickettsiae responsible for typhus, a disease that has ravaged mankind again and again down through the ages. Today, prompt treatment with antibiotics usually brings about a swift recovery from these diseases and others caused by rickettsiae.

Umbilical infection

Newborns can develop an infection of the severed umbilical cord's stump if it is not kept clean and dry. Contact your doctor if you notice that your baby's navel area is red or warm, or if there is any foul-smelling discharge from the stump. The problem is usually easily eliminated with antibiotics. Note that when the stump falls off, you may see a drop or two of blood. This in itself does not indicate an infection and is nothing to worry about.

Symptoms:
- unusual skin heat or redness in the child's navel area
- foul-smelling discharge

What to do:
- Keep the stump clean and dry.
- Wipe the navel twice a day with cotton swabs and alcohol.
- Fold diapers down in front to keep the navel area dry.
- If an umbilical infection is diagnosed, follow your doctor's instructions regarding treatment.

Call the doctor if:
- the navel area appears to be infected.
- the child's umbilical stump becomes inflamed or oozes a discharge.

Viral infections

Viruses are even smaller than bacteria and more difficult to combat. They cause such common childhood diseases as mumps, measles, chicken pox, roseola and German measles. In addition, more than 100 different viruses have been identified as causes of the common cold.

In contrast to bacteria, which damage the body by direct action or by releasing toxins, viruses are parasitic. They are the hijackers of the cell world and must actually take over and use living body cells in order to reproduce and cause disease. A virus attacks by attaching itself to the surface of a normal body cell and then seizing control of the cell's reproductive mechanisms. Some viruses are ingested by the targeted cell as that cell takes in food. Other viruses actually inject their own genetic material into a cell while clinging to the cell's wall. In either case, once inside, the virus alters the host cell's genetic code, reprogramming it to produce new virus particles. Often, the host cell then disintegrates, releasing thousands of newly created viruses into surrounding tissue, where they are free to attack other body cells. Some viruses — including herpes simplex, the germ that causes cold sores — go into hiding in the body for long periods, only to flare up again and again during periods of stress.

Unfortunately, antibiotics, which work so effectively against bacterial infections, are virtually useless against most viral infections. Many viral diseases, however, can now be prevented by immunization *(page 58)*. In some instances, the doctor will give the child an injection of gamma globulin — a blood serum protein especially rich in antibodies. For some viral infections, including infectious hepatitis, injections of gamma globulin can prevent the development of symptoms or make them less severe. In other cases, often all the physician can do is treat your youngster's symptoms and wait for her body's own immune system to knock out the intruders unaided.

Wound infections

When your child cuts or scrapes himself, his body reacts immediately by mobilizing the immune system to fight off any bacterial invaders and by pouring in protein to rebuild damaged skin and tissue. With first aid — and a parent's usual diligence in keeping the wound clean — healing is rapid, and in a few days to a week the skin should be as good as new.

Occasionally, however, bacteria do manage to establish an infection beachhead, causing the body to produce a fever and pus and swelling in the affected area as the immune system fights the invaders. In such cases, the child should see his doctor. Left untreated, the infection could spread to the bloodstream *(see Blood poisoning, page 99)*

Symptoms:
- pain or swelling around a cut or scraped area of skin
- oozing or discharge of pus
- fever
- red streaks around the wound
- swollen lymph glands

What to do:
- Wash a fresh wound with soap and water and apply an antiseptic or an antibiotic cream. Clean the wound daily thereafter.
- Change bandages frequently or leave the wound open to the air.
- Encourage your youngster to leave the scab alone.
- If a wound becomes infected, keep the child in bed with the affected area elevated above the level of the heart.
- Apply gauze dressing and keep it wet with warm (not hot) water until you can reach the doctor.

Call the doctor if:
- symptoms of infection appear.
- the infection persists after the prescribed treatment is over. ❖

Nervous System

Your child's ability to walk, talk, think and learn — indeed, to perform any physical or mental activity — is made possible by an intricate communications network known as the nervous system. The system consists of billions of nerve cells, or neurons, held together and protected by supporting cells called neuroglia, or glia. Masses of neurons and glia form the tissues of the central nervous system — the brain and spinal cord — and the peripheral nerves, which wend their way through all parts of the body, relaying messages to and from the brain.

Each nerve cell has a single nucleus and two types of branching fibers, called axons and dendrites, that work like a pair of "in" and "out" doors. Axons take messages away from the cell; dendrites bring messages to the cell. During the early months of life, however, this communications network is still in an incomplete state, which explains most of a young baby's motor and mental limitations.

While a child is born with a full complement of nerve cells, those in the brain are not fully developed at first. Many of the brain's dendrites have yet to sprout, and myelin, a chemical coating on the axons that speeds messages along, is also missing. Without these parts, the brain cannot transmit many messages. A baby, for example, will not be able to stand until her brain has enough dendrites and myelin to tell her legs to stand. Nor can this process be hurried in any way. Thus, trying to teach your child to walk before her nervous system is sufficiently developed will only lead to frustration and failure.

Although the process of sprouting dendrites and adding myelin continues until adolescence, the brain's greatest growth occurs during the first two years of life. By a child's first birthday, his brain will have gained about 75 percent of its adult weight. Good nutrition plays a key role in this growth. Too little protein in the diet, for example, can slow down the addition of dendrites and myelin, leading to permanent brain damage.

Most damage to the nervous system, however, occurs before birth. About 3 percent of all children are born with a nervous-system disorder. Common causes include poor prenatal nutrition, malformations of the brain and exposure through the mother to rubella, herpes and other infections that can impair developing nerve cells.

Although damage to the nervous sys-

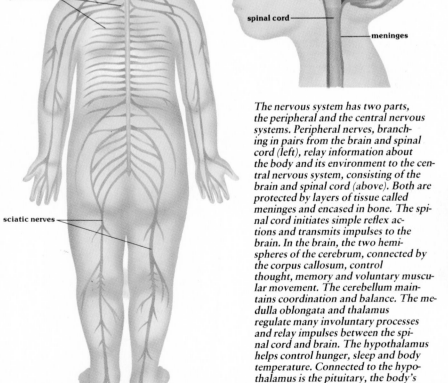

The nervous system has two parts, the peripheral and the central nervous systems. Peripheral nerves, branching in pairs from the brain and spinal cord (left), relay information about the body and its environment to the central nervous system, consisting of the brain and spinal cord (above). Both are protected by layers of tissue called meninges and encased in bone. The spinal cord initiates simple reflex actions and transmits impulses to the brain. In the brain, the two hemispheres of the cerebrum, connected by the corpus callosum, control thought, memory and voluntary muscular movement. The cerebellum maintains coordination and balance. The medulla oblongata and thalamus regulate many involuntary processes and relay impulses between the spinal cord and brain. The hypothalamus helps control hunger, sleep and body temperature. Connected to the hypothalamus is the pituitary, the body's master gland, which controls growth and many overall functions.

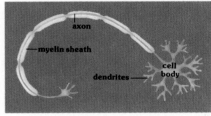

The work of the nervous system is done by nerve cells called neurons. Sensory signals travel from the dendrites, through the cell body and along the axon. From the end of the axon the signal jumps to an adjacent neuron and continues on. Axons are coated with myelin, a chemical that speeds the transmission.

tem is frequently permanent, many children can be helped to live more normal lives by early diagnosis and treatment. Children born with a nervous-system disorder often exhibit symptoms from birth, such as difficulty sucking or unusually limp or stiff muscles *(box, page 105)*. The major developmental milestones — for example, sitting alone by six months, crawling by nine months and walking by 12 months — may also be delayed. You should be alert for these symptoms in your child and bring them to a doctor's attention immediately.

Brain tumor

A brain tumor is an abnormal growth on the brain. It can be either cancerous or noncancerous. While rare, brain tumors are the most common type of tumor in children. The cause of brain tumors is unknown, although some are believed to result from nerve cells that fail to develop and instead grow into tumors.

Headaches, especially upon rising in the morning or at other times when the head changes position, are a common symptom of a brain tumor. Other symptoms range from nausea, vomiting and blurred vision to weakness on one side of the body, loss of coordination and a change in personality.

An infant with a brain tumor may have an abnormally large head, occurring when the tumor disrupts the normal circulation of cerebrospinal fluid out of the brain, causing hydrocephalus, or water on the brain. In infants up to a year old, whose skull sections have not yet fused, the fluid accumulation pushes apart the bones, enlarging the child's head.

Even noncancerous brain tumors can be life-threatening, because they compress and damage brain tissue as they grow inside the skull. Noncancerous tumors can often be removed by surgery. Cancerous ones are usually treated with both surgery and radiation therapy.

Cerebral palsy

Among illnesses that burden children with permanent handicaps, cerebral palsy is one of the chief offenders. It is caused by damage to the parts of the brain that control movement and balance. The damage usually occurs before, during or shortly after birth. Premature babies are at a particularly high risk for cerebral palsy because blood vessels in the central nervous system mature only within the last few weeks of pregnancy.

Although doctors once believed that the most common cause of cerebral palsy was a cutoff of oxygen to the baby's brain during delivery, they now think that the damage more often occurs before birth. The most probable cause is exposure of the developing fetus to a viral infection such as rubella or cytomegalovirus, or to certain parasites, especially those found in animal feces. After birth, a stroke or an injury to the head can cause brain damage resulting in cerebral palsy.

The muscles of a child with cerebral palsy may be either excessively stiff or excessively floppy, depending on which part of the brain has been damaged. The severity of the condition varies from child to child and often affects only part of the body. Some children have no additional physical or mental problems; but if areas of the brain other than those associated with motor development have been damaged, a child may develop seizures, learning disabilities, mental retardation or partial loss of sight, hearing or speech.

Symptoms of cerebral palsy are sometimes not apparent right after birth and may change as the child grows and develops. The tensing and stiffening of muscles, for example, may not begin until a child is several months old.

Although there is no cure for cerebral palsy, early diagnosis and treatment can prevent muscle deformities and help a child learn how to move more naturally. Treatment usually consists of physical therapy. Surgery is sometimes required to prevent or correct muscle deformities.

Symptoms:
- difficulty in sucking and swallowing
- prolonged drooling
- persistent arching of the back
- poor head control after three months
- unusually early preference — before 12 months of age — for using either the right or left hand
- limited movement of an arm or leg on one side of the body
- unusual manner of crawling, such as scooting along on the back
- persistent walking on toes
- tendency to fall easily
- delayed achievements of motor milestones *(box, page 105)*

What to do:
- If cerebral palsy is diagnosed, follow your physician's advice on treatment. Family counseling may also help parents adjust to raising a child with this lifelong condition.

Call the doctor if:
- your child shows any symptoms of impaired motor development.

Chorea

Chorea, a rare nervous-system disorder caused by an inflammation of blood vessels in the brain, is characterized by an involuntary jerking and twitching of the body. Among the several forms of chorea, Sydenham's chorea — also known as St. Vitus' dance — is the type most common among children. It may occur in a child who has been ill with rheumatic fever, an inflammatory disorder of the joints that occurs as a complication of strep throat. In addition to muscular twitching, the symptoms of chorea include clumsiness, slurred speech and a general loss of coordination. Although these symptoms may persist for weeks or months, most children recover completely from Sydenham's chorea with no permanent physical or mental damage.

Treatment usually includes bed rest as well as medication that stops the twitching and helps keep the youngster more comfortable.

Encephalitis

Encephalitis is an inflammation of the brain, a very serious condition that requires immediate medical attention. The cause of the inflammation is often unknown, although in many cases it is the result of a viral infection that has entered the body via the bite of a virus-carrying insect. In rare cases, encephalitis occurs as a complication of a viral disease such as herpes, measles, chicken pox, influenza, mumps or infectious mononucleosis.

Often, several days or weeks pass between the initial infection and the development of symptoms. The illness sometimes begins with a few days of flulike complaints — chills, fever, headache and sore throat — which soon develop into more serious symptoms of protracted vomiting, bizarre behavior, disordered thinking and extreme sleepiness. The most characteristic symptom is a stiff neck, which occurs when the back of the brain and the lining of the spinal cord become inflamed. The child may suffer intense pain when turning her head from side to side or bending her neck forward.

Since encephalitis is a life-threatening illness, the patient must be hospitalized as quickly as possible. The most serious cases can cause death within two to four days; in its less virulent forms, encephalitis usually runs its course in one to two weeks. Although the illness has no cure, careful monitoring can reduce the chance of permanent damage to the central nervous system and to other vital organs, such as the lungs and heart.

Symptoms:
- chills, fever, headache, sore throat
- stiff neck
- protracted vomiting
- extreme sleepiness
- disordered thinking or hallucinations
- bizarre behavior and movements
- loss of bowel and bladder control
- convulsions

What to do:
- Seek immediate medical help if your child shows a combination of any of the above symptoms.
- Give clear liquids in small quantities.
- DO NOT give any medication unless approved by a physician.
- DO NOT give the child any food unless told to by a doctor.

Call the doctor if:
- your child displays symptoms of encephalitis.

Epilepsy

Epilepsy is not a specific disease, but a term used to describe a person's tendency to suffer repeated, intermittent seizures *(see Seizure disorders, page 106).*

Headache

Headaches are a very common complaint among children and rarely indicate a serious medical condition. Most headaches in young children are caused by an infection such as influenza or strep throat, and they are often accompanied by fever, sore throat, chills and other symptoms of the infection. The headache usually goes away when the infection is treated. Dental and vision difficulties are other common causes of headaches in children. Be sure your child's teeth and eyes are checked regularly after the age of three.

Occasionally, stress, fatigue or tension can be the source of a child's headache. The dull, throbbing pain of a tension headache often starts in the muscles in the back of the neck and proceeds up to the forehead. A warm bath, acetaminophen and rest can provide relief. If such headaches recur frequently, your child may benefit from psychological counseling to deal with the source of the tension.

Migraine headaches, although rare in children under eight years of age, can also afflict very young children, particularly if the child's family has a history of these headaches. The intense, throbbing pain of a migraine, caused by the dilation of the arteries beneath the skull, usually comes on suddenly and is often confined to one side of the head. In young children, however, the pain may be diffuse. The child may vomit or complain of nausea and may ask to be left alone or to go to sleep. Although not considered dangerous to a child's health, a headache of this type should be reported to a physician for positive diagnosis and to rule out other, more serious illnesses.

In rare cases, a child's headache may be a symptom of a life-threatening medical condition, such as meningitis *(page 104)* or a brain tumor *(page 102).* Or the headache may indicate a serious injury after a fall or blow to the head. Always notify a physician when a child's headache is so severe that the child cries and clutches his head, or when it is accompanied by vomiting, mental confusion or excessive sleepiness. A headache that awakens a child from his sleep or that persists for more than three days also should be brought to a physician's attention.

Hyperactivity

Hyperactivity — sometimes called attention deficit disorder or minimal brain dysfunction — is a symptom rather than an illness. Often ascribed incorrectly to healthy children who happen to be exceptionally energetic, hyperactivity is characterized by excessive activity inappropriate to the age of the child. A hyperactive child is typically less attentive and more fidgety and impulsive than other children his age. He is easily distracted, has difficulty concentrating and darts from one activity to another. Some hyperactive children are also hostile and aggressive; many have learning disabilities. Four times more common in boys than in girls, hyperactivity usually subsides before a child reaches his midteens.

Doctors are not sure what causes hyperactivity, but it is probably a combination of several factors. Hyperactivity may be an inherited behavior, or it may be triggered by an emotionally stressful event in a child's life, such as divorce or death in the family (see Stress-related illness, page 107). Some doctors believe hyperactivity is the result of mild brain damage sustained before or shortly after birth, perhaps by exposure to an infection or toxic chemical or by the physical trauma of birth. Others, however, strongly disagree and believe no brain damage is involved. One of the more controversial theories attributes hyperactivity in children to food additives and salicylates, a form of salt found naturally in certain foods. However, studies have shown that only a small number of hyperactive children benefit from a change in diet.

Hyperactivity is usually not diagnosed until a child is in school and a teacher expresses concern about the child's inability to concentrate or follow directions in class. But parents can be alert to earlier signs of the disorder. Hyperactive children often have a history of having been demanding, especially active babies, with feeding and sleeping difficulties. Many were colicky as infants. As toddlers, they may have been particularly aggressive toward other children. Some physicians have observed that hyperactive children often reach developmental milestones, such as sitting up, standing or walking, at an earlier-than-average age.

Raising a hyperactive child can be an extremely difficult experience, and parents should seek professional help if they observe true hyperactive tendencies in a child. Treatment usually involves special behavioral modification techniques that teach the youngster how to focus his attention. Drugs — particularly stimulants, which, paradoxically, have a calming effect on hyperactive children — are also sometimes used in the treatment of the disorder. However, these medications can cause insomnia, loss of appetite, irritability and other side effects and are usually prescribed only to older children who are having difficulties in school.

Meningitis

Meningitis is an inflammation of the meninges, the delicate membranes that cover the brain and spinal cord. The infection usually spreads to the meninges through the bloodstream from an infection that has already started in the ears, sinuses, tonsils or upper respiratory tract.

This life-threatening illness, which requires immediate hospitalization, primarily affects young children: Some 90 percent of the infections occur in children under the age of six. Neonatal meningitis, a particularly virulent form of the illness that afflicts infants during the first month of life, is sometimes contracted before the baby leaves the hospital — either from someone who may unknowingly be a carrier of the illness or from contaminated equipment. The more common Hemophilus meningitis, named for the bacterium that causes it, accounts for 60 to 75 percent of meningitis cases in children between the ages of one month and five years. Other, rarer causes of meningitis in children include viruses, fungi and tumors.

Meningitis can be contagious, although not everyone who comes in contact with the infection will become ill with it. If you know your child has been exposed to meningitis, watch her closely for signs of the illness. The infection usually comes on suddenly after several days of a more common illness, such as an ear or respiratory infection. The initial symptoms are flulike — fever, headache, vomiting, fatigue and irritability — and may also include a stiff neck, an aversion to light and a red or purple rash. As the illness progresses, the youngster becomes lethargic and disoriented and eventually lapses into a coma. Without early medical intervention, brain damage and death can result.

If you suspect your child has meningitis, take her to a hospital immediately. Diagnostic tests probably will include a spinal tap — the sampling of the fluid in the spinal canal — to identify the specific cause of the illness. Treatment can range from simple bed rest for the less serious viral strain of meningitis to an aggressive therapy of antibiotics for bacterial meningitis. Severe cases of meningitis may require several weeks of hospital care and several years of follow-up examinations to watch for signs of neurological damage requiring further treatment and therapy. A vaccine is available for Hemophilus infections (see HIB disease, page 60).
Symptoms:
- chills, fever, headache and other flu-like symptoms
- vomiting
- aversion to light
- in infants, a bulge of the fontanel, the soft spot on the skull.
- stiff neck, shoulders or back
- red or purple rash
- lethargy and excessive sleepiness
- seizures or coma

What to do:
- Get immediate medical attention if meningitis is suspected.
- Give clear liquids in small quantities.
- DO NOT give any medication unless approved by a physician.
- DO NOT give any food by mouth.

Call the doctor if:
- your child displays any symptoms of meningitis.

Neuroblastoma

Neuroblastoma is a cancerous tumor that forms on nerve tissue. Although it is very rare, it is one of the most common types of cancers that afflict infants and chil-

Detecting a Disorder of the Nervous System

Symptoms of trouble in the central nervous system are often hard to distinguish from the normal movements and behavior of a healthy, active child.

Usually, it is a combination of some of the following symptoms, not a single one, that signifies a possible neurological problem.

Symptoms from birth to 12 months:
- unusually limp or stiff muscle tone
- unexplained irritability or crying
- tendency to startle easily
- difficulty sucking or swallowing
- unfocused staring

- twitching
- inability of eyes to follow a moving object after 3 months of age
- inability to respond to new sounds after 3 months of age

A delay in achieving key milestones of motor development may also signal a neurological disorder. Babies normally develop gross motor skills within the broad age ranges listed below.

Milestone	Age Range	Average Age
Smiling	2 weeks to 3 months	1 month
Rolling over	2 to 10 months	4 months
Sitting alone	5 to 9 months	6 months
Crawling	6 to 11 months	9 months
Creeping	7 to 13 months	10 months
Standing	8 to 16 months	11 months
Walking	8 to 18 months	12 months

Symptoms from 1 to 6 years:
- regression in motor abilities
- abnormal posture
- poor balance or coordination

- change in personality or alertness
- morning headaches
- seizures or staring spells

In toddlers and preschoolers, delayed language ability is another key indicator of a nervous-system disorder. A youngster usually masters language skills at the following pace:

Milestone	Age Range	Average Age
Speaks single words, understands "no."	12 to 18 months	12 months
Combines 2 to 3 words.	18 months to 3 years	2 years
Uses simple sentences.	3 to 4 years	3 years
Uses correct tenses, follows 3-step commands.	5 to 6 years	5 years

dren. The tumor may appear in the chest, neck or skull; but about 70 percent of them arise in the abdomen. The growth is usually small and thus often goes undetected until the cancer has spread to other parts of the body. Once it spreads, it is more difficult to treat. For this reason, parents should be alert to early signs of the illness. These include fever, diarrhea, vomiting, lethargy and loss of appetite. The child's skin may become pale, and small bumpy or bruiselike rashes may appear, especially around the eyes. The child may also complain of pain or tenderness in the abdomen or may have difficulty breathing.

Neuroblastoma is an extremely serious illness that can lead to spinal-cord damage and death if not diagnosed and treated early. Treatment usually consists of a combination of surgery, chemotherapy and radiation therapy.

Reye syndrome

Reye syndrome (also known as Reye's syndrome) is a rare but dangerous illness that causes inflammation of the brain and liver. It is most common in children between the ages of six months and 15 years; however, it has been known to strike younger babies and young adults as well. Reye syndrome usually occurs toward the end of a viral infection, particularly chicken pox or influenza. Typically, a child who develops Reye syndrome will appear to have partially or fully recovered from an infection, but then will suddenly begin vomiting persistently. She may show a personality change, becoming combative or excessively active. As the illness progresses, she will become disoriented, lethargic and sleepy. Her breathing may become fast and labored.

The cause of Reye syndrome is unknown, but children with a viral infection who take aspirin or other medication containing the salt called salicylate seem to be at greater risk. For this reason, doctors strongly advise against giving children aspirin during a viral infection, recommending acetaminophen instead.

Reye syndrome is a very grave illness that claims the lives of about one in five children who contract it. Of those who do recover, however, most suffer no permanent brain damage. If your youngster shows any symptoms of the illness, take her immediately to a hospital. Intensive care will be needed to relieve pressure on the brain and minimize damage to the central nervous system.

Symptoms:
- sudden, frequent vomiting following a bout of the chicken pox, flu, a cold or other ordinary viral infection
- hyperactive or combative behavior
- rapid breathing
- sleepiness, lethargy, disorientation, loss of coordination
- coma

What to do:
- Arrange for immediate hospitalization if your child shows any symptoms of the syndrome.
- Give clear liquids in small quantities.
- DO NOT give the child any food.

Call the doctor if:
- your child begins to vomit or complain of nausea, or otherwise takes a turn for the worse after seeming to recover from a viral infection.

Seizure disorders

Seizures, or convulsions — episodes of involuntary movement caused by a sudden electrical discharge of nerve cells in the brain — are among the most common neurological disorders seen in children. Some 4 to 8 percent of all children experience at least one seizure before adolescence. *(For advice on how to handle a child's seizure, see page 24.)*

The cause of many seizures in children is unknown. One of several exceptions is the febrile seizure, which is caused by a particularly high or fast-rising fever *(page 91).* Illnesses that irritate the brain and interfere with its blood supply — such as meningitis, encephalitis, nephritis and lead poisoning — sometimes cause seizures. Severe head injuries and complications during birth can also permanently scar the brain and lead to repeated convulsions. The tendency to suffer attacks repeatedly is called epilepsy.

There are several types of seizures. The most common — and most dramatic — is the grand mal convulsion, which in children is usually triggered by a fever. The child emits a startled cry, then falls unconscious to the floor. His eyes roll up into his head and a foam of unswallowed saliva may flow from his mouth. He may also lose control of the bladder and bowel. Within seconds, the child's body starts to shake rhythmically, often violently. The seizure typically lasts for two or three minutes. After the youngster regains consciousness, he may feel irritable and complain of a headache before falling into a deep slumber.

The petit mal seizure is a subtler convulsion, often mistaken for daydreaming. Typically, the child suddenly and unexpectedly stops talking or moving and stares ahead vacantly for a few seconds. He may drop what he is holding or even totter and fall. Petit mal seizures can occur as often as 20 to 40 times a day, yet go unnoticed or be passed off as inattentiveness. Most children outgrow these seizures, although medication may be needed to limit the number of episodes.

A psychomotor seizure, also called a temporal-lobe seizure, involves the part of the brain — the temporal lobe — where memories, feelings and perceptions of smells are stored. During the seizure, the child suddenly laughs, cries, runs around in circles or strikes out violently for no apparent reason. The seizure rarely lasts longer than a minute. Afterward, the youngster may appear to be confused or sleepy and will usually have no recollection of the episode. Psychomotor seizures often continue into adult life and require medication to keep them under control.

The Salaam, or jackknife, seizure afflicts babies and toddlers, typically between the ages of six and 12 months. During this type of seizure, all of the child's muscles contract at once, causing the head and knees to jerk together like a jackknife. The seizures, which last only two or three seconds, tend to occur in clusters — usually when the child is drowsy or has just awakened. These seizures are often associated with mental retardation or a serious neurological disease or disorder.

Less common forms of seizures in children include what are termed Jacksonian convulsions, characterized by a sudden and progressive jerking that initially affects one part of the body but may spread to other parts, and akinetic spells, which involve a sudden and complete — but very brief — loss of muscle tone and consciousness. Usually, a child recovers from an akinetic spell within a few seconds.

Although a seizure can be a frightening experience for parent and child alike, most do not harm the child's health. However, prolonged grand mal attacks — those lasting one hour or longer — can cause brain damage and result in mental retardation or cerebral palsy. Report all seizures promptly to your doctor. A seizure that is unrelated to a fever should be followed by medical tests to determine its cause. These tests may include an electroencephalogram to record electrical activity in the brain or a more sophisticated diagnostic procedure, such as a CAT scan, to detect abnormal structures in the brain.

Repeated episodes of seizures may require anticonvulsant medication, such as phenobarbital or phenytoin, which suppresses the abnormal electrical discharges in the brain.

Stress-related illness

Prolonged stress, whether emotional or physical, can lower a child's resistance to disease. When a child experiences stress, her brain sends impulses through the nervous system to all parts of the body. The heart, muscles and stomach tense, and the adrenal glands secrete hormones. These adrenal hormones weaken the body's fleet of lymphocytes — the white blood cells that create antibodies to fight viruses, bacteria and other harmful agents that invade the body.

Not all children who experience stress become ill, but research suggests that they are at greater risk than children who lead relatively stress-free lives: For example, studies have found that high-stressed children suffered three to four times as many illnesses and accidents as low-stressed children suffer. Colds, sore throats, neck and back pain, headaches and stomachaches have all been linked to stress. In some youngsters, epilepsy and asthma attacks are also believed to be exacerbated by stress.

A variety of situations can create stress in a young child — among them the death of a close family member and the separation or divorce of parents. Research also indicates that children from close, supportive families manage to cope better with whatever stress they do encounter. Effective stress-coping skills include talking openly with each other about problems and concerns, spending time together and reaching out to nonfamily members for emotional support and guidance during stressful times. Parents who as a rule reward their children for good behavior rather than punish them for bad behavior create a low-stress home environment.

Tic

The sudden, quick, repetitive movement of a select group of muscles is known as a tic. Symptoms of various tics include twitching, blinking, lip smacking, coughing, sniffing, throat clearing and shrugging. Vocal tics, such as grunts, barks or the repetition of phrases or words, may also occur, although these are rarer.

Up to 20 percent of all children develop transient tics at some time or other, but less than 1 percent have persistent or severe tics. Usually, the tic is mild and short-lasting and involves a facial movement, such as eye blinking. However, some tics — especially those that involve the head, trunk or limbs — may last for years and continue into adulthood.

While tics can be aggravated by illness, allergies and fatigue, they are most often associated with tension and stress. Once the source of the child's stress has been identified and dealt with, the tic usually goes away. Parents can help by making sure their child gets adequate rest, particularly during stressful times in his life. A child with a tic should also be reassured that the symptom is not his fault and that it will most likely go away with time.

Although few tics signal a serious neurological problem, a child who develops a tic should be examined by a physician to rule out such illnesses as chorea *(page 102)* and seizure disorders *(page 106)*. Because tics seldom last more than a few months, medicine is rarely prescribed to control them. The exception is in the case of Gilles de la Tourette syndrome, a rare and dramatic disorder characterized by multiple tics, compulsive barking and other utterances, and — in some cases — the shouting of obscene words. This malady, which may be inherited and occurs three times more often in boys than in girls, is sometimes treated with a prescribed tranquilizer. ❖

Reproductive System

The sexual organs of a child, whether male or female, are essentially complete at birth, though they will remain dormant until puberty. Some babies come into the world with genitals that appear overly large or mature — a temporary condition caused by the mother's hormones crossing the placenta during pregnancy. The hormone estrogen can stimulate a baby's reproductive organs, producing a whitish or blood-streaked vaginal discharge in girls and swollen, secreting breasts in infants of both sexes. These symptoms are common and no cause for concern or special care; they usually clear up within a few weeks.

Parents may also be surprised to see signs of sexual arousal in very young babies — penile erections in infant boys and vaginal lubrication in girl babies. This is a normal reaction to physical stimulation of the genitals, and it can also be caused by such physiological conditions as a full bladder or bowels.

As children grow older they discover quite innocently that touching or playing with their genitals brings pleasurable sensations, which then may prompt the youngsters to masturbate deliberately to produce these good feelings. Masturbation is normal at any age, and parents should not shame, frighten or punish children for playing with their genitals occasionally. Frequent or excessive masturbation, however, may be a sign that the child is experiencing emotional

problems, and the issue should be discussed with a physician.

Sexual abuse

Boys and girls of any age can be the victims of sexual abuse, which is defined as an adult's exploitation of a child for sexual gratification.

Physical sexual abuse occurs when a child is forced to play a passive or active role in a sexual act; it involves touching offenses that range from fondling to vaginal, oral or anal intercourse. In nonphysical sexual abuse, children may be exposed to exhibitionism, voyeurism, pornography or explicit language intended to shock or arouse a child. Many such forms of physical and nonphysical abuse are crimes punishable by law.

Studies have revealed that the majority of sexual abuse is inflicted by family members or acquaintances whom the child trusts. Because molesters typically intimidate a child into silence, detecting abuse may be difficult. Parents should be on the alert for such behavioral signals in their children as an avoidance of a particular person or place, social withdrawal, sudden self-consciousness about genitals, regression to babyish behavior, sleep disturbances or the acting out of sexual behavior with toys.

In some cases of sexual abuse there may be revealing physical signs as well: pain or irritation of the genitals or anus, a vaginal or penile discharge, vaginal

bleeding and frequent urinary tract or vaginal infections.

If you suspect sexual abuse for any reason, have your child examined by a doctor. Children seldom lie about harm of this sort, so if your child is able and willing to talk about such incidents, take her statements very seriously — and get in touch with the appropriate social agency.

To help prevent sexual abuse, discuss the subject frankly with your child. Tell her that if anyone touches her or talks to her in a way that makes her feel uncomfortable — if anyone touches the parts of her body that would be covered by a bathing suit, for instance — she should say "no" and tell you or another trusted adult right away.

Swollen scrotum

A swelling of the scrotum in male babies and young boys may be caused by infection, injury or a condition known as hydrocele. Hydrocele, which develops when fluid leaks into the scrotum from a small opening in the abdominal lining, is most common among newborns. The body will usually reabsorb the fluid slowly on its own by the child's first birthday, though your doctor may prefer to remove the excess fluid with a needle before that time.

A strong blow that bruises the genital area, such as a straddling injury suffered on a toy vehicle, will also produce swelling, which may be reduced with an ice

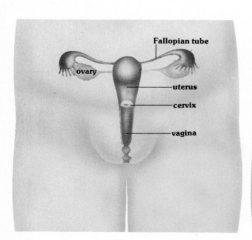

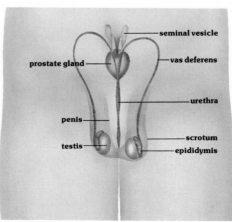

In the female reproductive system (far left), the ovaries produce eggs, or ova, and begin to release them at puberty. Ova travel through the Fallopian tubes to the uterus, where a fetus will develop during pregnancy. The cervix, at the base of the uterus, opens into the vagina, a muscular canal leading outside the body.

In the male (near left), the testes, encased in a sac called the scrotum, produce hormones and sperm at puberty. During ejaculation, sperm collected in the epididymis travel through tubes called vas deferens past the prostate gland, where they mix with fluid from the prostate and seminal vesicles before flowing down the urethra and out the tip of the penis.

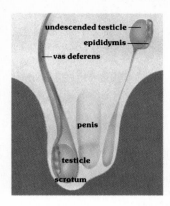

The testes form high in the abdomen of a male fetus and remain there until one to two months before birth. Then, along with the epididymis and vas deferens, the testes descend through a canal in the groin to take their place in the scrotum. The condition known as undescended testis — most frequently seen in premature infants — occurs when one or both testes fail to reach the scrotum.

pack. More serious causes of swelling in older children include a hernia *(page 68)*, an infection of the testicle or a rare condition called torsion of the testes, in which the testicular stem becomes twisted within the scrotal sac and cuts off the blood supply to the affected organ. All three problems demand the prompt attention of a doctor.

Undescended testis

A child whose scrotum appears lopsided, flattened or unusually small may have an undescended testis, the term for the failure of one or both of the testes to assume their proper position *(above, right)*. In most cases, an undescended testis will migrate normally into the scrotum before the boy's first birthday. If it has not done so by that time, however, discuss it with the doctor, who may advise treatment with hormones or surgery.

A condition often confused with an undescended testis is a retractile testis: The organ has descended normally to the scrotum, but from time to time it retreats to a position just inside the abdominal cavity. A retractile testis will descend again on its own and is no cause for alarm.

To tell a retractile testis from an undescended one, seat your youngster in a warm bath and have him draw his knees to his chest; this usually causes a retractile testis to descend.

Vaginal infections and inflammations

While an occasional clear vaginal secretion is normal throughout girlhood, a thicker, more profuse discharge may signal infection. Common sources of vaginal infection and inflammation are contamination from urine or feces, pinworms, irritation from bubble-bath chemicals that instigate an itch-scratch-infection cycle, or the presence of a foreign object such as sand or toilet paper in the vagina. Infection or inflammation may also develop when a child has been sexually abused.

If the child is taking antibiotics, a yeast growth is the likely cause of infection. Yeast, a fungus, can flourish when antibiotics kill the benign bacteria that normally keep it at bay. A mild vinegar sitz bath often brings relief: Fill a tub deep enough to immerse the child's bottom, add one cup of white vinegar and gently wash the youngster's outer genital surfaces; the

vinegar water will seep into the vagina. Redness and itching without discharge are more likely the result of a skin problem or infection of the outer tissues of the genitals only, and not a condition originating in the vagina.

Symptoms:
- in younger girls, rubbing and scratching; in older girls, complaining of itching and pain in the genital area
- reddish or swollen vulva (the external parts of the vagina)
- mild or profuse discharge, which is sometimes foul-smelling or cheesy-looking, and that may be yellowish, greenish or gray
- increased urge to urinate; pain during urination

What to do:
- For a hygienic problem, wash outer areas with mild soap and water.
- For a yeast infection, give a vinegar bath for 15 minutes twice a day.
- For a suspected object in the vagina, you should place your child in a kneeling posture with her chest down and inspect the vaginal opening with a flashlight. If an object is present but you cannot easily remove it, have the doctor remove it.
- Avoid bubble-bath solutions and tight-fitting synthetic garments, which impede ventilation.
- Teach your daughter the correct after-toilet wiping procedure — from front to back, so feces will not be wiped onto the vagina.

Call the doctor if:
- the discharge is thick and profuse.
- a mild discharge has not cleared up within five days.
- an object lodged in the vagina cannot be easily removed. ❖

The Decision to Circumcise an Infant Son

Parents of newborn boys are routinely offered the option of having the child circumcised — a surgical procedure to remove the flap of foreskin covering the head of the penis. The issue has become somewhat controversial in recent years: Though it was once believed that circumcision reduced the incidence of venereal disease and cancer, the American Academy of Pediatrics now officially maintains that routine circumcision has no proven medical benefits.

But for a variety of reasons, the practice is still widespread in the U.S. The brief and simple operation — usually performed by a doctor before mother and baby leave the hospital — consists of clamping the foreskin to restrict blood flow and then cutting off the tip of the flap with a scalpel.

Until the penis heals, wash it gently with mild soap and water, and coat it with petroleum jelly to prevent it from sticking to the diaper. Do not try to remove the thick, yellowish substance that appears in the first few days; it aids the healing process.

The foreskin of an uncircumcised infant cannot be pulled back, and you should not try to force it back to clean beneath it. But in most cases by the time the boy is one or two years old, you will be able to pull the foreskin back, wash the exposed glans of the penis with soap and water, then push the foreskin forward again. Teach your child to do this himself every time he bathes. If, after the boy is four or five years old, the foreskin is still too tight to be pulled back, discuss the condition with the child's doctor.

Skin

The skin is the largest organ of the human body, stretching over a total area of nearly two square meters and weighing up to 20 pounds, on average, by adulthood. Ranging in thickness from a mere half millimeter in the eyelids to five millimeters on the back between the shoulder blades, the skin protects the body from injury, bacterial infections and extremes in temperature. It also helps to regulate the body's own internal temperature and acts as a vast sensory receptor, receiving and transmitting a stream of sensations to the brain through millions of nerve endings embedded in the surface of the flesh.

Skin itself consists of three layers. The paper-thin outer layer, or epidermis, renews itself every four weeks through a continuous process of reproduction and shedding. New cells are manufactured at the base of the epidermis and gradually rise to the skin surface. As they do, they are transformed from living cells into a lifeless protein called keratin — the same substance that forms the building block of the skin's specialized structures, the nails and hair. These keratinized cells on the skin's surface are then imperceptibly shed in the course of everyday activities, by rubbing against clothing or bathing.

Beneath the epidermis is the dermis, or true skin. In this layer are blood vessels, nerve fibers, lymph channels and muscle tissue, as well as hair follicles, sweat glands and sebaceous, or oil, glands. Blood vessels and nerves also tunnel through the subcutaneous tissue, the bottommost layer of skin, which is responsible for the formation and storage of fat.

Like the other organs of the body, the skin is designed to withstand a lifetime of use. And like the other organs of the body, it undergoes numerous changes over the years. In fact, as your baby grows, she is likely to pass through many periods of peeling, spots and blotchiness — conditions that might be cause for alarm in the teenager or adult, but that are entirely normal for an infant. Moreover, few youngsters escape the occasional rash or skin infection on their way through childhood, although you can help prevent or relieve many minor skin conditions by keeping your child clean and by dressing her in loose-fitting clothing. If you are worried about a particular skin problem, by all means see your doctor. Probably, it is not serious and with proper care will clear up in a few days.

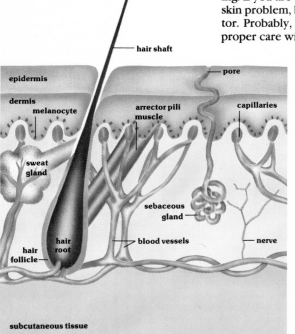

epidermis

dermis
melanocyte

sweat
gland

hair
follicle

hair
root

hair shaft

pore

arrector pili
muscle

capillaries

sebaceous
gland

blood vessels

nerve

subcutaneous tissue

A paper-thin sheath of cells called the epidermis forms the outermost of the skin's three layers. This layer contains melanocytes — cells that produce a dark pigment called melanin, which colors the skin and shields it from the sun's ultraviolet rays. The middle layer, the dermis, contains blood vessels and nerve fibers as well as sweat glands and hair follicles. A sebaceous gland, attached to each follicle, secretes an oily substance called sebum, which lubricates the hair shaft. Each follicle also has an arrector pili muscle that makes the hair stand on end. The third and deepest layer of skin is subcutaneous tissue, which produces and stores body fat.

Birthmarks

A birthmark is a discoloration or raised area on the skin. Nearly half of all babies are born with a birthmark, while many others develop one during the first few months of life. Some birthmarks may be unsightly, but most will disappear by the time a child reaches school age.

One common type of birthmark is a brown or black, raised or flat discoloration called a mole *(page 118)*. Another is a hemangioma — a network of dilated blood vessels beneath the skin. In some cases this may appear as nothing more than a faintly reddened area of skin; in others it forms a large, dense mass that rises from the skin surface. The most prevalent kind of hemangioma is known as a salmon patch, or stork bite; it looks like a cluster of small, red spots and appears most often on the back of a baby's neck or on the forehead, upper eyelid or bridge of his nose. No treatment is necessary for this, and the discoloration usually disappears by the age of one.

Another common hemangioma is the strawberry mark. This bright red, raised blemish looks very much like half a strawberry attached to the child's skin, usually to the face or neck. At birth, most strawberry marks are so small that they go unnoticed. Over the next few months, however, the birthmark grows rapidly — sometimes reaching four inches in width — before its growth finally slows and the strawberry begins to shrink. The most important thing to remember about strawberry marks is that no matter how large one might grow, virtually all of them disappear with no treatment, usually by the time the child is five. Large marks that do not fade may call for surgical intervention, but not until the youngster is at least six, to limit scarring.

A third and rarer kind of hemangioma is called a port-wine stain. This flat, irregularly shaped area on the face or elsewhere on the body may be pink, purple

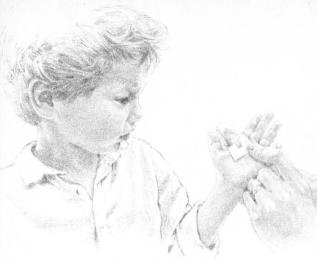

To protect an intact blister, arrange sterile gauze squares in a stack slightly taller than the blister. In the center of the stack, cut a hole just large enough to fit comfortably around the bubble, then lay the gauze over the area, positioning the blister within the opening. Cover the stack with several squares of uncut gauze and then tape the dressing in place.

or — in deeply pigmented infants — black in color. Unlike strawberry marks, port-wine stains are quite noticeable at birth and they generally persist into adulthood. Treatment is difficult, but laser therapy has proved useful for some patients who are in their teens or older. Excellent covering cosmetics are available and are the most dependable therapy.

Still another hemangioma is the Mongolian spot, a bluish, bruiselike discoloration of the lower back or buttocks, most prevalent among dark-complexioned children. Mongolian spots are harmless and usually disappear in one or two years.

While the majority of birthmarks will vanish if left alone, you should consult your doctor if you notice any oozing from the blemish or if the overlying or adjacent skin becomes red and inflamed. The skin covering a strawberry mark is especially fragile and, once broken, susceptible to infection. You may want to talk to your doctor about covering a strawberry mark to protect it if it is located in a place where it is likely to be bumped repeatedly. You should also contact your doctor if a birthmark seems to be growing at an abnormal rate or if you want to correct a port-wine stain.

Blisters

Blisters are fluid-filled bubbles on the surface of the skin — the result of an allergic reaction or of an injury to the skin caused by friction, burns or infection. These bubbles form a barrier against infection while the injured skin repairs itself and act as a cushion to protect the new skin growing beneath them. As the blister heals — usually in three to four days — the fluid inside is absorbed and the old skin overlying the blister either rejoins the underlying tissue or peels.

Ordinarily, no treatment is necessary for a blister. But to prevent the child from breaking the blister accidentally, you should cover it with a sterile dressing *(above)*. Never deliberately puncture a blister. Instead of speeding the healing process, that increases the risk of infection. If the blister should break, wash the area thoroughly with soap and water, then cover the wound with a bandage that has been treated with petroleum jelly to prevent the fabric from sticking. Notify your doctor if you notice any signs of infection, including increased pain, inflammation or redness.

Most children's blisters are caused by friction, especially friction resulting from ill-fitting shoes. But infants, too, develop blisters, and many nursing babies are likely to form sucking blisters along the middle part of their lips. These sometimes peel, but they require no treatment and will gradually disappear.

A similar skin problem, the blood blister, is not really a blister at all. The result of a pinch injury, it is actually a clot of blood trapped beneath the skin. It is nothing to be concerned about and will heal by itself in a short time.

Boils and carbuncles

A boil is a painful bacterial infection of a hair follicle or oil gland. The culprit is usually the staphylococcus germ, which infiltrates the follicle or gland and multiplies in its moist, damp environment. White blood cells then pour into the site to battle the bacteria, and gradually a walled-off pocket of pus accumulates — a mixture of white blood cells and destroyed bacteria and skin tissue. As the pressure in this pocket increases, the boil comes to a head, ruptures and drains. The pain subsides and the boil heals.

Cleanliness and daily changes of clothing will reduce the chances of your child's developing a boil. However, boils are very common and virtually everybody is afflicted at one time or another. Normally, a boil will burst and drain on its own in a few days to a week, and you can speed the process along by applying hot compresses to the site. If it does not burst, or if the boil is located on the child's face, where it is more likely to lead to a complicating infection, you should consult your doctor. The doctor will examine the child and, if necessary, lance and drain the infection. Any child who suffers repeatedly from boils should also be examined by a doctor, since recurrent boils can sometimes be an indication of lowered resistance due to an underlying disease, such as diabetes or anemia. A blood or urine test is often all that is needed to pinpoint the problem.

Much rarer and more serious than a boil is a carbuncle — a large abscess that is, essentially, a cluster of boils. A carbuncle has several heads and extends deeper into the skin than a boil. It may also be accompanied by fever and swollen lymph nodes. If you suspect your child is developing a carbuncle, you should contact your doctor immediately: Prompt medical attention is essential to prevent the spread of the infection.

Symptoms of a boil:
- red, painful lump beneath the skin
- increasing pain as pus is produced and the boil comes to a head

Symptoms of a carbuncle:
- a larger and deeper abscess than a boil, with several heads
- pain
- fever

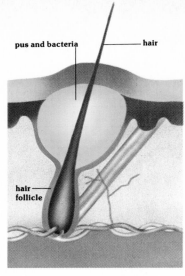

pus and bacteria — hair

hair —
follicle

A boil develops when bacteria infect a hair follicle (above). White blood cells surround and kill the bacteria, forming pus, which builds up to bring the boil to a head. The boil's eventual rupture drains the pus onto the skin's surface and relieves the pain.

- inflammation
- swollen lymph nodes

What to do:
- Apply hot, moist compresses for 10 to 15 minutes every few hours to encourage drainage and relieve pain. Soak the cloth every few minutes to keep it hot, being careful to avoid scalding the child.
- Keep the affected area clean by washing with soap and water. Disinfective soaps are useful in reducing the amount of bacteria on the skin.
- Once the boil ruptures, clean off the pus and continue to apply compresses, then cover with a sterile dressing.
- Discard all used compresses and bandages to prevent the spread of infection to other family members.
- DO NOT squeeze or puncture a boil or carbuncle, since the infection may then be spread beneath the skin or even into the bloodstream.

Call the doctor if:
- a boil is located on the child's face.
- your child develops a fever or red streaks branch out from the boil.
- the boil does not drain within a week.
- you suspect that your child is suffering from a carbuncle.

Canker sore

A canker sore is a small, painful ulcer in the lining of the mouth, covered with a gray membrane and surrounded by a bright red halo. The sores may occur singly or in groups, and once contracted, they are likely to recur.

A canker sore should not be confused with a cold sore, or fever blister, which is an infection caused by a virus *(see next entry)*. In contrast, the cause of canker sores is unknown, although dietary deficiencies, allergic reactions and hypersensitivity to some foods may all play a role. Stress, too, seems to be a predisposing factor in the development of canker sores and in their recurrence.

Canker sores are not serious, nor are they contagious. However, in some cases the sores may interfere with your child's eating and speaking, and it is probably best to avoid any foods that cause increased irritation. There is no effective cure for canker sores, but most cases heal on their own within one to two weeks.

Symptoms:
- small, shallow ulcers in the mouth, covered with a gray membrane and rimmed by a bright red halo
- pain

What to do:
- Have your child rinse his mouth with salt water (one-half teaspoon of salt to eight ounces of water) three times a day after meals.
- Avoid hot or cold foods if they increase pain, and any other foods that seem to aggravate the condition.
- Encourage your child to drink plenty of liquids to prevent dehydration.

Call the doctor if:
- the child needs a prescription to reduce pain or if the condition does not improve after two weeks.

Cold sore

A cold sore is a small, painful blister or cluster of blisters that develops on or around the lips or inside the mouth as the result of a viral infection. As the infection progresses, these blisters rupture, form shallow ulcers and then encrust.

Cold sores are caused by the herpes simplex type I virus, a relative of the germ responsible for chicken pox. This is not, however, the same strain that causes genital herpes in adults.

Cold sores are a very common and contagious condition; researchers estimate that 70 percent of the U.S. population has been exposed to the virus by the age of 14. The virus is spread by close bodily contact and can affect mucous membranes or broken skin anywhere on the body. A child's initial attack, which lasts one to three weeks, can be severe — with fever and swollen lymph nodes — although in most children a first attack will produce symptoms so mild that they go unnoticed, or no symptoms at all. In either case, once the attack passes, the virus retreats into nearby nerve cells and remains there in a dormant state until it is reactivated by exposure to sunlight or wind or by emotional stress, a cold or a fever. Recurrent episodes of the disease are usually milder and generally clear up within 10 days. Complications rarely ensue, but the virus can spread to other tissues, including the eyes.

There is no known cure for herpes simplex, although a new antiviral compound called acyclovir has proved effective in limiting the spread of the virus. The medicine is generally not recommended for children, however. For youngsters, treatment usually consists of relieving local discomfort while waiting for the condition to heal by itself.

Symptoms of first attack:
- in noticeable cases, fluid-filled blisters on or around the lips or inside the mouth that dry in a few days to form yellowish crusts
- fever
- pain
- in more severe cases, swollen lymph glands, difficulty in eating

Symptoms of recurrent attacks:
- tingling or burning feeling before the blisters appear, usually on lips only
- fever

What to do:
- To prevent the spread of the infection, tell your child not to put her fin-

gers in her eyes, on her genitals or on a cut after touching her mouth.

- Make certain your youngster gets enough liquids. Give her soft foods, ice pops and cold drinks to soothe her mouth; older children can use a straw to bypass the sores.
- Use acetaminophen to reduce fever and relieve pain.
- Apply cool compresses to any crusts that form, to help loosen them.

Call the doctor if:

- the infection does not improve within one to two weeks.
- your child complains of pain in the eyes or shows signs that the infection has spread to other parts of the body.
- the sores are so painful the child does not eat or drink.

Cradle cap

Cradle cap is the common term for seborrheic dermatitis, a temporary scaliness that can appear on a child's scalp. Though most prevalent among newborns, it can also affect toddlers and even older children. The condition begins as thin, dry scales, which turn into yellow, greasy, scaly patches. It is often aggravated by inadequate cleaning of a baby's scalp by a parent who is hesitant to scrub the area over the fontanel, the soft spot on top of the infant's head. Remember that the fontanel, while softer than the surrounding bone, is still covered by a tough membrane and will not be harmed by a good cleansing of the scalp.

Cradle cap usually does not bother or harm the baby, though in rare cases the condition may become infected, signaled by a yellowish discharge oozing from the scaly patches. If this occurs, see your doctor, who will recommend an appropriate treatment. But in nearly every case, simple daily washing with soap and water will help to relieve the condition.

Symptoms:

- thin, dry scales on the scalp that en-

crust to form yellow, greasy patches

What to do:

- Wash the baby's scalp daily with soap or baby shampoo and water.
- For heavier build-ups, use a soft baby-toothbrush moistened with baby oil to loosen the scales, or rub baby oil into the scalp and cover with a warm towel for 15 minutes. Uncover, then comb the scales loose and rinse.
- Follow directions for a prescribed shampoo or ointment.

Call the doctor if:

- you notice a yellowish fluid oozing from the scales.
- the condition persists despite several weeks of home treatment.

Diaper rash

Since nearly all babies wear diapers, nearly all babies will eventually suffer from diaper rash. Even with the best of care, a rash is inevitable; a baby's naturally sensitive skin is simply no match for the irritation posed by a wet diaper. Nor are babies who wear disposable diapers immune to diaper rash: In most cases moisture is the villain, and a wet diaper is a wet diaper, no matter what kind of material it is made of.

The most common type of diaper rash appears as patches of red, rough skin, sometimes dotted with small red pimples, in the diaper area. Sometimes the skin is raw and moist. In boys, the rash may also spread to the foreskin. The cause is primarily the build-up of ammonia, which is produced when bacteria from bowel movements break down a substance in urine. Traces of laundry detergent in cloth diapers that have not been thoroughly rinsed can also irritate the baby's skin.

Left untreated, a diaper rash may become complicated by a secondary yeast or bacterial infection. A yeast infection will appear as bright red spots, which may join to form a single large, inflamed

area bordered by red spots. Pus-filled pimples may indicate an infection of staphylococcus bacteria, especially if the eruptions are accompanied by fever. A very red, scaly rash appearing behind the ears, under the arms or in the folds of the skin, as well as in the diaper area, could be caused by seborrhea, an inflammatory scaling disease. Any one of these complications or secondary infections should be brought to your doctor's attention.

Fortunately, simple diaper rash is easily treated at home and normally does not require a doctor's care. Treatment is aimed at relieving the current condition and preventing future occurrences. Ideally, the baby suffering from diaper rash should be allowed to go without diapers as much as possible, since exposure to the air is the fastest, surest cure. Otherwise, diapers should be changed frequently and the baby's bottom kept dry. A stubborn rash that fails to respond to home treatment should be brought to your doctor's attention. To prevent future outbreaks, you can apply a zinc-based ointment or petroleum jelly, which forms a barrier against moisture, or use baby powder or cornstarch to keep the baby's skin dry. Be sure to wash and rinse all cloth diapers thoroughly.

Symptoms:

- red, rough skin in the diaper area, sometimes accompanied by small red pimples or raw, moist patches

What to do to prevent diaper rash:

- Change diapers often, whether you use cloth or disposable diapers. Keep use of plastic pants to a minimum.
- Thoroughly wash cloth diapers, avoiding the use of fabric softeners or other harsh chemicals, and rinse in plain water to remove all traces of detergent. Running them through a second rinse is also advantageous. To help kill bacteria, add one-half cup of vinegar to the rinse water or dry the diapers in the sun, or both.

- Use diaper liners to keep moisture away from baby's skin.
- Apply a zinc-based ointment or petroleum jelly to protect your baby's skin from wetness, or use baby powder or cornstarch. Be sure to put the powder or cornstarch in your hand first, before applying to the baby's bottom, to avoid having the infant inhale a cloud of dust particles.

What to do to treat diaper rash:

- If at all possible, allow the baby to go diaper-free to expose the rash to the drying effects of the air *(below).*
- Change diapers more frequently and discontinue the use of plastic pants until the rash has cleared up.
- Gently wash the affected area with water when you change the baby. Do not use soap, which may cause further irritation. Dry his bottom thoroughly (or allow him to air-dry) and lightly sprinkle the area with baby powder or cornstarch. It is best not to use creams or lotions once a rash has developed, since these only seal off the area from air.
- For a secondary infection complicating a case of diaper rash, follow the antibiotic treatment that your pediatrician recommends.

Call the doctor if:

- you notice any signs of infection, including blisters, pus-filled pimples, increased inflammation or fever.
- the diaper rash does not clear up within three to four days.

One method of treating diaper rash is to remove diapers altogether for a few hours each day in order to expose the rash to the air. Keep the room warm and let the baby play or sleep on a towel-covered waterproof sheet.

Eczema

Infantile eczema, or atopic dermatitis, is an itchy, scaling skin condition that is most frequently found in children with a family history of either eczema, hay fever or asthma. Eczema is not contagious, and although its exact cause is unknown, it is believed to be a manifestation of hyperreactivity or sensitivity of the skin. Occasionally an attack can be traced to exposure to a certain fiber or food — especially one that you may have recently introduced to your child.

Whatever the cause, eczema prevents a child's skin from retaining adequate levels of moisture. The resulting dry skin triggers a vicious itch-scratch-itch cycle that aggravates the condition and invites secondary infection. The itching is so intense that even small babies try to relieve it by rubbing against the bedclothes or crib. Sweating caused by excessive heat or synthetic fabrics worsens the itching, as do rough fabrics, such as wool.

In children, eczema usually makes its first appearance by the age of three months, starting almost always as red, weeping eruptions on the child's cheeks. The rest of the face and the arms, legs and neck may also become inflamed. Sometimes the disorder will disappear after a few months, but more often it comes and goes over the next few months or years, spreading to the hands and forearms and to the bends of the elbows and knees. In persistent cases, the affected skin becomes thickened and leathery. Happily,

most children tend to outgrow the disorder by puberty.

Successful treatment of eczema depends on breaking the itch-scratch-itch cycle and preventing future flare-ups. A doctor's care is essential, and you should contact your pediatrician if you suspect that your child may be suffering from eczema. Home treatment is aimed at relieving the itching by keeping the skin moist and lubricated and at helping your child to cope emotionally with the disorder. In addition, your doctor may prescribe one or more topical preparations or oral antihistamines to reduce itching and, when necessary, antibiotics to control any secondary infection. Even though a specific substance cannot be proved to cause your child's eczema, an incidental food allergy can cause a very red, itchy flare-up of the affected skin. If you can pinpoint the offending substance, it is best to remove it from the child's diet.

Symptoms:

- in infants — red, weeping patches on the cheeks, followed by inflamed arms, legs and neck
- in children older than two to three years — red, weeping patches in the bends of the elbows and knees, on the wrists, forearms and neck
- sometimes, spread of patches to other areas of the skin
- itching
- swelling, blistering, oozing and crusting of patches
- very dry skin
- in long-term cases of the condition, thickened, leathery skin

What to do:

- If eczema is diagnosed, administer prescribed medication according to your doctor's instructions.
- Bathe your youngster no more than three times a week, using a superfatted soap. Add baby oil or vegetable oil to the bath water after the child has soaked for 20 minutes, to lubricate his

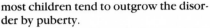

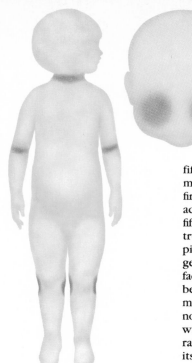

When an infant develops eczema, the characteristic red, scaly skin is likely to appear first on the baby's cheeks (near left). In older children, the condition usually affects the skin on the neck, inside the elbows and behind the knees (far left). The rash often appears on the forearms, hands and skin behind the ears in later episodes.

dry skin. After bathing, blot the skin dry with a towel.

- Keep skin moist by using oil-and-water lotions or creams after bathing.
- Keep the child's nails trimmed short to discourage scratching.
- Avoid wool and rough synthetic fibers when choosing clothes for the eczematous child. And dress him in light, cotton clothing at night and during hot weather.
- Because of possibly serious complications that can result from infection by the herpes simplex virus, eczematous children should not be exposed to anyone with weeping cold sores.

Call the doctor if:
- you suspect eczema.
- the condition changes suddenly.
- a secondary infection develops, signaled by fever or inflammation.
- you or your child is having difficulty coping emotionally with the disorder.

Fifth disease

Rubella, measles, scarlet fever and a rare, mild form of scarlet fever called Filatov-Dukes disease are four of the five most common contagious rashes that affect children. The fifth is called erythema infectiosum or, as it is more widely known,

fifth disease. The only symptom of this mild viral infection is a rash that erupts first on a child's face, giving him the characteristic "slapped cheek" appearance of fifth disease. The rash will spread to the trunk and limbs before at last fading into a pink, lacelike pattern. This rash may linger for up to a month, while seemingly fading and intensifying from hour to hour before it gradually disappears. No treatment is necessary and there is absolutely no need to limit the activities of the child with fifth disease, especially since the rash can persist for weeks and the illness itself is so mild. You should, however, contact your doctor if the rash is accompanied by a fever, which might indicate the presence of a more serious illness than fifth disease.

Hair loss

Although hair loss is not usually associated with childhood, it does happen for various reasons and can be a matter of great concern to parents. In rare cases, children lose hair as the result of a serious illness or emotional stress that interferes with the normal growth cycles of hair. Once the underlying disorder is treated, the hair will grow back naturally. Hair loss can also be caused by diseases that affect the scalp — such as ringworm *(page 121)* — or strike the hair follicles themselves. Such conditions require a doctor's attention.

Often, however, in the absence of a rash or other symptoms, the cause of a child's hair loss is obvious: The youngster is nervously pulling or plucking at her hair, causing individual hair fibers to break off or come out altogether. Tight barrettes or ponytails can have the same effect. The treatment in such cases is just as obvious: The parent should encourage the child to leave her hair alone, or loosen the barrettes or ponytail. A small baby may lose hair from the back of his head from rubbing against the sheet while

sleeping on his back. Putting the baby to sleep on his stomach most of the time will prevent the rubbing and allow the hair to regrow.

Another cause of temporary hair loss — when the scalp and hair are otherwise healthy — is alopecia areata. This disorder, the cause of which is unknown, is characterized by the loss of hair in round or oval patches. Although there is no appropriate treatment, alopecia areata is normally a self-limiting disease and almost always the child's hair grows back completely within 12 months. Patience seems to be the most effective cure for this baffling disorder.

Heat rash

Heat rash, sometimes called prickly heat, is a very common skin condition characterized by tiny red pimples that erupt in skin folds and on the neck, chest and diaper area in babies. It occurs when the pores that carry sweat out of the body become obstructed — usually by two skin surfaces rubbing together or by clothing. The trapped sweat causes the inflammation and rash. The condition is ordinarily triggered by excessively hot, humid weather, but it can also be caused by a high fever or by overdressing an infant or child. Infants who are too warmly dressed have been known to develop a heat rash even during the winter.

Heat rash is not harmful, and the best way to deal with it is to avoid it in the first place by keeping your child cool and dry. Make sure that your baby is not overdressed for the weather and choose light cotton clothing rather than synthetics. If your child does develop a heat rash, the treatment for it consists of cooling the youngster's skin in order to encourage the obstructed pores to open.

Symptoms:
- dry, bright red rash — usually appearing in skin folds or on the cheeks, neck, chest or diaper area — of tiny

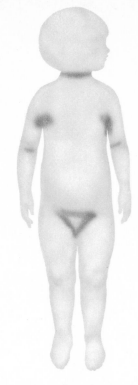

Heat rash appears when sweat is trapped under the skin's surface. This may occur wherever skin surfaces touch or overlap — usually at the neck, under the arms or in the creases where the legs join the trunk (right). Heat rash may also show up under tight-fitting or overly warm clothing.

red pimples surrounded by blotches of pink skin that may itch or produce a prickling or burning feeling

What to do:
- Check to see that your youngster is not overdressed.
- Give the baby a cool bath or sponge the child with cool water to encourage obstructed pores to open.
- Sprinkle cornstarch or baby powder on the baby to help keep skin dry. To avoid having the child inhale a cloud of dust particles, put the cornstarch or powder into your hand first before applying it to the baby's skin.
- Dress your child in loose-fitting cotton clothing; let a baby go without clothes altogether.
- If possible, place the child in an air-conditioned room.

Call the doctor if:
- blisters appear on the pimples.
- the heat rash does not improve with home treatment.

Hives

Hives are a very common skin reaction in the form of raised, red bumps called wheals. These range in size from half an inch to a few inches across. Larger wheals may have white centers.

Hives usually cause intense itching and can occur anywhere on the body. Allergies are among the most likely causes of hives. Many foods — including shellfish, eggs, milk, chocolate and strawberries — or food additives can trigger an outbreak of hives. Drugs, especially penicillin, can provoke hives, as can exposure to pollen and the bites of certain insects *(see Bites and Stings, page 12)*. If your child is subject to hives, you should try to isolate the cause and avoid exposing the youngster to that particular allergen in the future. Somewhat less commonly, hives can be caused by parasitic or viral infections, or by exposure to the sun or cold temperatures. Doctors disagree as to whether

or not stress and anxiety cause hives.

During any one attack, crops of hives will appear and disappear at different places on the skin. If an individual wheal remains in the same place for longer than 18 hours, the rash is probably not hives and you should consult your physician for treatment. Otherwise, given a mild case of hives, no treatment is necessary — except to relieve the itching it causes — and the wheals should clear up within several days.

In more serious cases, the swelling can occur in the lining of the mouth or throat and can lead to difficulty in breathing. If you notice that your child's breathing is impaired, call the doctor immediately or take the child to the emergency room *(see Breathing Difficulties, page 16)*.

Symptoms:
- intense itching, followed by raised, red bumps, or wheals, on the skin, with sharp borders and sometimes with white centers
- successive appearances and disappearances of the wheals, which rarely persist for longer than 18 hours in the same place
- in more serious cases of hives, swelling of the lining of the mouth or of the throat, difficulty breathing

What to do:
- Apply ice-water compresses to relieve itching. Calamine lotion is also effective in easing discomfort. Or check with your doctor about various over-the-counter antihistamines.
- Try to determine what triggered the attack and avoid exposing the child to it in the future.

Call the doctor if:
- swelling affects the mouth or throat or if breathing is impaired.
- the condition worsens or home treatment fails to ease itching.

Impetigo

Impetigo is a highly contagious skin infection caused by streptococcus and staphylococcus bacteria. It is most prevalent during the summer months and in warm, moist climates. The bacteria enter the skin through a scratch or insect bite, and a local inflammation quickly ensues. This inflammation progresses to tiny blisters that rupture and ooze and then dry to form yellowish brown crusts. The disease is readily and rapidly spread by contact from one part of the body to another or from child to child.

Except in newborns, for whom it can be a debilitating illness, impetigo is not serious in itself. It can, however, occasionally lead to a complication called glomerulonephritis — a rare kidney disorder whose symptoms include cola-colored urine, headaches and elevated blood pressure. For this reason, you should treat impetigo early and vigorously in cooperation with your doctor. With antibiotics and proper care, the condition should be cured in seven to 10 days.

In treating impetigo, it is essential to follow your doctor's instructions carefully regarding prescribed medication and hygiene measures to prevent the spread of the condition. Since impetigo is easily passed on to other children, you should keep your child home from school or day care until the infection is cleared up.

Symptoms:
- in newborns — a tiny, pus-filled blister, which does not develop a thick crust as it does in older children, surrounded by reddened skin, usually in the diaper area or armpit
- in older children — small red spots that form blisters, then break and ooze a yellowish fluid that dries to form thick, yellowish brown crusts
- itching

What to do:
- If impetigo is diagnosed, follow your doctor's instructions regarding any oral antibiotics he may prescribe.
- Clean the affected skin with an antibacterial soap.
- Rub away any crusts, soaking first with warm, soapy water to loosen.
- Keep the affected child's diapers, clothing, towels, washcloths and bedding separate from the family's. Disinfect them daily by washing them in boiling water or by adding chlorine bleach to the wash cycle.

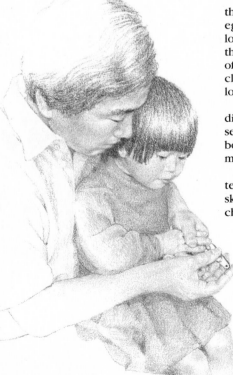

To prevent a child from scratching her skin raw during an itchy rash, cut her fingernails quite short. Hold the youngster on your lap to keep her still and, using clippers or small blunt-edged scissors, trim the fingernails to just below the fingertips.

- Keep the affected child home from school or day care until the infection has cleared up.

Call the doctor if:
- your child shows signs of impetigo.
- the illness does not respond to prescribed treatment.
- you notice any signs of complications, including headaches, fever or dark-colored urine.

Lice

Lice are tiny insects that feed on blood and lay their eggs on hair. Three kinds of lice affect humans, but only two of them — head lice and body lice — are common among children. The third kind, pubic, or crab, lice, affects youngsters only rarely. Infestations of head lice, however, are especially prevalent among children, since the insects are spread easily from child to child and even from jacket to jacket on a school coatrack. Outbreaks of lice are not unusual and not a reflection of neglect on the part of parents, the school or the day-care facility.

Head lice are too small to be seen with the unaided eye, but you can spot their egg cases, called nits. The adult head louse lays its grayish, seedlike nits near the base of hair shafts, often on the back of the head and around the ears. The nits cling to the hair and are not easily dislodged, even with vigorous brushing.

The body louse infests clothing or bedding, depositing its eggs in the fabric itself, especially along the seams. The adult body louse only visits the skin of its human host to feed on blood.

Once the eggs hatch, the lice cause intense itching by biting and irritating the skin. Usually, this is the first sign that a child is infested. You may also notice a

redness on the scalp when head lice are the culprits, or scratch marks or hives on the abdomen or back if the offenders are body lice. Unfortunately, as with many other skin conditions, scratching increases the risk of a secondary infection, so it is best to contact your physician, who can recommend treatment to relieve the itching and to eradicate the adult lice and their nits.

Ordinarily, treatment involves the use of a special antilice shampoo. Other family members should also be examined for signs of infestation, and the affected child's clothing, bedding and hair-care implements should be discarded or sterilized by washing in boiling water. Hats and stuffed animals should be stored in a tightly sealed plastic bag for at least three weeks — long enough for the eggs to hatch and die.

Symptoms of head lice:
- intense itching
- inflammation of the scalp
- nits along hair shafts

What to do for head lice:
- Keep the child from scratching, to prevent a secondary infection.
- Wash the affected child's hair with an over-the-counter nonprescription antilice shampoo, carefully following the instructions on the package to ensure that you kill the nits as well as the adult lice. If your doctor prescribes a special shampoo, follow his advice.
- Use a fine-tooth comb dipped in vinegar to remove nits from the hair.
- Inspect other family members for infestation and treat them, if necessary.
- Discard or disinfect any items that might harbor the adult lice or their nits, including the affected child's clothing, bedding, towels, hairbrushes, combs, barrettes, curlers and hats. To disinfect, wash such items in boiling water. Alternatively, wash the items in water at least 120° F. to remove the lice, and then iron the items

to kill the nits. Dry cleaning is also effective, as is storing the articles in a tightly sealed plastic bag for three weeks or more.

Symptoms of body lice:
- itching
- scratch marks, hives or small red pimples, usually on the abdomen or back

What to do for body lice:
- Use an antilice preparation with your doctor's guidance.
- Disinfect clothing and bedding as for head lice. Use a lice-killing powder or spray on mattresses.

Call the doctor if:
- you suspect your child has lice.
- you notice any signs of a secondary infection, including fever, inflammation or swollen lymph glands.

Moles

Moles are small brown, black or flesh-colored spots on the skin. They are usually the size of freckles and can be flat or raised, smooth or warty, or hairy. Sometimes moles are present at birth. More often, they develop during childhood. In either case, moles usually do not disappear on their own, although they can be removed for cosmetic reasons or if they are located where they will be subject to frequent irritation. Removal is a safe and simple procedure that can often be performed in a doctor's office.

Moles are rarely harmful, although some can become malignant. Your doctor may recommend that any moles your child was born with be removed as a precaution, since congenital moles are more likely to cause trouble than moles that appear later.

One type, known as the giant hairy nevus, has a particular tendency to develop into a form of skin cancer. This mole may be brown, blue or black. It may sprout long, coarse hairs and may vary in size from less than half an inch to eight inches or more across. Physicians usually rec-

ommend having this type of mole removed by surgery.

You should also consult your doctor if you notice any change in a mole's color or if the mole enlarges rapidly, itches, develops a sore or bleeds.

Molluscum contagiosum

Molluscum contagiosum is a common but harmless skin condition that produces raised, firm, waxy nodules, sometimes with a crater in the center. Usually flesh-colored or pearly white, these nodules appear most often on the child's face, trunk, lower abdomen, inner thighs and penis. They can appear singly or in clusters. Caused by a contagious virus, the infection is spread by direct contact with an afflicted person or through contact with contaminated clothing. Although molluscum contagiosum is normally a self-limiting disease that clears up on its own in six to nine months, it can persist for months or even years longer.

Since it can be so persistent and is so easily spread to others — or to other parts of the body — it is best to have the illness treated by a doctor. The treatment of molluscum contagiosum consists of removing the virus-laden plug within the blemishes, either by freezing with liquid nitrogen, using prescribed medication or lancing with a needle or curette.

Symptoms:
- raised, waxy, dome-shaped nodules, sometimes with a central depression, either singly or in clusters

What to do:
- If molluscum contagiosum is diagnosed, use prescribed medication according to your doctor's instructions.
- Disinfect clothing and bedding by boiling in water or by adding chlorine bleach to the wash cycle.

Call the doctor if:
- you suspect molluscum contagiosum.
- the ailment spreads to other members of your family.

- you notice any signs of secondary infection, including pus, pain, inflammation or fever.

Newborn rashes

Nearly half of all infants suffer from a newborn rash at one time or another during the first few weeks of life. Although it can be upsetting to watch a pimply rash erupt on your newborn baby's face or neck, rest assured that such rashes are entirely normal and harmless.

Three different kinds of rashes are common among newborns. The first, sebaceous hyperplasia, appears as tiny white or yellow pimples over the baby's forehead, nose and cheeks. This rash is thought to be caused by the baby's exposure to maternal hormones in the womb. The result is that the infant's oil glands overproduce — much as a teenager's do during puberty — clogging the pores and causing the newborn version of acne. The second kind of rash, milia, which appears as white bumps on the face, is caused by plugged sweat glands. The third type, erythema toxicum, produces small yellow-white bumps in the midst of flat red splotches that usually appear by the second day after birth. None of these rashes call for any special treatment, nor is it necessary to visit the doctor, since in most cases the conditions clear up on their own within a few weeks.

Pityriasis rosea

Patches of pale red, crinkled spots on your child's skin may signal a case of pityriasis rosea, which is a fairly common rash thought to be caused by a viral infection. Despite the itching that it produces, this mildly contagious illness is harmless and disappears in four to eight weeks, leaving the child with lifelong immunity against a recurrence.

In up to 80 percent of cases, the onset of pityriasis rosea is announced by a herald patch — a large spot, up to four inches

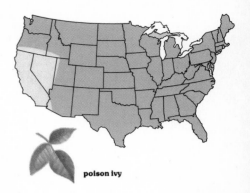

poison ivy

in width, which can appear anywhere on the body. About a week later, a more widespread eruption of smaller spots occurs, generally on the trunk and on the arm and leg surfaces nearest the trunk, or on the face, hands and feet. Pityriasis rosea affects both the left and the right sides of the body equally, appearing in more or less symmetrical patterns. No treatment is necessary, other than to relieve itching.

Symptoms:
- initially, appearance of a pale red spot up to four inches in diameter somewhere on the body
- five to 10 days after initial spot, eruption of small spots that are pale red to brown, round or oval, flat or slightly raised, usually with a crinkly surface and rimmed with scales
- symmetrical distribution of the rash on the right and left sides of the body
- mild itching of the skin at first, which diminishes over time

What to do:
- Apply calamine lotion to relieve the youngster's itching.
- With your doctor's approval, try to relieve severe itching with over-the-counter antihistamine tablets.
- Expose the child to sunlight to speed the healing process.

Call the doctor if:
- you are unsure that the rash is due to pityriasis rosea.

Poison ivy, oak and sumac

Exposure to poison ivy, oak or sumac is the most common cause of skin irritation. It is estimated that about half the people in the United States are allergic to urushiol, an oily substance found in the leaves, stems, flowers, roots and berries of these three related plants in the sumac family. For those people, contact with the plants need not even be direct for an allergic reaction to take place: The urushiol-bearing oil from the plants can produce the same irritating effects when it is picked up from the fur of pets, from clothing and even from the smoke of burning plants.

Poison ivy, the most widespread of the three plants, is a woody vine or trailing shrub that grows in woods, fields, vacant lots and in backyards. It is found throughout most parts of the United States, with the exception of California and Nevada. Each of the plant's reddish stems bears three shiny green leaves *(top right)* from spring through summer. In the fall the leaves turn vivid red, and creamy white berries may also be present, even through the winter.

Its cousin, poison oak, appears in two varieties. The eastern poison oak is a low shrub that thrives in the southeastern United States. Pacific poison oak, as its name implies, is found in the states on the West Coast. Like poison ivy, they have three shiny green leaves — in this case, shaped like oak leaves *(center right)*. The third member of this poisonous triumvirate is poison sumac, which grows as a bush or small tree in the swampy areas of the eastern U.S. Each of its stems bears two opposing rows of leaflets with a single leaflet at the tip *(bottom right)*.

No matter which of the three plants is the culprit, the result is the same for the susceptible child who comes into contact with it: Usually within 24 to 48 hours of contact — though sometimes after a delay of up to 10 days — the exposed skin will become reddened, swollen and blistered. These symptoms will usually be accompanied by intense itching and burning. The blisters burst, leaving weeping sores that soon crust over.

Contrary to popular belief, the fluid from these blisters will not spread the inflammation to others or to other parts of the body. Only the offending plant's oil can spread the inflammation, and for that reason it is essential that you remove the oil from your child's skin, clothing and shoes as soon as possible after exposure.

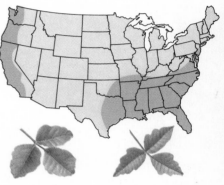

Pacific poison oak   **poison oak**

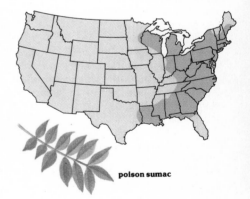

poison sumac

Looking Out for Plants in the Poison Ivy Family
Widespread throughout the United States, poison ivy is distinguished by three pointed, smooth-edged leaflets per stem. Poison-oak leaflets, also three-per-stem, are rounded and slightly lobed in the western, or Pacific, variety, but the eastern variety has pointed tips and deeply lobed edges. Poison sumac, which has seven to 13 smooth-edged leaflets per stem, grows in swampy areas of the eastern United States.

If you can remove the urushiol within five minutes of contact, you may be able to avoid an allergic reaction. Instructions for removal of the oil appear under "What to do" *(below)*. Treatment, once the rash appears, is limited to relieving the youngster's itching; in most cases, plant-induced contact dermatitis heals by itself within one to two weeks without any further complications.

But the best treatment is, of course, prevention. Dress your child in a long-sleeved shirt and long pants or high socks if you know she will be playing in an area where these plants might grow. Teach her what the plants look like so she can avoid them in the future. And have her memorize the cautionary jingle, "Leaflets three, let it be."

As a footnote: Those people who are allergic to poison ivy are also likely to be sensitive to other plants in the same family — including the cashew and pistachio plants and the mango, Japanese lacquer and ginkgo trees — and should take appropriate precautions.

Symptoms:
- reddish rash and blistering, generally appearing in a line where the plant touched the skin
- swollen, reddened skin
- intense itching and burning

What to do:
- Wash immediately with soap and water to remove the oil from the skin and to prevent or reduce the inflammation. After washing, rub the affected skin area with alcohol, and then rinse it with water.
- Trim your child's nails and encourage her not to scratch.
- Apply calamine lotion to relieve itching, or give over-the-counter antihistamine tablets.
- Apply compresses soaked in Burow's solution (available from your pharmacist) or in a solution of one tablespoon of baking soda mixed with one quart of cool water; repeat the process four times daily for 15 minutes to one hour.
- Wash any exposed clothes thoroughly or send them to be dry-cleaned. Decontaminate shoes by wiping them with cleaning fluid.
- Teach your child to avoid the plants in the future.
- In severe cases, follow your physician's instructions if he prescribes any medication to reduce the itching or inflammation.

Call the doctor if:
- there is any swelling around the eyes, mouth, nose or genitals.
- the itching is severe and does not respond to home remedies.
- the youngster exhibits indications of secondary infection, including increased inflammation, fever or swollen lymph nodes.

Purpura

Purpura is a disorder in which tiny hemorrhages in the upper layers of the skin produce areas of purple discoloration. There are several kinds of purpura, but the most common form among children is known as anaphylactoid purpura.

Anaphylactoid purpura occurs most often in boys between the ages of two and eight. Its cause is unknown, although allergies are suspected of playing a role, and the disease sometimes follows in the wake of an upper respiratory infection. Whatever its cause, this form of purpura can affect the small blood vessels of the skin, joints, intestines and kidneys, resulting in the rupture of the blood vessels themselves and the outbreak of a characteristic rash on the skin *(below)*. The child with purpura may also complain of abdominal or joint pain and, in some cases, the youngster may have bloody bowel movements.

There is no specific treatment for anaphylactoid purpura; the illness usually disappears on its own in several days to a few weeks. Occasionally, complications may occur, the most serious of which are intussusception *(page 70)* — the telescoping of a segment of intestine into itself — and nephritis *(page 126),* a kidney inflammation. If you notice signs of complications, you should contact your doctor right away.

Symptoms:
- rash consisting of large hives and purple discoloration, particularly on the legs, thighs and lower abdomen
- swelling of the scalp and of the skin over the backs of the hands and the tops of the feet
- low-grade fever
- arthritis of large joints, including the knees, ankles, hips, wrists and elbows
- abdominal pain, vomiting
- blood in stools

What to do:
- Use the glass test illustrated below to help determine whether your child's rash is the result of purpura.
- If purpura is diagnosed, follow your doctor's recommendations regarding treatment for relief of symptoms.

Call the doctor if:
- you suspect your child may have anaphylactoid purpura.
- such symptoms as fever, abdominal

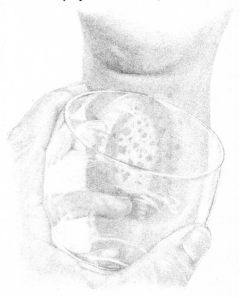

To see if a rash is caused by purpura, press a clear glass against it. A surface rash will disappear; a purpura rash, caused by inflamed or broken blood vessels under the skin, will remain visible.

pain, bloody urine or vomiting continue once treatment has begun.

Ringworm

Ringworm is a fungal infection of the skin, hair or nails that in fact has nothing at all to do with worms. The disorder, which is more common among children than it is among adults, produces small, round, red spots that grow larger and gradually form the characteristic ring- or horseshoe-shaped lesions that give the ailment its name.

There are actually three kinds of ringworm, two of which affect children: tinea corporis, or ringworm of the body; and tinea capitis, or ringworm of the scalp. The third type is tinea pedis, more commonly known as athlete's foot, a condition that is rare in young children.

Tinea corporis often causes no symptoms other than minor itching. It is transmitted by direct contact with contaminated floors, benches or shower stalls, or by touching infected pets. Treatment for this highly contagious ailment consists of keeping the skin dry and using topical medications to kill the fungus.

Tinea capitis is also transmitted by direct contact. It is a painless inflammation of the scalp that causes patchy hair loss and scaling. More stubborn and difficult to cure than tinea corporis, the condition must be treated by a doctor with oral antifungus medication.

Because of the contagious nature of these forms of ringworm, it is essential that you disinfect the child's clothing and bedding and discard any hairbrushes, combs or other items that might harbor the fungus. You should also keep your child home from school or day care until the infection has healed, to prevent the spread of the disease to others.

Symptoms of tinea corporis:
- small, round, red spots that enlarge and form ring-shaped lesions
- itching

What to do for tinea corporis:
- Scrub the affected skin with an antiseptic soap to remove scales.
- Keep the skin dry to discourage the growth of the fungus.
- Apply an over-the-counter antifungal medication to the affected skin.
- Sterilize clothing and bedding by washing in boiling water.
- Keep your child home from school or day care until the infection is cured.

Symptoms of tinea capitis:
- inflammation of the scalp
- patchy hair loss
- broken hairs
- scaling

What to do for tinea capitis:
- Shampoo the child's hair daily.
- If tinea capitis is diagnosed by your doctor, administer prescribed oral medication according to instructions.
- Discard such items as hairbrushes, combs, barrettes and curlers, and sterilize all clothing and bedding by washing in boiling water.
- Keep your child home from school or day care until the inflammation is completely cured.

Call the doctor if:
- you suspect tinea capitis.
- any fungal infection fails to respond to treatment.

Rocky Mountain spotted fever

Rocky Mountain spotted fever is a serious illness caused by microbes called rickettsiae and transmitted by infected ticks, most often in the spring and summer months. (See Bites and Stings, page 12). It is a true medical emergency, and you should contact your physician immediately if you suspect that your youngster may be suffering from this potentially life-threatening disease.

Despite its name, which derives from the Montana laboratory where the disease was studied at the turn of the century, Rocky Mountain spotted fever is to-day most common in the southeastern and south-central states. Three to 10 days after being bitten by an infected tick, the victim will develop a high fever accompanied by headaches, chills and muscle pain. Within three to four days, the disease causes an inflammation of the lining of the small blood vessels, which presents itself as a rash. Unlike the rashes of measles or chicken pox, which erupt first on the child's face or chest, the rash of Rocky Mountain spotted fever begins on the ankles and wrists before spreading to other parts of the body.

Left untreated, Rocky Mountain spotted fever can lead to the spread of the infection to the central nervous system, or to circulatory and lung complications, coma and, ultimately, death. The greatest danger lies in delay of diagnosis, since once the victim is in a doctor's care, he can be easily treated with antibiotics. Happily, one attack confers immunity against a recurrence of the disease.

Symptoms:
- high, unremitting fever up to 104° F.
- chills
- headache
- bone and muscle pain
- flat, red rash that appears first on the ankles and wrists before spreading to other parts of the body
- in untreated cases, delirium, convulsions and coma

What to do:
- Prevent tick bites by dressing your child in clothing that fits tightly at wrists, ankles and waist when he is playing in tick-infested areas.
- Inspect your child for ticks after any outing in the woods or other places inhabited by ticks.
- If you find a tick attached to or embedded in the skin, remove it by covering it with alcohol, petroleum jelly or any oil that will make the tick relax its hold. If the tick does not release its hold, remove it carefully, using

tweezers. If no oil is at hand, grasp the tick as close to the skin as possible and pull it off gently, trying not to crush it.
- Wash the affected area thoroughly with soap and water.
- Be alert for signs of Rocky Mountain spotted fever — including fever, rash or headache — during the two weeks after removing the tick.

Call the doctor if:
- you notice any combination of the above symptoms in your child, whether or not you are aware of a previous tick bite. DO NOT delay.

Roseola

Roseola is a common viral infection that most often affects children under the age of three. It begins suddenly with a high fever that persists for three to five days. The fever stage of the illness is followed, once the temperature falls to normal, by the development of a rosy red rash, usually on the chest, abdomen and back. This rash fades quickly, often in a day. Although it is contagious, roseola is not a serious illness and generally clears up on its own within a week. In rare instances, it may be accompanied by convulsions or complicated by a nasal or ear infection. There is no treatment for roseola other than measures to reduce the fever.

Symptoms:
- high temperature of up to 105° F. for three to five days
- flat, rosy red rash that develops on the youngster's chest, abdomen or back after the fever breaks

What to do:
- Use acetaminophen to reduce fever.
- Be alert for the development of any other symptoms that might indicate a more serious illness.
- Do not confine the child to bed if she feels like getting up to play.

Call the doctor if:
- the youngster's fever lasts for longer than four or five days.

- the youngster develops complications, including convulsions or a nasal or ear infection.

Scabies

The contagious skin condition called scabies, once relatively rare in this country, has been on the rise in recent years. It is caused by mites, small parasites that burrow into the outer layer of skin. The resulting inflammation is easily spread by contact with infected persons or with their clothing, bedding, towels or other contaminated items.

The irritation caused by the scabies mite produces an extremely itchy red rash that can affect any part of the body — especially in folds of skin. Infants, however, are more likely to be affected on the face and neck. If you look closely you may even be able to see the linear tracks that are caused by the burrowing of the parasites, especially if the tracks have not been obscured by the youngster's own scratching.

The diagnosis of scabies is confirmed by scraping the involved skin and examining the scrapings under a microscope for the telltale mite. There is no effective home remedy. The doctor may order the use of a prescription ointment or lotion. The doctor may also want to examine other family members for signs of infestation. As with other skin infections, the affected child's clothing, bedding and any other articles that could harbor the mites must be discarded or disinfected by washing in boiling water.

Symptoms:
- red rash anywhere on the body, but especially in the skin folds between the fingers and toes, under the arms and behind the knees
- small blisters that appear at the ends of linear tracks
- severe itching that is worse at night

What to do:
- If scabies is diagnosed, apply medicat-

ed cream or lotion according to your doctor's instructions.
- Wash the affected skin area, using an antiseptic soap.
- Trim the youngster's nails to discourage scratching.
- Keep the affected child home from school or day care for at least one day after treatment has begun.
- Disinfect the child's clothing and bedding by washing in boiling water.

Call the doctor if:
- you suspect scabies.
- you notice any signs of secondary infection, including increased inflammation, swollen glands or fever.

Warts

Children commonly develop warts — which are harmless, though somewhat contagious, growths of skin tissue caused by a virus. Warts may occur singly or in clusters and be large or small in size. Their texture may be smooth or rough, raised or flat. The growths can appear anywhere on a child's body, but the most likely sites are on the fingers, hands and soles of the feet. Most warts are painless, although those growing on the soles of the feet — plantar warts — can be painful because of their location.

The best treatment for warts is to leave them alone. Studies show that 65 percent of all warts will disappear on their own within two years, and up to half of all plantar warts affecting young children are gone within six months of first appearing. The youngster should not pick at a wart, since this will increase the risk of spreading the virus or developing a secondary infection.

Warts that are painful, enlarge rapidly or are cosmetically disfiguring require a doctor's attention. In such cases, the doctor can remove the growth by applying caustic medication or by freezing it with liquid nitrogen. Such treatment is almost always effective. •ː•

Recognizing Common Skin Rashes

The chart below offers a quick-reference guide to various skin rashes and the illnesses or conditions that cause them. The common problems of cradle cap, newborn rash and diaper rash are not included because of their easily recognized, localized symptoms. Complete information on those three conditions, as well as those included in the chart, is presented elsewhere in this book.

CONDITION/ ILLNESS	Skin Appearance	Other Symptoms	Area Affected	Duration
CHICKEN POX	flat red spots, then tiny blisters that break and crust over	low fever, fatigue, intense itching	back, chest and abdomen first, then rest of body	about seven days
ECZEMA	dry, red, cracked skin; blisters that ooze and crust over	itching	in infants, on cheeks; in older children, on neck, inside elbows and knees	until controlled by medication; intermittent flare-ups
FIFTH DISEASE	red rash of varying intensity that fades to a flat, lacy pattern	none	face first, then trunk and limbs	up to one month
HEAT RASH (PRICKLY HEAT)	small red pimples, pink blotchy skin	occasional itching	skin folds, neck, chest, diaper area	until irritants are removed
HIVES	raised, red bumps, or wheals	itching; in extreme cases, swelling of throat, difficulty breathing	any area	a few minutes up to a day
IMPETIGO	in infants, pus-filled blisters, red skin; in older children, oozing spots that crust over	itching	arms, legs, face or trunk	until controlled by medication
HEAD LICE	inflammation of scalp, nits (egg cases) visible along hair shaft	itching	head	until controlled by medication
BODY LICE	scratch marks, hives or small red pimples	itching	usually back or abdomen	until controlled by medication
MOLLUSCUM CONTAGIOSUM	raised waxy nodules, may have sunken center; appear singly or in clusters	none	face, trunk, lower abdomen, inner thighs, penis	six to nine months, or longer
PITYRIASIS ROSEA	initial splotch up to four inches wide; five to 10 days later, reddish spots with crinkly surface rimmed with scales	mild itching	trunk, arms, legs	four to eight weeks
POISON IVY, OAK, SUMAC	red, swollen skin, rash and blistering	intense itching and burning	exposed areas	one to two weeks
PURPURA	rash consisting of large hives and purple discoloration	fever; swelling of scalp, skin covering hands and feet; abdominal or joint pain; blood in stools	legs, thighs, lower abdomen	several days to three weeks
RINGWORM	red spots that become ring-shaped lesions; on scalp, inflammation, scaling, hair loss	minor itching	any area of body	until controlled by medication
ROCKY MOUNTAIN SPOTTED FEVER	flat, red rash	high fever, headache, muscle pain, chills	affects ankles and wrists first, then spreads to rest of body	until controlled by medication
ROSEOLA	flat, rosy red rash	high fever for three to five days, then rash appears	chest, back, abdomen	about seven days
SCABIES	red rash with blisters at the end of linear tracks	intense itching	any area, but most often in folds of the skin	until controlled by medication
SCARLET FEVER	rough, bright red rash	high fever, sore throat	neck, groin, armpits; then rest of body	five to seven days

Urinary System

The urinary tract is one of the body's cleansing systems, a delicate and efficient mechanism that removes wastes from the blood and disposes of them through urination. It consists of six organs: a pair of kidneys, a pair of ureters leading from the kidneys to the bladder, the bladder itself and the urethra *(below)*.

The kidneys are the beginning of the urinary tract; they are also its most complex organs. Blood that has circulated through the body and picked up wastes from cells surges through the kidneys with each heartbeat. There it passes through about a million tiny filtering units called nephrons. These filter out poisons, excess salt and water, and send them down the ureters as urine. Nutrients and useful fluids, meanwhile, are recirculated back into the bloodstream.

Because the kidneys are intimately associated with the bloodstream and fluids, kidney disorders may be signaled by a change in blood pressure or fluid retention. A youngster who has high blood pressure, or one who develops a puffy face or swollen ankles, should always be seen by a physician.

The urine produced by the kidneys trickles down the ureters to the bladder. Because an infant's bladder is small and the muscle at its base is relatively weak, babies urinate frequently. In time, the bladder grows and the sphincter muscle at its base strengthens. This, together with a maturing nervous system, makes voluntary bladder control possible. Nighttime bed-wetting can sometimes be caused by a lag in the development of this part of the urinary tract.

Urine ultimately leaves the body via the urethra. This tube — which is several inches long in a boy and less than an inch long in a girl — is subject to a number of mild infections. These infections become more serious as they spread up the tract toward the kidneys. Fortunately, however, such ailments almost always succumb to antibiotics.

Bed-wetting

Bed-wetting brings distress to both parent and child, but the problem is actually a minor one that almost always vanishes with time. Doctors no longer believe that bed-wetting by itself indicates serious psychological problems or that it requires psychiatric attention. Patience and a positive parental attitude are the best prescriptions.

You should not consider bed-wetting a problem at all until long after a child has mastered daytime bladder control, or

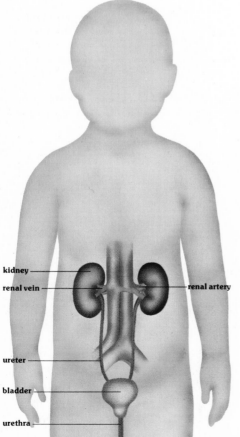

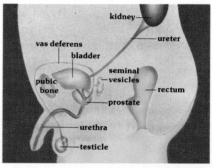

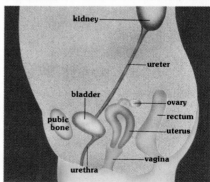

The urinary tract removes wastes, excess salt and water from the blood, expelling them from the body as urine. The main work of this system is performed by the kidneys. Situated at the upper rear of the abdominal cavity, these twin organs cleanse the blood by passing it through filtering units called nephrons. Approximately one quarter of the body's blood goes to the kidneys each minute, entering by way of the renal arteries, then circulating back into the bloodstream via the renal veins. Tubes called ureters carry the resulting trickle of urine down from the kidneys to the bladder, which rests in the pelvis behind the pubic bone. From the bladder, urine passes out of the body through a tube called the urethra.

Male and female urinary tracts include the same organs but are structured differently. In males (top), the urinary system is linked to the reproductive organs. In females (bottom), the urethra is short and ends near the vagina and the anus, making a girl's urinary tract more susceptible to infection.

even until he has entered school. When nighttime wetting seems to have progressed beyond ordinary accidents in a child of five years old, it acquires a medical name, enuresis, and only then might it merit a visit to the doctor.

Bed-wetting, however, is rarely the result of disease or a physical abnormality. In those cases, children have trouble with daytime control, too, and usually show other signs of an illness such as diabetes or urinary infection. Evidence of this sort, of course, does require a call to the child's physician.

In most cases, however, the causes of enuresis are poorly understood. The problem afflicts mainly boys and it often runs in families. Authorities differ on how much of the problem is psychological and how much of it is caused by a simple delay in the development of a youngster's urinary tract.

Whatever the reason, the problem is common. Ten percent of five-year-olds wet their beds regularly, 15 percent occasionally. Many continue for years beyond this age, but in nearly all cases the problem stops spontaneously before the child reaches adolescence.

Experience has indicated that bed-wetting follows patterns. When a child moves into a new home, has a particularly exciting experience or is confronted with a new baby brother or sister, he may begin a bout of bed-wetting. Bed-wetters may also be children who have had toilet training impatiently thrust upon them. Insecure boys are more likely than others to be bed-wetters; if you suspect that your child has problems aside from bed-wetting that merit treatment on their own, you may wish to seek counseling for the youngster.

Maintain a low-key, reassuring attitude toward bed-wetting. When you rouse your child in the morning and see the wet bedclothes, treat it as a natural event and tell your child that you know he will be dry soon enough. Occasionally tell him that many others have had this problem and that they all finally grew out of it. It is important to remember that bed-wetting is involuntary. Scolding and shaming are counterproductive.

Waking a child so that he can empty his bladder may work with some light sleepers, but not most heavy ones, who naturally will feel groggy and resentful. In fact, much bed-wetting is associated with deep sleep. Other children tend to wet the bed first thing in the morning, so you can try taking the child to the toilet immediately after he wakes up. Restricting liquids in the evening might also help, but stay within the bounds of reason; if your youngster is thirsty, you should let the child drink.

Medically prescribed remedies for bed-wetting include drugs that contract the sphincter at the base of the bladder. These usually work only temporarily. You might try lining the child's bed with moisture-sensitive pads that set off alarms when wet. These may eventually cause the child to develop a reflex action, waking when he needs to urinate. But they are useful only when the youngster himself strongly wants to end the problem. You should use alarms only under a doctor's supervision.

The simplest solutions are usually the best. Praise dry nights. Post stars on a calendar. Give presents as rewards early in your child's training, rather than dangling them in the future. They will show the child that you are confident he will master his problem.

A waterproof pad beneath the bottom sheet helps the cleanup. You can also give your child a feeling of responsibility by laying out clean pajamas and sheets and telling him to care for himself if he wakes up wet in the middle of the night. With matter-of-fact measures such as these, you will almost certainly find that the problem solves itself in time.

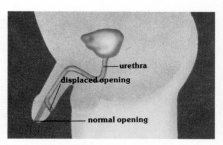

In hypospadias, a relatively common birth defect, the opening of the urethra is located on the underside of the penis rather than at its tip. The displacement causes an inability to direct the urine stream in the usual manner and may interfere with normal sexual functioning in adulthood. The problem can be corrected by surgery, though multiple operations are sometimes necessary.

Hypospadias

Hypospadias is a birth defect in which the urethra terminates at an abnormal point. In boys, it exits somewhere on the underside of the penis rather than at the tip *(above)*. A related but rarer defect called epispadias is the termination of the urethra on the upper side of the penis. Girls, too, can suffer a short urethra, which may end at the separation of the labia minora or inside the vagina, but such cases are very rare. Hypospadias occurs in one to three out of every 1,000 children born in the United States.

Doctors classify hypospadias in boys into three types, depending on where the urethra ends. When the opening is the penis tip, the child has first-degree hypospadias; this minor problem may require no treatment. If the urethra ends near the middle of the penis, the condition is called second-degree hypospadias and may merit simple reconstructive surgery. Third-degree hypospadias is defined by an opening close to the scrotum. This condition may require two operations, one when the boy is a toddler and one before he is four years old. Surgery often involves using the foreskin of the penis to construct an extension of the urethra; for this reason, boys with hypospadias are not circumcised. The surgery is nearly always successful.

Nephritis

Nephritis, also called glomerulonephritis, is an inflammation of the kidneys that occurs most often in children over four years old. The most common form of this relatively rare condition attacks the kidneys' million or so tiny filtering units, or nephrons, and arises one to three weeks after the child recovers from a streptococcal bacterial infection, such as strep throat, scarlet fever or impetigo. The kidneys cease to regulate fluids properly. They reduce their output of urine, allow blood to seep into what urine they do produce and cause the body to retain too much fluid elsewhere.

The severity of nephritis varies widely, from a mild case with few symptoms to one involving dangerously high blood pressure and kidney damage. The type preceded by a strep infection usually vanishes without complications in a few weeks. Other, rarer forms of nephritis can be chronic and lead to slow, progressive kidney failure. These may be related to purpura *(page 120).*

Any child who shows symptoms of nephritis, particularly puffy skin and the characteristic trickle of dark urine, should see a doctor. The physician normally will order urine and blood tests and may prescribe antibiotics to fight any remaining strep infection. There is no treatment for the inflammation itself, which must run its course, but the symptoms can be successfully treated and the child made comfortable. Rest, even bed rest or hospitalization, may be called for, as well as a special diet that restricts salt, liquids and sometimes protein (meat, fish, eggs) in order to relieve strain on the kidneys. Most children recover quickly and completely from nephritis.

Symptoms:
- at first, puffy skin around the eyes; later, a bloating of skin on the face and ankles caused by fluid retention
- decreased amounts of urine
- urine that is smokey-colored or reddish brown
- loss of appetite
- in some cases of the condition, vomiting, headache, or fever
- in some cases, convulsions and increased blood pressure

What to do:
- Be alert for symptoms following a streptococcal infection.
- Be prepared for your youngster to stay in a hospital.
- Once your child is home from the doctor or hospital, keep her to her diet and schedule of medicines. Allow her plenty of rest.

Call the doctor if:
- you suspect nephritis based on the symptoms listed.
- your child has been diagnosed as having nephritis, and her blood pressure rises or she has a convulsion.

Nephrosis

Nephrosis, or nephrotic syndrome, is a rare chronic kidney disease that is closely related to nephritis *(previous entry).* It is thought sometimes to be a complication of untreated nephritis. In nephrosis, the kidney's filtering membranes are so damaged that protein — normally recirculated into the bloodstream — escapes in the urine. At the same time, the body retains too much salt and fluid. Bloating and protein deficiency result.

Most cases of nephrosis develop in children from one to six years old. Its outward symptoms resemble those of nephritis: reduced urine output and puffy skin around the eyes, followed by general swelling of the face, ankles and belly. These symptoms should always prompt a visit to the doctor, who will probably prescribe blood and urine tests. She also may order a needle biopsy of the kidneys, in which a small sample of kidney tissue is extracted from the patient by needle and then examined.

Treatment often involves hospitalization for a time and a special diet high in protein and low in salt and fluids. The doctor may prescribe a variety of drugs, including corticosteroids. Some drugs that are effective against the disease also suppress the body's immune system, so the child may be given antibiotics as well, to fight any invading infections. A child with nephrosis is also especially susceptible to infections because the disease has weakened his body.

Caught early, nephrosis can be cured in several weeks. In some children, the symptoms linger or recur, requiring treatment over the course of months or even a few years. In these cases, parents may wish to get counseling on ways to protect the child from infections without unduly restricting his social life. In very rare cases, the disease leads to kidney failure; however, even this serious condition can be treated successfully with dialysis or a transplant, so that the child can lead a relatively normal life. For most children, the disease will disappear completely and without further effects.

Symptoms:
- puffy skin around the eyes, ankles and belly due to fluid retention; possibly accompanied by a slow, steady weight gain as well
- reduced amounts of urine
- possibly, vomiting and diarrhea

What to do:
- Be prepared for your youngster to stay in a hospital.
- When your child is home from the doctor or hospital, allow him plenty of rest; mild activities are acceptable.
- Keep your child to his schedule of prescribed medicines.
- Keep your child to the diet prescribed for him.

Call the doctor if:
- you suspect nephrosis.
- your child has been diagnosed as having nephrosis and shows any sign

of infection, such as fever, skin sores, cough or a burning sensation that occurs during urination.

Urinary-tract infections

Childhood urinary-tract infections are common, but most cases are easily treated and do not indicate serious illness.

Bacteria are the chief culprits. Germs from the intestine can travel through the bloodstream to any portion of the urinary tract, but for the most part, bacteria invade the urethra and bladder from outside the body. These bacteria usually originate in fecal matter. Girls are much more likely than boys to suffer these infections because their urethras are so much shorter — allowing germs faster passage to the bladder — and because the opening to the urinary tract is much nearer the anus than in boys. Obstructions in the tract, such as an unusually tight sphincter or kidney stones, may promote infections in stagnant urine.

Bacterial infections can be vanquished by antibiotics. But since viruses do not respond to antibiotics, viral urinary inflammations must run their course. In addition, other problems may cause the same symptoms as do urinary-tract infections — especially frequent and painful urination. Vaginal infections *(page 109)* and physical irritation of the urethra, caused by an injury or by detergents in bubble baths, are two examples.

The severity and symptoms of urinary-tract infections vary widely. In general, infections increase in seriousness as they rise toward the kidneys. Mild infections of the urethra and bladder may have no noticeable symptoms at all, or they may produce symptoms that do not directly implicate the urinary system, such as un-

explained malaise or fever. High fever, diarrhea and vomiting can indicate a more serious infection, one that has reached the kidneys.

Usually, however, the problem will show up with frequent or painful urination or discolored urine. You should report any suspected urinary-tract infection to a doctor, who may have your child's urine analyzed to identify the bacteria or other source of trouble. If bacteria are discovered, antibiotics will probably be prescribed for a week or two.

Most children who suffer one of these infections are stricken by a second one within a year or two and after that remain clear. If a girl has a third occurrence, the doctor may want to use X-rays and other tests to check for underlying troubles, such as partial blockages. Boys are frequently X-rayed after a first infection, because it is so often caused by some anatomical abnormality.

Symptoms:
- in a newborn — listlessness, a reluctance to feed, jaundice
- in an infant — squirming, irritability, frequent or dribbling urination, fever, failure to thrive
- in children who are older than one year of age — frequent or painful urination, dribbling urine flow, urine that is bloody or foul-smelling
- resumption of bed-wetting after a period of dryness
- puslike discharge in the urine
- unexplained fever or malaise
- if the child's kidneys are affected, fever, abdominal pain, back pain, chills, nausea and diarrhea

What to do:
- For infants and toddlers, change diapers frequently.

- Encourage your child to drink plenty of liquids. Cranberry juice is a good choice because its high acid content counteracts the alkaline environment in which bacteria thrive. Carbonated drinks should be avoided, because they are alkaline.
- Encourage your youngster to empty her bladder completely each time she urinates. Going a second time after a few minutes helps.
- Eliminate spicy foods, which can irritate the bladder.
- Give acetaminophen for pain.
- Teach your daughter to wipe herself from front to back after using the toilet, in order to keep fecal matter away from the urethra.

Call the doctor if:
- you suspect a urinary-tract infection.
- your youngster has a urinary-tract infection and develops a temperature higher than 101° F.

Wilm's tumor

Wilm's tumor is a very rare, solid and malignant tumor of the kidney. It rarely affects a child older than five. Parents often spot the tumor by noticing a palpable swelling on one side of the abdomen while bathing the child. Fever, pain and blood in the urine are other symptoms. If you suspect a tumor, do not poke it — pressure may dislodge malignant cells and send them to other body organs.

Call a doctor immediately if your child has symptoms of Wilm's tumor. If a tumor is discovered, your child will need surgery to remove it. Radiation therapy and drugs may follow. Fortunately, such methods are highly successful. Ninety percent of children treated for Wilm's tumor are cured completely. ❖

3 Keeping Children Healthy

The best medicine you can ever give your child is a sound program of preventive care. In large measure, it is the attention a youngster receives when he is well — the regular medical and dental checkups, the full round of vaccinations, concern for diet, rest and exercise — that lays the foundation for physical well-being and good health habits throughout life. Your youngster's physician will play a big part in this effort, but the responsibility is primarily yours.

As in all things, parents are the role models when it comes to attitudes about health: Your actions will shape your youngster's feelings about being sick just as they teach him how to stay well. Parental love and comfort are a powerful tonic when your little one is ill, but be careful not to coddle him too much. Keep your mood upbeat and make clear to the child that the goal is to get over the sickness, not dwell on it. A youngster should never arrive at the conclusion that being sick is fun or a way to get special attention.

This section of the book touches upon many general health concerns regarding children, including the proper use of medication for babies, toddlers and pre-schoolers. While you don't want your child to grow up thinking of medicine as a cure-all, there are a few basic over-the-counter drugs and supplies that will come in handy when the routine sniffles, rashes and fevers of childhood strike. A prescription for a well-stocked household medicine chest, along with guidelines for safe use of its contents, appears on the following pages.

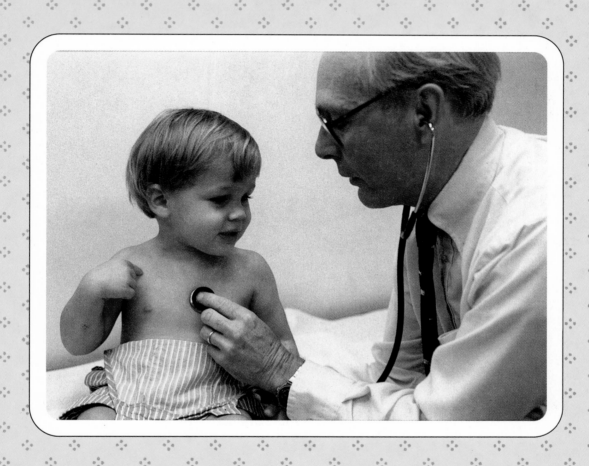

The Home Pharmacy

You can ready your medicine chest for childhood illnesses by stocking it with a few basic nonprescription medicines and all-purpose health supplies *(right)*. Aside from drugs prescribed for specific problems, however, you should use medicines sparingly, for several reasons. Over-the-counter products do provide symptomatic relief, but they will not affect a disease's course. Some produce side effects — such as nervousness or sleepiness — that may be as bad as the disease. And a few drugs, such as those that suppress coughing or vomiting, can interfere with the body's natural defenses. For many childhood ailments, good nursing — giving fluids, back-rubs and love — is the best kind of treatment.

When your child does need a drug, read the label before giving it and ask your doctor about these points:

- Exactly what schedule is necessary? If the label specifies six- or eight-hour intervals, can the drug be given at bedtime and breakfast, so you and your child need not get up at night?
- Should the drug be taken on a full or an empty stomach?
- Should any foods be avoided?
- What side effects are likely? Which ones require phoning the doctor or discontinuing the drug?
- Should your youngster avoid vigorous activities?

Giving a young child medicine is often a good test of parental ingenuity. Be calm, firm and fast, and resist any urge to threaten a resistant child. Bribes can be useful, but once you use this ploy be prepared for your child to demand payment for every dose. Never pretend that medicine is candy; your child could later poison himself with such a treat. And above all, be honest: Do not promise a magical cure or say a bitter drug tastes sweet.

How you administer a drug depends on its form and on your child's age. Most medicines are available as syrups; a few come in tablets or capsules or in suppositories for times when your child cannot take medicine by mouth. For best results, follow these guidelines:

- Always give drugs in a lighted room, so you can see the label.
- To prevent possible choking, you should hold your child upright or at an angle while giving the medicine.
- Measure liquid medicines precisely with a calibrated spoon, oral syringe, drug cup or dropper. If your child prefers a kitchen spoon, make sure to measure out the prescribed amount of syrup into it.
- Grind nonchewable tablets between two spoons, then mix the resulting powder with a bit of a slippery food such as jam or applesauce.
- Babies can suck small doses of liquid medicine from a detached bottle nipple. Larger doses can be blended with a few tablespoons of water and sucked from a bottle. Do not mix in large amounts of liquid; the medicine may separate or your child may drink only part of it.
- You can also give liquids to babies and toddlers with an oral syringe. Put it into the corner of the mouth to prevent the child's inhaling the medicine, and let it trickle in slowly.
- Give syrups or chewable tablets to youngsters who are over three years of age — use your judgment about your child's chewing ability.

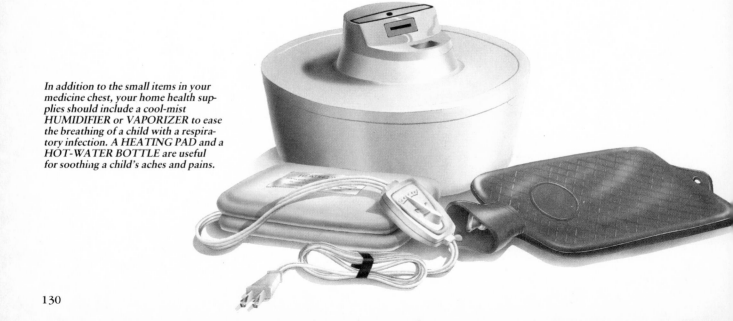

In addition to the small items in your medicine chest, your home health supplies should include a cool-mist HUMIDIFIER or VAPORIZER to ease the breathing of a child with a respiratory infection. A HEATING PAD and a HOT-WATER BOTTLE are useful for soothing a child's aches and pains.

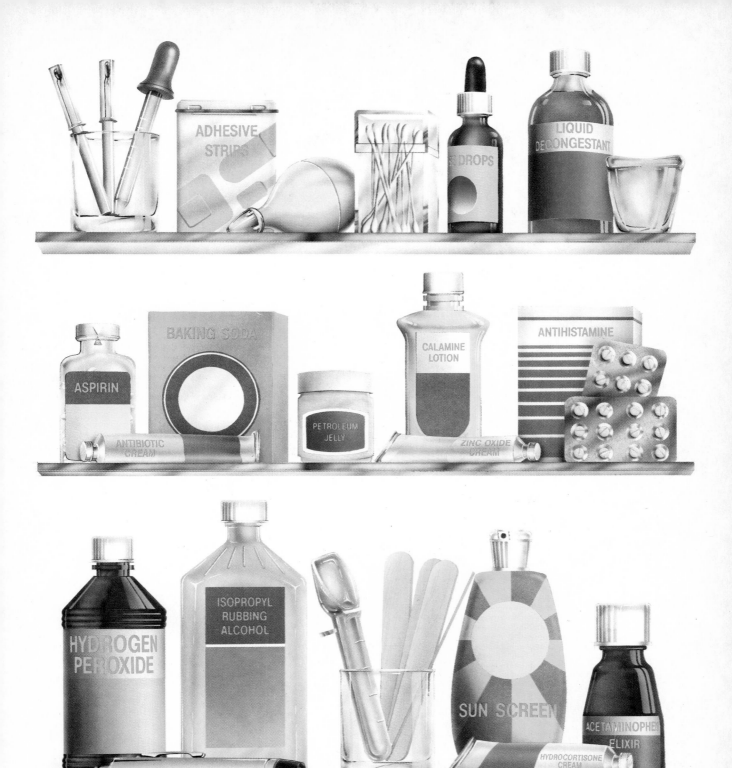

First row: rectal and oral THERMOMETERS; a calibrated
DOSAGE DROPPER; ADHESIVE STRIPS for small cuts;
a NASAL ASPIRATOR for clearing clogged mucus; COTTON-
TIP APPLICATORS for holding eyelids open; NOSE DROPS
for stuffed-up noses; LIQUID DECONGESTANT for colds; an
EYECUP for irrigating the eye. Second row: ASPIRIN for fever, pain and inflammations (check with your doctor before use);
ANTIBIOTIC CREAM, such as neomycin or bacitracin, to
prevent infection in cuts; BAKING SODA for soothing baths;

PETROLEUM JELLY; CALAMINE LOTION for rashes; ZINC
OXIDE for diaper rash; ANTIHISTAMINES for allergic skin reactions. Third row: HYDROGEN PEROXIDE, a nonstinging
antiseptic for small cuts; a small FLASHLIGHT for checking eyes
and throat; isopropyl RUBBING ALCOHOL for disinfecting
instruments; a calibrated DOSAGE SPOON and TONGUE
DEPRESSORS; SUN SCREEN; HYDROCORTISONE CREAM
for minor skin irritations; ACETAMINOPHEN ELIXIR, a liquid
medication for pain and fever.

Caring for a Sick Child

The Nature of Childhood Ills

The prevalence of illness in early childhood is not a parental illusion: Young children do come down with illnesses more often than grownups and older children, because their immune systems take a few years to mature fully. But if youngsters are more susceptible to disease, they are also more resilient. The typical toddler, for example, will suffer milder physical effects and bounce back more quickly than his mother or father would if struck by the same ailment.

In fact, as a parent, you should be aware that your child may suffer more emotionally than physically when a fever, cold or case of chicken pox has him down. Unable to understand the source of the bumps and aches or the reasons for the bad-tasting medicine, he needs your reassurance more than ever.

The first signs of illness
A parent's trained eye can usually tell that a child is coming down with something well before overt symptoms begin to show. Because you are so attuned to your youngster's normal appearance and behavior, you will probably be the first to spot the subtle changes that serve as early warning signs of illness. Perhaps her skin seems pale or flushed, or her eyes look tired. She may play more listlessly than usual, become whiny or take a voluntary nap at an odd time of day.

When vague signals such as these are precursors of illness, they will usually give way to more specific symptoms within a day or two. One of the major symptoms of childhood illness is fever *(see Fever, page 91)*. Other clues that something is amiss are vomiting, diarrhea, persistent and unexplained crying, and loss of appetite.

If your child shows any of the symptoms listed above, or any substantial deviation from her normal behavior patterns,

you should also check her for swollen glands, a stiff neck, a rash or any localized swelling or inflammation, and report the findings to your doctor.

Dispelling the sickroom myths
In recent years, a number of myths and attitudes about children's illness have gone the way of mentholated chest rubs and near-mandatory tonsillectomies. Most doctors now feel that, in general, the less fuss you make over your child's illness, the better.

Strict bed rest for the sake of recovery, for example, is now considered unnecessary. A youngster often does not feel terribly sick during a routine illness, and when she is feeling tired she will generally seek out her bed voluntarily. If she feels like it and the doctor hasn't advised you otherwise, let your child get dressed and play quietly about the house.

In fact, in many cases a child who is ill need not be kept indoors. Common sense should be exercised, of course, but if the temperature outside is mild, there is usually no harm in allowing even a child with a low fever to play quietly in the shade.

You also should not hesitate to take a feverish child out to the doctor in cold weather — dressed in appropriate outerwear, of course, but not too warmly. The most common mistake made in dealing with a fever is to bundle the child up excessively, when she really needs to be kept cool. Inside, air conditioners and fans can be used to make a feverish child more comfortable, as long as she is not directly in the path of the air flow.

Finally, doctors today seldom recommend isolating a sick child to prevent other family members from catching the bug. With many communicable diseases, a child is most contagious during the incubation period — before symptoms ap-

pear — which means that family members will already have been exposed. Although certain hygienic steps should be taken to prevent the spread of illness *(box, page 98)*, keeping a sick child separated from other family members serves very little purpose.

Antidotes to boredom
Toddlers and preschoolers may be frightened by their symptoms or such sickroom rituals as having their temperature taken rectally. You can ease these anxieties by explaining the illness and treatment in simple terms and by projecting a positive attitude about getting well.

Boredom is much more likely to be a problem: Cut off from his usual routine and companions, your child will probably want to stay near you for company and diversion. If he prefers to lie down to rest, you can settle him in a central location, such as on the living-room couch, where he can watch the activities of the household. Naturally you will need to make extra time to read aloud or play games while he is sick. But you should also urge him to amuse himself some of the time — and provide him with ways to go about it — so that you can accomplish your own tasks.

Coloring books, puzzles and drawing paper are always good bets for keeping a child occupied. But a special treat might be a box of toys that is brought out only when the child is ill. The contents of the box need not be elaborate; the simple fact that they are toys the child has not seen for a while should be enough to hold his interest. Be sure to add new items to replace the toys that he outgrows.

For a younger child, the company of a "sick friend" — a doll, stuffed animal or toy that also needs to be nursed back to health — can be a pleasant way to occupy slow-moving time.

When Illness Disrupts Routine

For most parents, nursing a sick baby, toddler or preschooler through routine childhood maladies soon becomes second nature. Nevertheless, because children generally require more attention when they are sick, any illness that lasts more than a few days will certainly interfere with your usual schedule, as well as that of your child. During an illness, children have a tendency to regress — usually to a stage of behavior just past. A baby who is weaned may refuse to drink from anything but a bottle; a toddler recently toilet-trained may begin having accidents again. You should anticipate such temporary backsliding and make allowances for it. Things usually return to normal automatically once the child is well.

Sleep disturbances

It is also not unusual for a child's sleep to be disturbed during an ailment — even one as minor as a cold or diaper rash. More serious conditions, such as croup or ear infection, will almost certainly interfere with sleep. At such times it is best to respond quickly to the child's need, even if it is just a sip of water or a comforting word and hug. If your youngster is sick enough to need frequent checks during the night, you may find it convenient to sleep in his room or to bring his bed into your room. However, if the illness is not particularly serious, it will be less disruptive to stick to your normal sleeping arrangements.

In fact, while your child is ill, it is a good idea to adhere to regular nap and bedtime schedules as closely as possible, allowing for the possibility that he may need more sleep than usual. Bear in mind that if the child's illness turns out to be lengthy or requires bed rest during the day, the resulting tedium and monotony may make it difficult for him to fall asleep at night. In those cases, a change of scene

from his bed to the couch, perhaps coupled with a regimen of light physical activity, can help get him to bed more readily at the end of the day.

Though your youngster's sleep patterns should return to normal once he has recovered, he may resist if he has been allowed to be near you while he was ill. If he cries more than usual the first or second night alone, you might try comforting him without picking him up. Within a day or two he will most likely settle into his former routine without further resistance. But if he continues to have difficulty adjusting after a week, call the doctor — his irritability may signal a relapse of the illness.

Feeding a sick child

The old adage "Feed a cold and starve a fever" is another baseless myth about home nursing care, as is the notion that forcing a sick child to eat gives her strength to fight the illness. The fact is that sick children generally have less of an appetite than usual, and should be allowed to choose the type and amount of food they feel like eating. Most child-

hood illnesses are short-lived, and if your youngster does not eat a balanced diet for a few days she will not suffer from malnutrition or have a slower recovery. Even indulging special food requests is fine, as long as it doesn't interfere with any special diet the doctor may have prescribed *(box, below)*. Don't worry that giving in to a passion for milk shakes will create lasting mealtime problems. As soon as the illness has run its course, your child's appetite will probably return with gusto. In fact, she may eat ravenously for a week or so, and any weight lost during the illness will be quickly regained.

More important than food during an illness is sufficient intake of fluids: Don't force your child to eat if she isn't hungry, but make sure that she drinks plenty of liquids. With babies and young children, dehydration can be a serious threat — especially if fever, vomiting or diarrhea is present. Every half hour or so the child should be offered water, juice or some other clear liquid. If she is reluctant to drink, you may have to try a few creative ways of providing the fluids she needs *(box, page 93)*. ❖

Special Diets Your Child May Need to Follow

Doctors frequently suggest particular foods for children who are ill. A child suffering from bouts of vomiting, for example, will usually be prescribed a liquid diet until those symptoms have passed. Then the child may progress to soft, bland food that is easily digested. If diarrhea is present, a diet known as BRAT — an acronym for the foods that form it — may be suggested. For constipation, the child should eat foods high in fiber or bran content. Following are some examples of food allowed in each type of diet:

- Liquid — water, weak tea, clear broths, gelatin water, juice, flat soda
- Bland — poached eggs, soft cereals, toast soaked in milk, mashed vegetables, bananas, applesauce, noodles, bland soups, gelatin desserts, yogurt
- BRAT — bananas, rice, applesauce and toast
- High fiber — prune juice, bran, beans, fresh fruits, fresh vegetables, whole-grain cereals

Your Child's Physician

Selecting the Right Doctor

The choice of a physician for your child is an extremely important one that requires methodical investigation and thought. Your first concern will be to locate a person who is thoroughly qualified professionally to monitor your child's health, growth and development. But equally important are personal characteristics such as compassion, patience and an ability to communicate clearly. All parents, especially those who are having their first child, will want a doctor who can provide routine advice, reassurance and moral support along with good medical care.

Your child's physician should be either a pediatrician, whose practice is restricted to children, or a family practitioner, who is trained to care for adults as well as children. The best time to conduct your search for the right doctor is before your child is born, when you are not pressured by an immediate medical need.

Gathering recommendations

Ask the following professional sources to recommend qualified physicians:
- a doctor whom you respect
- the department of pediatrics or family practice at the nearest medical school
- the local medical society
- a reputable local hospital

You should also ask friends or family for suggestions. Although they are not necessarily reliable judges of medical competence, they can provide information about the personal characteristics of doctors and how they run their practices.

It is a good idea to check the credentials of the doctors who have been suggested to you by looking up their names in the *American Medical Association Directory of Physicians* or the *Directory of Medical Specialists* at your local library. Either book will provide such information as the physician's age, the medical school attended, institutions where post-graduate training was completed and all hospital affiliations. Make sure these hospitals and schools are reputable, fully accredited institutions.

Evaluating a practice

Once you have assessed the candidates' qualifications, pare your list down to a few names. Telephone their offices, and ask the office manager or a nurse about office practices and procedures. You will want to know about:
- the type of practice. Does the doctor work alone, in a partnership or group, or for a health maintenance organization? When he is unavailable, would a colleague treat your child?
- office hours. Are there special hours to accommodate working parents?
- office location. Is it convenient to your home? Does the physician have multiple office locations?
- fees for well-child checkups, sick visits, immunizations or care outside of normal office hours.
- whether the physician or a nurse answers routine telephone inquiries, and whether certain hours are set aside for routine calls.
- the arrangements for 24-hour coverage, including the names of the doctors who cover for him when he is on vacation or not on call.

If a doctor's qualifications and the way the practice is operated appear satisfactory, arrange an interview.

Interviewing the doctor

As you wait to talk to the doctor, observe the physical arrangement and general atmosphere in the waiting room. Is it a cheerful place? Are there toys, games and books for children of various ages? Are there separate waiting areas for sick and for well children? Do staff members appear efficient and courteous?

When you talk with the doctor, you will want to ask the following questions:
- How many well-baby checkups does he recommend during the first three years? What observations and procedures does he include in a checkup? Do checkups last at least 15 minutes?
- What is his attitude toward breast-feeding and bottle-feeding? (Is it compatible with yours?)
- Does he handle emergencies in his office or ask you to take the child to a hospital emergency room? Would he meet you there?
- If he is affiliated with more than one hospital, where would he admit your child if the youngster needed to be hospitalized?
- If you are a working mother, does the doctor have a positive attitude about your holding a job?

You may have areas of special concern to discuss. If, for example, you plan to raise your child as a vegetarian, find out whether the doctor is prepared to give you sound nutritional guidance.

As you interview the doctor, assess his personal characteristics as well. Does he answer your questions willingly, without making you feel rushed or patronized? Does he explain things clearly and listen to your point of view? In short, do you feel comfortable with the doctor and confident of his ability?

The choice you ultimately make will depend on how you weigh and balance the answers to all of these questions. Even if you have taken great care in selecting a doctor, however, you may find after several visits that your expectations are not being met in some important way. Discuss your concerns with the doctor. If the problem does not seem solvable, do not settle for an unsatisfactory doctor-parent or doctor-patient relationship. Instead, start the search process over again.

Warnings That Your Child Needs Medical Care

The exact symptoms of many illnesses and disorders are described in the entries on pages 46-127. Here is a general summary of symptoms and behaviors that indicate your child may be ill and you should call the doctor. (Signs that tell you your child needs emergency help are presented on page 10.)

- Fever: Any temperature above normal in a baby under four months old. A rectal temperature of 101° F. in an infant between four and 12 months old. In a youngster between one and two years old, a rectal reading of 103° F. or more. At any age, a rectal temperature of 104° F. or an oral one of 103° F. Any temperature lasting longer than 24 hours with no other symptoms, or lasting three days even if other symptoms are present.
- Pain: Any severe pain, or any pain recurring at regular intervals. Pain that is accompanied by loss of appetite. Pain localized in the lower right quadrant of the abdomen — which could indicate appendicitis.
- Diarrhea, vomiting: One episode of either in an infant younger than six months old. Three or more episodes of either within six hours' time in an older child.
- Listlessness, unresponsiveness or marked irritability.
- Headache that is especially severe, recurs frequently or lasts more than two hours. A headache that is accompanied by a stiff neck and fever or by dizziness.
- Any loss of appetite or difficulty feeding in a child younger than six months; a sudden refusal to eat or a moderate appetite loss lasting four days in an older child who is normally a good eater. Any loss of appetite accompanied by pain.
- Abnormal discharge issuing from any body opening.
- Blood in stool or vomit. Prolonged or excessive bleeding from a cut.
- Unusual rash.
- Earache.

Telephoning the Doctor

When you are worried about your youngster's physical well-being but are unsure whether the problem warrants the doctor's attention, it is best to call her. The problem may prove to be minor — in fact, pediatricians generally find that three out of four health concerns during early childhood can be cleared up with a telephone call rather than an office visit — but a caring doctor would prefer that you call whenever you are in doubt. Physicians expect more frequent telephone calls from first-time parents and from the parents of infants.

You should have key pieces of information at hand before you pick up the phone. Write down the principal reason for your call and the behavior or symptoms that concern you most. Be as precise as possible. If there is fever, for example, describe its onset, degree and duration. Have the names of any medication your child is taking, along with the phone number of your pharmacist. Be prepared to write down any instructions the doctor may give you.

If you are calling the doctor outside of office hours, your call may be taken by an answering service. Give the person your name, telephone number, the name and age of your child and a brief message. Ask him to repeat the information to be sure he has recorded it accurately. If the doctor has not returned your call within an hour, you should call the service and leave your message again.

Going to See the Doctor

To make the most of the brief time you will actually spend with the doctor during an office visit, you should organize yourself in advance. Before a routine visit, write down any questions you have or information that you think the physician would find useful.

If your child is sick, take along a written list of symptoms, in order of their appearance, and include anything unusual about the youngster's behavior. Note any recent changes in his routine, such as a new food or a different baby-sitter. Such details are easily forgotten in the flurry of the examination.

Preparing your child

Nearly all young children feel some apprehension when it comes to going to the doctor. You can help ease any such anxieties your youngster may have by using the following approach:

- Always give a child who is old enough to understand a few days' advance notice when you have planned a routine visit to the doctor.
- Read your youngster a story about a visit to the doctor or act out a visit to the doctor's office, using a toy medical kit or dolls.
- Explain to your youngster what the doctor or nurse will do. Be honest. Do not tell your child that a shot or some other painful procedure will not hurt when you know it will.
- Do not threaten that the doctor will be angry if the youngster is frightened or uncooperative. It is perfectly normal for children between six months and about three years of age to fear

Playing patient and letting your child be the doctor helps her act out fears and feel less anxious about an impending checkup. Your realistic reaction to a pretend shot reminds her that pain is sometimes a part of medical care.

doctors and other people whom they do not know well.

- Do not portray the doctor or nurse as a person with magical powers who can cure illness.

The routine visit

If you are going for a well-child checkup or other routine visit *(page 140),* write down the doctor's answers to the questions you have prepared. Listen carefully to advice or instructions, and ask for clarification of anything you do not understand. If you are charting your youngster's development in a baby book or fam-

ily medical record, make sure that you get the exact information you need before leaving the doctor's office.

The sick visit

When the physician has to examine your youngster because of illness, you should find out the answers to the following basic questions:

- What are the diagnosis and the cause of the illness?
- How long is its normal course? What, if any, changes in symptoms should you expect as the illness progresses?
- What is the treatment? If medicine is

prescribed, is there any information you need that is not explained on the pharmacy label?

- Could other symptoms develop that should be reported to the doctor as possible signs of complications?
- Is the disease contagious? If so, for how long? How can you prevent the disease from spreading to the rest of the members of your family?
- Can a recurrence of the youngster's illness be prevented?
- What home care techniques, such as a special diet or limits on activity, are called for? ⁂

Medical Specialties

A pediatrician or a family practitioner has the expertise to treat all the common ailments of childhood. If your child develops a severe or unusual condition, however, the doctor may decide to refer you to a specialist for diagnosis or treatment. Along with pediatric surgeons, who specialize in operating on children, physicians who limit their practice to the areas described below may also be called on to care for children with unusual health problems. The designations by which specialists are called are generally formed by substituting the suffix "ist" for the last letter or letters of the name of the specialty. If your doctor says she is referring your child to an otolaryngologist, she means a specialist in otolaryngology — ear, nose and throat problems. Surgeons also often concentrate their work in one or more of the following specialty areas.

Allergy: abnormal reactions to substances that are ordinarily harmless, such as certain foods or pollens.
Cardiology: diseases of the heart and blood vessels.
Dermatology: disorders of the skin.
Endocrinology: disorders of the organs and tissues that produce hormones.
Gastroenterology: disorders of the esophagus, stomach and intestines.
Hematology: blood disorders.
Neonatology: care of premature babies or other newborns with unusual problems.
Nephrology: kidney problems.
Neurology: disorders of the brain and nervous system.
Oncology: tumors and cancer.
Ophthalmology: diseases of the eye; vision disorders.
Orthopedics: disorders or injuries of bones, joints, tendons.
Otolaryngology: problems of the ear, nose and throat.
Psychiatry: mental and emotional disorders.
Pulmonary medicine: disorders of the lungs.
Urology: urinary-tract and male-genital-tract disorders.

Allied Health Workers

In addition to physicians, there are several other groups of professionals within the health-care system. You should be familiar with their titles and the nature of their work in case you need to call on their services for your child.

Audiologists administer tests and provide nonmedical treatment for ear problems. They frequently work with speech-language pathologists.
Child-life specialists help children cope with traumatic events such as surgery by encouraging them to play out their anxieties with dolls or mock hospital equipment.
Emergency medical technicians perform immediate lifesaving procedures.
Nurse practitioners or **nurse clinicians** are registered nurses with special training in preventive care, techniques of physical examination and health counseling.
Nutritionists use their specialized knowledge of diet to maintain health and to manage certain diseases.
Optometrists examine eyes, diagnose vision problems and prescribe corrective lenses. **Opticians** prepare prescribed lenses and fit patients with glasses.
Physical therapists use techniques such as exercise to develop strength and mobility in disabled patients and to maintain functions threatened by disease.
Physician assistants perform routine physical examinations, laboratory tests and other technical tasks under the supervision of a physician.
Psychologists administer tests and provide counseling in the field of mental and emotional health.
Registered nurses are trained in the care of the sick and in health maintenance. They work in physicians' offices, hospitals, clinics and many other types of health facilities.
Social workers assist a family with financial difficulties or any social problems that may arise after illness.
Speech-language pathologists diagnose and treat speech disorders through corrective exercises.

In the Hospital

Early Preparations

Statistics suggest that your child is unlikely to need hospitalization: In an average year, only five or six children in 100 enter hospitals. Despite these reassuring figures, however, you should be prepared to handle a hospital visit with your child in the event that she suffers an accident or illness requiring special care. Whether it involves a stay of hours or weeks, hospital care is a stressful, often painful and frightening experience for a youngster. You can make it easier for all concerned if you take steps in advance to choose a good facility, to inform yourself about what is likely to happen to your child and to give the youngster the emotional support she is sure to need.

Your first step should be to make sure that hospitalization is really necessary for the child. Sometimes hospitals can administer tests or treatments on an outpatient basis. This is ordinarily preferable for the child, though it may be less convenient for the doctor.

In many situations, of course, a stay in the hospital is unavoidable. These include any procedure requiring general anesthesia, serious head injuries, dangerous infections and other conditions that can change abruptly for the worse. Treatments impossible at home, such as intravenous fluid therapy, also call for hospitalization.

If your child must go to the hospital, you should make the best of the experience. Months afterward, your youngster may recall the positive aspects of her hospital stay — the ward's friendly staff and the interesting new toys she played with, or a postoperative diet of ice cream and gelatin desserts — while the negative memories fade away.

Choosing a hospital

On one of your regular visits to your child's pediatrician, you should ask her which hospital she recommends for emergency care and where she prefers to admit patients. Two hospitals close to your home may vary considerably in emergency-room care. And if you are scheduling hospitalization for your youngster for tests, treatment or surgery, where proximity is less important than it is in emergency care, you may have even more facilities to choose from.

Your doctor or her staff may be able to furnish much of the information you will need when choosing a hospital. You can also talk to the public-relations departments of the hospitals themselves or to people in your community who have personally dealt with the facilities. Some important questions to ask are:

- What is the overall reputation of a particular hospital?
- Is the emergency room fully staffed around the clock?
- What percentage of the hospital's patients are children?
- What special facilities, such as a playroom, does the pediatric unit have?
- Does the hospital offer a special preadmission tour or provide any information on preparing a youngster for hospitalization?
- Are parents allowed to visit their children 24 hours a day?
- Are there liberal visiting hours for siblings of hospitalized children?
- Does the hospital allow a parent to room in, or remain with the child throughout his hospitalization?
- Is a parent allowed to be with the child during tests and treatments, including the administration of anesthesia before surgery?
- Is the hospital a center for treating a particular type of disorder?
- What is the hospital's record in caring for patients with the same problem your youngster has?

Scheduling admission

When hospitalization is not urgent, you may be able to help your child by choosing an advantageous time to schedule his treatment. Some kinds of eye surgery, for instance, and certainly cosmetic surgery will probably not demand immediate scheduling. Try to postpone hospitalization when there is unusual stress in the family, such as the illness of a parent. A young child may believe he has caused the problem and that being sent to the hospital — which children often view as banishment — is a way of punishing him.

Take age into account. A very young child may be unable to understand why he's going to the hospital. If the procedure can wait until he is older, it is likely to be less upsetting. An older child may also be mature enough to tolerate a procedure as an outpatient, under a local, rather than general, anesthetic.

Finally, make sure that your child is admitted no earlier before a scheduled procedure than is absolutely necessary. This will ensure that his stay in the hospital is as short as possible.

Preparing yourself and your child

Before your child leaves for the hospital, learn as much as you can about what will happen there by asking the doctor to explain upcoming tests and treatments. Have him recommend some clearly written books or articles on the subject.

Then inform your child. If she is under the age of six, two or three days' advance notice of a hospital stay is about right; a week is appropriate for an older child. Tell her simply and honestly what will be done. It may help to read her a story about a child who goes to the hospital. If possible, take her on a tour of the building where she will stay. At the same time, be attuned to her fears of pain and separation. Encourage her to talk about or act out her anxieties and reassure her, focusing on the solution to her problem rather than the problem itself.

You can also help your child feel more comfortable at the hospital if you let her take some familiar and beloved possessions. If she is being hospitalized for a contagious disease, however, you should leave home any irreplaceable items, as everything the youngster uses in the hospital will be either destroyed or sterilized before she is discharged.

The items listed at right are usually acceptable to a hospital, but you may wish to check first:

- pajamas; several changes of underwear; one or two outfits for wearing between treatments
- toilet articles, such as a toothbrush, hairbrush and comb
- toys, games and books
- blanket or other comfort object
- photographs of family members

While Your Child Is Hospitalized

Rooming in
A child under six copes with hospitalization much better if a parent rooms in — is admitted with her, shares her room and stays with her as much as possible. If the hospital offers a rooming-in program, take advantage of it, your circumstances permitting. If not, you should do the next best thing and spend as much time at the hospital as you can. When you end a visit, do not try to sneak away unnoticed. Tell your child you are leaving and when you plan to return. Try not to let the youngster's tears distress you. It is normal for her to cry when you arrive as well as when you leave.

If you do room in with your child, take only the necessities, as space will be limited. You may have to sleep on a cot or in a chair. Find out beforehand what the hospital's eating arrangements are for parents. If you cannot order food from your child's room, take snacks to tide you over until you can get out for a meal.

Some hospitals allow rooming-in parents to participate in or take over some aspects of their youngster's care. Ask the hospital staff how you can help out while you are there.

Protecting your child's rights
Hospitals belonging to the American Hospital Association support the Patient's Bill of Rights, which ensures respect and consideration, privacy and information about treatment. A child is due the same rights as an adult patient.

Look for the Patient's Bill of Rights posted in public areas of the hospital, or ask for a copy from the public-relations department. Among the key provisions is the right to know the diagnosis of the child's condition and what his physician plans to do. Explanations should be given in clear language that you can understand. You also have the right to know in advance the name of a treatment or procedure, its purpose and any risks that it may pose. The parent should also be told about any alternative.

Your youngster has the right to privacy and confidentiality. Information about his case should be shared only among the people caring for him or with other medical personnel they consult.

Although patients' rights are policies, not laws, you as a parent should talk to the youngster's physician or other staff members if you feel the policies are not being followed.

On occasion the rights of the child may conflict with the parent's wishes. If a parent denies permission for a treatment and the physician believes the refusal endangers the youngster, the doctor may act on the child's behalf and ask a court to overrule the parent.

When your child comes home
Children commonly show some aftereffects of a hospital stay. These may include disturbed sleep and nightmares, regressive, fearful or disruptive behavior, and a change in eating habits.

You can help your child bounce back to normal by reestablishing his usual routines quickly. Don't fuss over him or allow your normal discipline to lapse because of his illness, but do encourage the youngster to talk about his experience if he seems willing to do so.

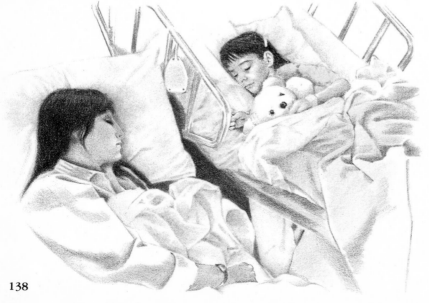

Your child will suffer less fear and stress over a hospital stay if you can arrange to spend the night in her room. Your accommodation may be an adjacent bed, a cot or just a pillow and a chair; but any inconvenience is minor compared with the comfort your youngster draws from your presence.

Emergency Care
Traveling to the hospital

For fast action, learn in advance the best route from your home to the emergency room. If your child's condition allows it, call her doctor before departing. Take the following things along or have someone bring them as soon as possible:

- health-insurance and hospitalization cards; your social security number and other personal identification
- your child's immunization record
- any medication your child is taking
- containers of any dangerous substance swallowed
- a blanket or other comfort object
- bottle and formula, diapers
- the telephone number of your youngster's physician

On the way to the emergency room, tell your child where she is going and why, and reassure her that the strangers there will be helping her get better.

If an ambulance or helicopter takes your child to the hospital, medical treatment may begin during the ride. Since both the treatment and the ride may frighten her, you should stay with her if possible. Prepare her for the loud siren and the speed of an ambulance.

If medical procedures do begin en route to the hospital, try to minimize any feeling of force or coercion. For instance, you might volunteer to hold an oxygen mask in place instead of its being strapped over the child's face.

At the emergency room

When you arrive at the emergency room, your child's condition will quickly be assessed. If she is in no immediate danger, there may be a wait before treatment. In this interval you will be asked to sign a standard legal release and other forms.

Learn the names and titles of the people treating your child. Find out what procedures are being carried out, why they are necessary and whether you can stay with your child throughout her treatment *(see box, below)*. In a crowded emergency room a staffer may ask you to restrain your youngster or to do something that would cause her pain. You may decline and ask that someone else do it if you find this too upsetting. Remember, though, that all emergency-room procedures, however distressing they may seem, are a necessary part of assessing and treating your child's condition.

If you would like to consult with your child's regular doctor or a specialist about tests or treatments recommended by the emergency-room staff, inform the attending physician. An emergency room should have a list of specialists on call. If a doctor you do not know is going to be called in to consult or to admit your child to the hospital, make sure you write down his name for later reference.

Emergency-room staff members are always on the alert for child abuse, so do not be surprised if you are asked probing questions about an accident.

Before taking your child home, be sure you understand the diagnosis and what further care your child will need. ❖

Helping Your Child Weather Tests and Treatments

Panic often surpasses pain when a child is approached by a needle-bearing stranger or a mysterious machine. Here are some common procedures your child might face in the emergency room, and how you can help.

Drawing blood for diagnostic purposes invariably upsets children old enough to know what a needle means, and the sight of blood itself can be distressing. For very young children a heel prick may suffice; for older children, the technician taps a large vessel in the inside forearm. Hold the child in your lap if possible, and try to keep her eyes — and yours — off the needle. Tell her it will sting "like a bee" but will soon stop hurting. Allow the youngster to protest or cry, but you should warn her not to move.

Sutures are needed to hold lacerated skin together when a cut is long or deep. The doctor may use local anesthesia, unless she feels the injection would be just as painful as the sutures. Metal staples are often used for a straight, clean cut; otherwise the doctor sews small stitches with a special needle and nylon thread. Either technique may traumatize your child; your role as comforter and calmer may be especially valuable. Tell the child she can cry or shout if it hurts, but that she must stay very still.

Splints or casts will be applied to immobilize a fracture. In many cases this can be done without an anesthetic. Be aware that a young child may see a cast as a mutilation or a new limb replacing the one that has seemingly vanished. Reassure her that the cast will be gone "before vacation" or "in six Saturdays" and in the meantime it will make her "special" among her friends.

X-rays taken by a huge metal machine with robot-like moving parts often frighten a child. Explain it as a big camera that will take a picture inside her body. Any pain will come from preliminaries such as the injection of a dye or the twisting of the affected part into proper position. To help keep the child calm and motionless, the operator may allow you to stay with her if you wear a protective lead apron.

A Program of Preventive Care

Well-Child Checkups

Keeping a child in good health demands consistent attention on the part of the parents and regular examinations by a physician. The foundation of your program of preventive medicine should be a schedule of well-child visits with your family physician or pediatrician.

These visits will generally begin with a preliminary interview, if you are new to the doctor, or with a prenatal visit if the baby is to be your first. When the baby is born, the doctor will usually administer a newborn examination within 24 hours of delivery, following up with a discharge exam before you leave the hospital. The first office checkup usually takes place at two weeks of age. After that the doctor will examine your child when she is two, four, six, nine, 12, 15, 18 and 24 months old, then annually until the age of six.

The checkups should reinforce your own preventive care in a number of ways. For one, regular examinations of the child allow the doctor to monitor physical, emotional and intellectual development, so that potential problems can be detected early. Well-child checkups also include screening tests for several rare but potentially serious physical problems, such as congenital hip dislocation or undescended testes, and immunizations against a range of childhood diseases, including polio, measles and whooping cough *(box, page 58)*.

Regular checkups also expose your child to doctors and nurses, so that if she becomes ill, the medical system will seem more familiar and less ominous. In addition, visits to a doctor underscore the importance of routine health care, encouraging the youngster to develop good health habits and, eventually, to take responsibility for her own health.

Getting answers to your questions

Perhaps most important, regular checkups give you an opportunity to ask the doctor about whatever concerns you. You may want to make a list of questions before each visit, in case they slip your mind in the course of the examination.

Your concerns will no doubt change as your child grows and changes. After a newborn exam you may want to discuss skin rashes, the umbilical cord or sleep patterns, for example, whereas at the stage known as the "terrible twos," your questions will more likely involve toilet training, temper tantrums or naps. Whatever your child's age, your questions and concerns should be central to the agenda of a well-child visit.

Eye care

The physician will evaluate the state of your youngster's vision and eye movement at each well-child checkup, testing visual acuity beginning about the age of three. Such examinations detect poor vision — usually nearsightedness — in about 20 percent of preschool children, who are then referred to an ophthalmologist or optometrist for corrective glasses. Some pediatricians also recommend a routine ophthalmological evaluation between the ages of three and four, when children are old enough to cooperate in a full visual examination.

But none of these tests is a substitute for parental observation. Your vigilance for signs of vision problems is particularly important with defects such as crosseye and nearsightedness, which can block normal development of the brain's visual pathways and cause permanent vision loss *(see Eyes, page 87)*.

Early Dental Care

The foundations for your child's dental health are actually laid months before birth, when the teeth are beginning to form in the fetus. A well-balanced diet of foods containing calcium, phosphorus and vitamin D is necessary during pregnancy for building strong teeth in the baby. The mother's diet should also contain fluoride, an element that reinforces the crystal structure of tooth enamel. If the water in your area does not contain adequate levels of fluoride, your pediatrician, obstetrician or dentist can prescribe a fluoride supplement for use during pregnancy and nursing. The pediatrician may also prescribe fluoride supplements for your baby's first months or years of life.

When the first teeth appear

The sequence in which baby teeth emerge from the gums is relatively predictable *(chart, opposite)*, but the timing is quite variable. The first tooth usually appears between five and seven months of age, but it is not uncommon to see teething begin as late as 15 months. Teething pains, which precede the appearance of each tooth by one or two months, are signaled by periods of drooling, fussiness and compulsive chewing. The pain is worst during the emergence of the first four molars.

Children continue to cut baby teeth intermittently over a period of two years, and parents often mistakenly assume that teething is to blame for the colds, vomiting, diarrhea or fevers that their child may suffer during this time. These are symptoms of real illnesses that have no connection with teething, and they should be evaluated in the ordinary way;

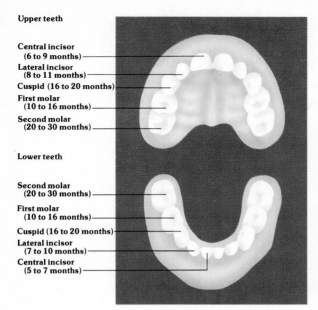

Upper teeth

Central incisor
(6 to 9 months)

Lateral incisor
(8 to 11 months)

Cuspid (16 to 20 months)

First molar
(10 to 16 months)

Second molar
(20 to 30 months)

Lower teeth

Second molar
(20 to 30 months)

First molar
(10 to 16 months)

Cuspid (16 to 20 months)

Lateral incisor
(7 to 10 months)

Central incisor
(5 to 7 months)

How Baby Teeth Come In

A baby's first tooth — usually one of the two lower incisors in the front of the mouth — begins to appear around the sixth month, on average. From then on baby teeth will gradually erupt from the front to the back of the mouth, roughly following the sequence indicated at left. The second molars are the last baby teeth to appear, usually when the child is between two and three years of age.

if your teething child's behavior indicates illness, you should call the doctor.

Dealing with teething problems

When your child is teething, do not let him chew on furniture or woodwork, which may be coated with poisonous lead-based paint; also be watchful with plastic toys, which can break into sharp splinters. To ease teething pains, give him something hard and cold to chew on, such as a teething ring or a washcloth tied around an ice cube. Do not attempt the impossible task of keeping teething rings sterile; you may, however, want to rinse them off if they fall in the garden or are mouthed by the family dog.

If the teething pains are severe, ask your doctor about giving acetaminophen. Some children are also comforted by having their gums rubbed.

Preventing tooth decay

The moment your child's teeth emerge you must begin the battle against cavities. These holes in the tooth enamel are caused by bacteria that reside in the mouth, producing a film called plaque that covers the teeth. When the bacteria encounter sugars — present not only in candy but in milk, fruit and many other foods — they secrete acids that corrode the tooth enamel and eat through the soft underlying pulp, eventually destroying

the entire tooth. Such damage threatens not only the baby teeth but the permanent teeth that lie beneath them.

You can combat oral bacteria in two ways. First, limit consumption of sugar. Cavity growth depends on the stickiness of sugary foods, the concentration of the sugar and the frequency and duration of exposure. In practice, this means avoiding sticky foods such as caramel and cotton candy; ice cream and fruit juice are less harmful. Diluted sugar, such as that in fruit or soda, is safer than the concentrated sugar in candy. And an occasional sweet snack or dessert — quickly eaten and done with — is preferable to candies such as lollipops, which coat the teeth with sugar for prolonged periods. For the same reason, you should never use bottles of milk, fruit juice or sugar water as pacifiers or sleeping aids.

The second action you should take is to clean your child's teeth regularly to remove bacteria. When your baby first cuts teeth, wipe the teeth along with the gums every evening after dinner, using a clean washcloth or a gauze pad. When your youngster is between the ages of one and two, encourage him to brush his teeth after meals while you brush your own. Use a child's toothbrush with soft, rounded bristles and a small amount of fluoride toothpaste approved by the American Dental Association. Avoid toothpastes that contain abrasives. Teach

your child to spit out the toothpaste, so he does not swallow too much fluoride.

For the first year or so, a child's tooth-brushing will be enthusiastic but ineffective. After letting him brush on his own, tactfully offer assistance and do the real work yourself. After the child is two, when motor coordination has improved, you can begin teaching correct techniques: Brush vertically, away from each gum, on the outside and then the inside surfaces of the teeth. Then scrub the chewing surface vigorously to remove food particles and bacterial plaque.

First visits to the dentist

When your child is three years old, it is time to begin regular visits to a dentist. Choose either a pedodontist — a pediatric dentist with specific training in children's dental problems — or a licensed dentist who enjoys young patients. Such dentists try to make each visit a happy experience, using show-and-tell methods and terms such as "tooth-feeler" and "tooth-shiner" to explain their probes and drills. Try to schedule appointments with the dentist for the morning, when your child is alert and cooperative, rather than at times when he is likely to be grouchy or hungry.

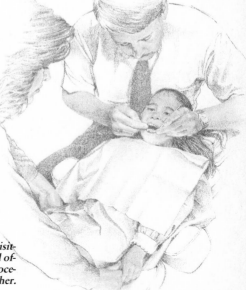

Your child may feel better about visiting the dentist if you stay with her and offer reassurance during dental procedures that are new or frightening to her.

Nutrition

Sound dietary principles for children are much the same as those for adults. Your child should eat a variety of fresh foods from the four major groups — meat, dairy products, fruit and vegetables. The diet should be high in fiber and low in salt, cholesterol and fat — particularly the saturated fats in animal products such as butter and red meat.

These simple rules belie the difficulties of feeding a temperamental toddler or preschooler. To minimize problems, prepare foods that your child likes to eat and give him small portions; he will ask for seconds if he is still hungry.

In fact, your child's appetite is your best guide to how much he needs. Before the age of three, children are creatures of instinct where eating is concerned: Given access to a variety of foods, they will naturally select the items that make up a healthy diet. After three, children fall into family- and social-eating patterns and will need guidance in choosing a diet.

Even then, however, avert mealtime confrontations whenever possible. It is better to avoid serving a food your child does not like for a few weeks than to engage in battle whenever it is presented.

Vitamin and fluoride supplements

Generally, a child who is getting a wholesome diet does not need vitamin supplements, but there are a few exceptions. Premature babies or those afflicted with metabolic defects, malabsorption problems or food allergies do occasionally require supplements. Some pediatricians prescribe vitamin D for all breast-fed babies. In most cases, however, even the pickiest two-year-old eater gets enough vitamins from an ordinary, balanced diet. It is best to ask your doctor about giving vitamin supplements.

Fluoride supplements, like vitamins, are usually unnecessary. But if the water your child drinks is unfluoridated, you may need to provide fluoride to keep his teeth healthy.

Height and weight

At each well-child checkup, your doctor will measure your youngster's height, weight and — until the child reaches six months — the head circumference. The resulting figures may then be plotted on standard percentile curves that indicate whether the youngster's development is average, below average or above average for her sex and age.

Such information can provide clues to medical problems, but it should be interpreted carefully, with an understanding of the many other factors involved in a child's health. There are substantial natural variations in growth patterns and height-weight proportions. And because the charts include only overall weight, an active, muscular child and a sedentary, chubby one may have the same percentile weight rating.

Underweight children seldom suffer ill effects, but childhood obesity is a serious problem that often starts in infancy and persists for life. You can avert weight problems by feeding your child as much food as she wants, but no more.

To keep the process of eating in proper perspective, do not use food as a bribe or pacifier. Beginning when your child is about six to nine months, set regular mealtimes, with perhaps one morning and afternoon snack rather than frequent, unlimited snacks. If your child becomes overweight despite your best efforts, do not restrict her mealtime food intake without first consulting your doctor. ❖

Maintaining Medical Records

Your child's doctor will keep complete medical records in his office, but you should keep at home your own health history of your youngster. This will ensure that you have the information you need to complete forms for school or summer camp when the time comes, and it will simplify switching doctors or moving. It may also help eliminate unnecessary shots. Most important, a child's detailed health history is vital in the emergency room, where her pediatrician's records may not be immediately available. Your records should include these key facts, with dates where appropriate:

- names, addresses and phone numbers of current and previous doctors
- allergies the child has, including reactions to drugs and insect stings
- any drugs the child is taking
- the youngster's height, weight and head circumference
- immunizations for polio, diphtheria-tetanus-pertussis (DTP), measles-mumps-rubella (MMR) and influenza
- results of hearing tests, eye exams or tests for tuberculosis, and any lab procedures such as urinalysis, X-rays and blood tests
- common childhood illnesses such as chicken pox, recurrent earaches or tonsillitis
- any serious illnesses or injuries the child suffers, especially injuries to the head and fractures
- major or minor surgery
- any incidences of hospitalization
- a summary of your child's prenatal life, birth and health during the newborn months, including any health problems the mother experienced during pregnancy
- a family medical history, which should include summaries of any problems of the youngster's siblings, parents, aunts and uncles or grandparents — particularly a history of allergies or asthma, diabetes, high blood pressure, tuberculosis, kidney disease, heart disease, congenital malformations, seizures, anemia or bleeding problems

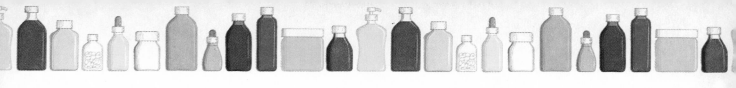

A Reference Guide to Medicines

In this chart, drugs commonly used to treat young children are arranged alphabetically by their generic chemical names, with brand names following. Drugs are available over the counter unless marked "Rx," in which case they require a prescription. Those available both ways are marked Rx/OTC. Drugs that contain more than one active ingredient appear with an asterisk. Each entry lists the drug's intended effect along with side effects that may occur; the "Special cautions" column describes symptoms of the most harmful side effects and advises you when to notify your child's doctor. Occasionally, for instance, a drug will have a so-called paradoxical effect and cause a reaction that is the opposite of the intended one. Remember that any medicine is a potentially dangerous substance for a young child. If you have a question regarding a medication, do not take chances; call your pharmacist or physician right away.

DRUG	Intended effect	Minor side effects	Serious side effects	Special cautions
ACETAMINOPHEN CHILDREN'S TYLENOL TEMPRA SYRUP & DROPS INFANTS' TYLENOL DROPS	Relieves pain and fever	Upset stomach	Reduced blood cell counts; skin rash; liver damage in overdose (rare)	Inform doctor if child develops sore throat, bruising, bleeding or weakness. Inspect drug packaging for signs of tampering (broken seals, discolored solution).
AMOXICILLIN (Rx) AMOXIL LAROTID	Treats bacterial infection.	Nausea; vomiting; diarrhea	Inflammation of the colon (colitis); allergic reactions, such as skin rash, wheezing or itching; reduced blood cell counts.	Child should take as directed until drug is gone. Consult doctor before use if child has stomach or intestinal disorders, kidney disease or allergies, particularly to penicillins. Notify doctor if child develops sore throat, bleeding or bruising, or persistant stomach cramps and diarrhea.
AMOXICILLIN AND CLAVULANIC ACID (Rx) AUGMENTIN	Actions similar to AMOXICILLIN			
AMPICILLIN (Rx) PRINCIPEN AMCILL	Actions similar to AMOXICILLIN			
ASPIRIN ST. JOSEPH'S ASPIRIN FOR CHILDREN	Relieves inflammation, pain and fever; treats juvenile rheumatoid arthritis	Upset stomach	Ringing in ears; severe nausea, stomach pain or vomiting; bleeding from stomach; hearing loss, drowsiness or confusion (overdose); allergic reactions, such as skin rash, itching or wheezing; anemia; bleeding due to slowed blood clotting; Reye syndrome	Consult doctor before use if child has stomach problems, ulcers, anemia, kidney or liver disease, bleeding disorders, asthma or allergies. Do not use for influenza-like illnesses or viral infections: Aspirin has been linked with Reye syndrome. Acetaminophen is an alternative. Stop taking aspirin five days before surgery. Avoid if tablets smell like vinegar. Give with milk or food. Notify doctor if child develops severe stomach pain or bloody or tarry stools. Consult doctor before use if child is taking other drugs.
BACITRACIN (Topical) BACIGUENT	Prevents or treats skin infections	Minor skin irritation or burning	Allergic reactions, such as skin rash or itching	Inform doctor if skin irritation or rash develops. Clean affected area of skin prior to application.
BENZOCAINE (Topical) AMERICAINE SOLARCAINE	Relief of minor burns, itching, bruises and sunburn	Burning; stinging; skin irritation	May impair oxygen-carrying capacity of blood in infants; skin rash or itching (allergic reactions); restlessness or drowsiness, irregular heartbeat or convulsions (overdose)	Notify doctor if child develops a blue color of the skin or displays weakness or breathing problems. Inform doctor of excessive restlessness or drowsiness — signs of overdose. Do not exceed recommended dose on label. Avoid use in the eyes. Consult doctor before use if child is allergic to any local anesthetic.
BROMPHENIRAMINE DIMETANE DIMETAPP*	Relieves symptoms of allergies, colds, sinusitis and hay fever	Drowsiness; dizziness; dry mouth or throat; difficulty urinating; nervousness; restlessness; insomnia	Rapid heartbeat; nightmares or hallucinations; convulsions; shortness of breath; decreased blood cell counts	Consult doctor before use if child has heart disease, urinary obstruction or seizure disorders. Inform doctor if child develops weakness, sore throat, bleeding or bruising. Excessive drowsiness can occur if taken with other antihistamines or depressants.

DRUG	Intended effect	Minor side effects	Serious side effects	Special cautions
CALAMINE LOTION CALAMOX CALADRYL*	Eases itching and pain of poison oak, poison ivy, insect bites, other skin irritations	None	Allergic reactions, such as worsening of skin rash or irritation	Avoid use in eyes, mouth or on genitalia. Consult doctor if condition worsens or if rash or irritation develops.
CARBAMAZEPINE (Rx) TEGRETOL	Controls seizure disorders	Drowsiness; clumsiness; nausea; vomiting; lightheadedness; diarrhea; dry mouth	Blurred or double vision; reduced blood cell counts; severe skin rash; liver damage; irregular heartbeat; inflammation of the nerves (neuritis); kidney problems; abnormal eye movements; hallucinations	Consult doctor before use if child has heart problems, blood disorders, or kidney or liver disease. Notify doctor if child develops sore throat, weakness, bruising or bleeding. Inform doctor if child develops dark urine or yellowing of the whites of the eyes or skin, or if blurring of vision occurs. May reduce the effects of theophylline, an antiasthma drug. Erythromycin may increase the side effects of carbamazepine.
CARBAMIDE PEROXIDE DEBROX* MURINE EAR DROPS*	Softens ear wax	None	None	Consult doctor if child's ear develops redness, irritation, swelling or pain that persists or increases while this medicine is used.
CEFACLOR (Rx) CECLOR	Treats bacterial infection, particularly ear infection (otitis media)	Diarrhea; nausea; vomiting	Allergic reactions, such as skin rash, itching or wheezing	Consult doctor before use if child has any allergies, particularly to penicillins, or if child has stomach disorders. Give with food if upset stomach occurs. Child should take as directed until drug is gone.
CEFADROXIL (Rx) DURICEF ULTRACEF	Actions similar to CEFACLOR			
CEPHALEXIN (Rx) KEFLEX	Actions similar to CEFACLOR			
CHLORPHENIRAMINE CHLOR-TRIMETON	Actions similar to BROMPHENIRAMINE			
CLOTRIMAZOLE (Topical) (Rx) LOTRIMIN MYCELEX	Treats ringworm and other fungal infections	Stinging; burning; itching	Severe skin rash; hives; blistering or peeling of skin; severe skin irritation	Avoid application to the eyes. Check with doctor if skin problem has not improved after four weeks of treatment.
CODEINE (Rx) TYLENOL WITH CODEINE ROBITUSSIN-AC SYRUP* TUSSI-ORGANIDIN LIQUID*	Suppresses cough; relieves mild-to-moderate pain	Constipation; drowsiness; loss of appetite; nausea; vomiting; dizziness	Difficulty breathing; restlessness or excitement (paradoxical effect); slowed heartbeat; confusion; physical dependence with high doses over prolonged periods; allergic reactions, such as skin rash and itching	Consult doctor before use if child has asthma, lung disease, liver disease or a heart condition. May cause excessive depressant effects when given with other sedatives, including antihistamines.
CROMOLYN (Rx) INTAL	Prevents asthmatic attacks	Coughing; hoarseness; watery eyes; dry mouth; stuffy nose	Skin rash; chest tightness, difficulty breathing or swallowing; dizziness; severe skin rash; pneumonia	Consult doctor before use if child has liver or kidney disease. This medication will not relieve an acute asthmatic attack. Gargling or rinsing of the mouth after use may help prevent dry mouth, hoarseness and throat irritation. Notify doctor if child develops chest pain, difficulty breathing or chills.
CYPROHEPTADINE (Rx) PERIACTIN	Treats allergic conditions; increases appetite	Drowsiness; irritability, excitation or nervousness (paradoxical effect); dry mouth; nausea; diarrhea; difficult urination; increased appetite or weight gain	Reduced blood cell counts; hallucinations or delirium; difficulty breathing; severe drowsiness; convulsions	Consult doctor before use if child has seizure disorders or respiratory disease. Not for use in premature or newborn infants. Notify doctor if child develops sore throat, fever, bleeding or bruising. Excessive drowsiness can occur when given with other sedative-type drugs or antihistamines.

DRUG	Intended effect	Minor side effects	Serious side effects	Special cautions
DEXAMETHASONE (Rx) DECADRON	Actions similar to PREDNISONE			
DEXAMETHASONE (Ophthalmic) (Rx) DECADRON PHOSPHATE OPHTHALMIC	Effects similar to HYDROCORTISONE (Ophthalmic)			
DEXTROMETHOR-PHAN CONGESPIRIN FOR CHILDREN PEDIA CARE #1 ROMILAR CHILDREN'S ROBITUSSIN-DM*	Suppresses coughing	Dizziness; drowsiness; upset stomach; vomiting	Difficulty breathing with large doses; confusion, restlessness or excitement (overdose)	Consult doctor before use if child has asthma or other respiratory disorders or liver disease. Notify doctor if cough persists after use for seven days or if skin rash, fever or headache is present with the cough.
DIAZEPAM (Rx) VALIUM	Relieves excessive anxiety; useful in some types of seizure disorders	Drowsiness; slurred speech; clumsiness; weakness	Excitement, irritability or hallucinations (paradoxical effect); confusion and behavioral problems; weakness; reduced blood cell counts; liver damage; difficulty breathing	Consult doctor before administering if child has liver or pulmonary disease. Consult doctor before discontinuing the medication after extended use, since withdrawal symptoms can occur (agitation, confusion, seizures). Enhanced depression of the central nervous system can occur when this drug is combined with other sedatives or narcotics. This medicine may interfere with the effects of phenytoin, a drug used to control seizures.
DICLOXACILLIN (Rx) DYNAPEN PATHOCIL	Actions similar to AMOXICILLIN			
DIMENHYDRINATE DRAMAMINE	Prevents motion sickness	Drowsiness; dizziness; nervousness; dry mouth	Confusion; excitation, restlessness or hallucinations (paradoxical effect); nightmares; rapid heartbeat	This drug should be taken at least one hour before travel for maximum effect. Extreme drowsiness can occur if taken with antihistamines or other sedatives. Tablets should not be chewed. Meclizine (Bonine®) is an alternative drug for motion sickness that can be given to a child who needs a chewable preparation.
DIPHENHYDRAMINE BENADRYL BENYLIN	Relieves allergies, hayfever and skin problems; used as a mild sedative	Drowsiness; dry mouth; dizziness; difficult urination	Irregular heartbeat; hallucinations; confusion; delirium	Consult doctor before administering this medication if child has heart disease, urinary obstruction or high blood pressure. Extreme drowsiness can occur if diphenhydramine is given in combination with sedatives or with other antihistamines.
EPINEPHRINE (RX/OTC) ADRENALIN CHLORIDE (OTC) MICRONEFRIN (Rx) MEDIHALER-EPI (OTC) SUS-PHRINE (Rx)	Treats acute attacks of asthma and other allergic conditions	Rapid heartbeat; nausea; headache; nervousness; tremors; dizziness	Irregular heartbeat; chest pain; increased blood pressure	Consult doctor before use if child has high blood pressure, heart disease, diabetes, thyroid disease or a neurological condition. Do not use if solution is cloudy or pink-brown in color.
ERYTHROMYCIN (Rx) PEDIAMYCIN ERY PED ERYTHROCIN ILOSONE	Treats bacterial infection	Nausea; vomiting; diarrhea	Liver damage (more frequent with Ilosone®)	Consult doctor before use if child has liver disease. Child should take as directed until drug is gone. Inform doctor if symptoms worsen or do not improve after several days. This drug may increase side effects of carbamazepine, a drug used for seizure control. The side effects of theophylline, a drug used to treat asthma, may be enhanced with this medication.

145

DRUG	Intended effect	Minor side effects	Serious side effects	Special cautions
ERYTHROMYCIN AND SULFIOSOXA-ZOLE (Rx) PEDIAZOLE	Treats ear infections (otitis media) and acute sinusitis	Nausea; diarrhea; vomiting; appetite loss	Allergic reactions, such as skin rash or wheezing; reduced blood cell counts; severe skin reactions; liver or kidney damage; muscle aches or pains	Consult doctor before administering if child has porphyria or liver disease. Child should drink plenty of fluids with this medication and should take as directed until drug is gone. Do not give to infants under one month of age. Inform doctor if child develops sore throat, fever, bruising or bleeding, pain on urination or blood in the urine, or yellowing of the whites of the eyes or of the skin. This medicine may enhance the side effects of theophylline, which is a drug used for asthma.
FERROUS SULFATE, FUMARATE AND GLUCONATE FER-IN-SOL FERGON FEOSTAT	Treats anemia	Appetite loss; nausea; vomiting; constipation	Severe stomach pain or cramps, decreased blood pressure, shock (overdose)	Consult doctor before use if child has hemochromatosis, liver disease, stomach disorders or blood disorders. Child should take with food to minimize stomach upset. Avoid concurrent use with antacids or tetracycline — take at least two hours apart.
HYDROCORTISONE (Rx) CORTEF HYDROCORTONE	Actions similar to PREDNISONE			
HYDROCORTISONE (Ophthalmic) (Rx) HYDROCORTONE OPHTHALMIC OPTEF NEO-CORTEF*	Relieves severe eye inflammation	Stinging; burning; watery eyes	Increased pressure in the eye (glaucoma), vision difficulties, eye infections; cataract formation (all with prolonged use)	Consult doctor before administering if child has any eye disorders or viral infections of the eye. Inform doctor if no improvement occurs after five to seven days, or if condition worsens. Notify doctor if child develops blurring of vision or pain in the eye or sees halos around lights.
HYDROCORTISONE (Topical) (Rx/OTC) CORTAID (OTC) CALDECORT (OTC) HYTONE (Rx) CORTISPORIN* (Rx)	Relieves minor skin irritations, itching and rashes; treats insect bites, poison ivy, poison oak or sumac	Itching; irritation; dryness; burning	Aggravation of local infection; skin eruptions; blistering of the skin; suppression of adrenal gland function with prolonged use	Do not use for chicken pox and fungal infections. Consult doctor before use if child has any skin infection. Avoid eye contact. Avoid plastic pants or tight-fitting diapers on areas being treated. Do not exceed recommended dose. Inform doctor of excessive pain, redness or blistering of skin. Do not apply for more than a two-week period.
HYDROXYZINE (Rx) ATARAX VISTARIL	Relieves itching, allergies, nausea and vomiting; produces mild sedation	Drowsiness; dry mouth	Severe drowsiness; tremors; severe skin rash; convulsions	Combined use with other antihistamines, sedatives or narcotics may result in extreme drowsiness.
IBUPROFEN (Rx/OTC) ADVIL (OTC) NUPRIN (OTC) RUFEN (Rx) MOTRIN (Rx)	Treats pain, fever and inflammation; used for juvenile rheumatoid arthritis	Nausea; vomiting; diarrhea or constipation; dizziness; lightheadedness; drowsiness	Ringing in the ears; decreased blood cell counts; fluid retention; ulcers; vision disturbances; severe skin rash; kidney damage	Do not give to children under six years of age unless authorized by doctor. Consult doctor before use if child has asthma, blood or stomach disorders, kidney impairment, or if child has had unusual reactions to aspirin or other drugs used to treat inflammation. Child should take with food or milk to lessen stomach upset. Risk of stomach irritation or ulcers is increased when ibuprofen is taken with aspirin or other anti-inflammatory drugs. Notify doctor if child develops sore throat, weakness, bleeding or bruising, swelling of legs or feet, or if pain on urination or blood in urine occurs. Notify doctor of black, tarry stools.
INSULIN (Rx) REGULAR ILETIN HUMULIN NOVOLIN	Treats diabetes mellitus	Local reactions at injection site	Nervousness, shakiness, rapid heartbeat, nausea, sweating, difficulty breathing, pale skin (due to low blood sugar from overdose); severe allergic reactions	Parents must thoroughly understand the disease and how to administer insulin properly. They must be able to differentiate symptoms of low and high blood sugar. Child should not take any other medication unless authorized by doctor.

DRUG	Intended effect	Minor side effects	Serious side effects	Special cautions
IPECAC SYRUP (AVAILABLE GENERICALLY)	Produces vomiting in cases of poisoning or overdose	Possible diarrhea and drowsiness after vomiting	Persistent and severe nausea or vomiting; difficulty breathing; rapid and irregular heartbeat; unusual weakness	Consult a poison-control center, doctor or emergency room before use. Do not give concurrently with activated charcoal. Avoid use if child is unconscious or convulsing. Unused bottles should be stored out of reach of children.
LINDANE (Rx) KWELL SCABENE	Treats lice and scabies infestation	Itching of skin	Coordination difficulties, rapid heartbeat, restlessness or nervousness, dizziness, convulsions (due to absorption of large amounts of drug through skin); severe skin rash	Infants and children are particularly susceptible to serious side effects. Do not apply more than the amount prescribed. Consult doctor before use if child has a seizure disorder. Do not apply to face, eyes or open cuts. Inform doctor if condition worsens or if skin rash or itching occurs.
MAGNESIUM HYDROXIDE MILK OF MAGNESIA	Relieves constipation; treats upset stomach	Diarrhea; nausea; stomach cramps; chalky taste in mouth	Irregular heartbeat, dizziness, behavioral changes, weakness (with large doses)	Consult doctor before giving this medication to a young child. Particular care must be taken if child has kidney disorders. This medication may alter the effects of other drugs; therefore, notify doctor if child is taking any other medications.
MEBENDAZOLE (Rx) VERMOX	Treats pinworm, roundworm and whipworm infestations	Diarrhea; stomach pain; nausea; vomiting	Severe skin rash	Consult doctor before use if child has liver disease or stomach disorders. Child should take as directed until drug is gone.
MECLIZINE BONINE	Actions similar to DIMENHYDRINATE			
METAPROTERENOL (Rx) ALUPENT	Treats asthma and other breathing disorders in children	Nausea; restlessness; nervousness; trembling; rapid heartbeat	Increased blood pressure; nausea or vomiting; headache; irregular heartbeat	Consult doctor before use if child has heart disease, high blood pressure or diabetes. Notify doctor if child develops persistently rapid heartbeat.
METHYLPHENIDATE (Rx) RITALIN	Treats hyperactivity in children	Appetite loss; insomnia; restlessness or nervousness; dizziness; nausea; headache; weight loss	Jerking movements of the body; irregular heartbeat; vision changes; behavioral changes; reduced blood cell counts; convulsions	Consult doctor before use if child has high blood pressure or a seizure disorder. Notify doctor of sore throat or weakness. Weight loss may occur with prolonged use. Extensive nervousness, insomnia or irritability may occur when drug is used with cold preparations.
METRONIDAZOLE (Rx) FLAGYL	Treats giardiasis and other infections	Diarrhea; nausea; vomiting; metallic taste in mouth	Severe skin rash; inflammation of the nerves (neuritis); reduced blood cell counts; coordination difficulties; behavioral changes; convulsions with high doses	Consult doctor before use if child has any neurological or blood disorder or liver disease. Child should take as directed until drug is gone, Take with food to minimize upset stomach. Inform doctor if child develops sore throat, fever, tingling sensations or numbness in hands or feet. The drug may cause darkening of the urine; this is harmless. The intended effects of this drug may be reduced when given with phenobarbital. Notify doctor if symptoms worsen or do not improve after a few days.
MINERAL OIL	Treats constipation (oral); helps remove earwax (otic)	Diarrhea (oral use)	Pneumonia, if oil enters airways following oral use; itching around rectal area	Do not use except on advice of doctor. Given orally, may reduce absorption of vitamins and other medication; consult doctor before combining with other drugs.
NEOMYCIN (Topical) (Rx/OTC) MYCIGUENT (OTC) NEOSPORIN* (OTC) MYCOLOG* (Rx) CORTISPORIN* (Rx)	Treats minor burns, cuts and skin abrasions	Burning or stinging	Allergic reactions, such as itching, swelling or skin rash; hearing loss due to absorption of large amounts	Avoid using in eyes or in deep cuts or serious burns to prevent excessive absorption. Consult doctor if no improvement is seen in one week.

DRUG	Intended effect	Minor side effects	Serious side effects	Special cautions

NEOMYCIN (Ophthalmic) (Rx)
  MYCIGUENT
  OPHTHALMIC
	Treats bacterial eye infections	Stinging or burning of eyes	Allergic reactions, such as swelling, itching or skin rash	Child should use as directed until drug is gone, even if eye feels better in a few days.

NEOMYCIN (Otic) (Rx)
  OTOBIOTIC OTIC
  CORTISPORIN
  OTIC*
	Treats bacterial infections of outer ear	None	Allergic reactions, such as itching, skin rash or swelling	Consult doctor before use if child has a perforated eardrum. Child should use as directed until drug is gone, even if ear feels better in a few days.

NITROFURANTOIN (Rx)
  FURADANTIN
  MACRODANTIN
	Treats or prevents urinary-tract infections	Nausea; vomiting; diarrhea	Inflammation of the nerves (neuritis); breakdown of red blood cells (hemolytic anemia); liver damage; pneumonia; unusual weakness, dizziness or drowsiness	Not to be used in infants under one month of age. Consult doctor before use if child has any respiratory disease, kidney disease or nerve damage. Inform doctor if child develops coughing, chills, fever, tingling sensations, numbness or burning of face or mouth, or yellowing of the whites of the eyes or skin. Child should take as directed until drug is gone. Give the medicine with milk or food in order to minimize stomach upset.

NYSTATIN (Oral/Local) (Rx)
  MYCOSTATIN
  SUSPENSION
  NILSTAT
  SUSPENSION
	Treats fungal infection of oral cavity, throat and intestine (candidiasis)	Nausea; upset stomach; diarrhea with large doses	Allergic reactions, such as skin rash	Child should take as directed until drug is gone. The drug should be retained in the mouth for as long as possible before the child swallows.

NYSTATIN (Topical) (Rx)
  MYCOSTATIN
  NILSTAT
	Treats fungal infection of skin and genital area	Burning or irritation	Allergic reactions, such as worsening of skin rash or swelling	Child should use as directed until drug is gone. Notify doctor if relief has not occurred after several days.

OXYMETAZOLINE
  AFRIN PEDIATRIC
  NOSE DROPS
  NEO-SYNEPHRINE
  12 HOUR
  CHILDREN'S DROPS
	Relieves nasal congestion due to colds, hay fever, allergies or sinusitis	Burning sensation; sneezing; dryness	Rebound nasal congestion; tremors; lightheadedness; headache; fast or irregular heartbeat; nervousness; insomnia; increased blood pressure	Consult doctor before use if child has heart disease, diabetes, high blood pressure or thyroid disease. Do not exceed recommended dosage. Avoid prolonged use, which can result in rebound congestion and swelling of the nasal mucous membranes.

PENICILLIN V (Rx)
  V-CILLIN K
  PEN-VEE K
	Actions similar to AMOXICILLIN			

PHENOBARBITAL (Rx)
  LUMINAL
  MANY GENERIC
  PREPARATIONS
	Treats seizure disorders; provides sedation	Drowsiness; dizziness; clumsiness; nausea; difficulty sleeping	Severe skin rashes; reduced blood cell counts; excitation, restlessness or extreme irritability (paradoxical effect); allergic reactions, such as swelling of the lips or eyelids or wheezing; liver damage; slurred speech, extreme drowsiness, troubled breathing (overdose)	Consult doctor before use if child has porphyria or liver or respiratory disease. Dependence may occur with prolonged use of high doses. Physical dependence is rare with usual doses to treat seizures. Do not discontinue abruptly after extended use of high doses, as withdrawal symptoms may occur (agitation, seizures). Notify doctor if child develops sore throat, fever, bleeding or bruising, or yellowing of whites of the eyes or of skin. Extreme drowsiness or breathing difficulty may occur if this drug is given with sedatives, narcotics or antihistamines.

PHENYLEPHRINE (Nasal) NEO-SYNEPHRINE	Relieves nasal congestion due to colds, hay fever or allergies; helps reduce discomfort of ear infections by reducing congestion	Dryness, burning or stinging of nasal mucous membranes	Rebound nasal congestion; tremors; insomnia; fast or irregular heartbeat; dizziness; headache; nervousness; increased blood pressure	Consult doctor before use if child has heart disease, high blood pressure, thyroid disease or diabetes. Avoid prolonged use or higher than recommended dosage to prevent side effects and rebound nasal congestion.

DRUG	Intended effect	Minor side effects	Serious side effects	Special cautions
PHENYLPROPANOLA-MINE PROPADRINE NALDECON PEDIATRIC SYRUP*	Treats nasal congestion due to colds or allergies	Nausea; nervousness; headache; restlessness; insomnia; sweating; vomiting	Increased blood pressure; irregular or rapid heartbeat; chest tightness; hallucinations; behavioral disturbances	Consult doctor before use if child has heart or thyroid disease, high blood pressure or diabetes. Inform doctor if no improvement within seven days or if fever is present. Give several hours prior to bedtime. Avoid high doses for long periods — may cause mental changes resembling psychosis.
PHENYTOIN (Rx) DILANTIN-30 PEDIATRIC DILANTIN-125 DILANTIN INFATABS	Treats seizure disorders	Nausea; vomiting; drowsiness; dizziness; constipation	Reduced blood cell counts; liver damage; allergic reactions, such as enlarged lymph glands, fever or rash; bleeding gums; slowed bone growth or fractures; confusion or behavioral changes; worsening of convulsions; clumsiness; slurred speech; tremors; erratic movement of eyes	Consult doctor before use if child has heart disease or blood, liver or kidney disorders. This drug should be taken daily, as directed, to maintain seizure control. Child should take with or after meals to reduce stomach upset. Notify doctor of darkened urine, stomach pain, yellowing of whites of eyes or skin, sore throat, fever, bleeding or bruising. Combined use with theophylline, an asthma drug, may reduce intended effects of both phenytoin and theophylline. Many other drug interactions can occur; therefore, consult doctor before use if child is taking other medication.
PIPERAZINE (Rx) ANTEPAR VERMIZINE	Treats pinworm and roundworm infestations	Nausea; diarrhea; stomach cramps	Tremors; weakness; abnormal jerking movements; visual disturbances; severe skin rash	Pinworm infestations are easily transmitted and all family members should be treated. Take drug on empty stomach. Consult doctor before use if child has liver or kidney disease or seizure disorders.
PREDNISOLONE (Rx) DELTA-CORTEF STERENE	Actions similar to PREDNISONE			
PREDNISONE (Rx) DELTASONE ORASONE METICORTEN	Treats bronchial asthma and other severe inflammatory conditions; treats juvenile rheumatoid arthritis	Congestion; nausea; insomnia; weight gain; nervousness	Emotional disturbances; decreased growth; potassium loss; persistent nausea or vomiting; acne; increased blood pressure; ulcers; bone disease; pancreas inflammation; impaired immune response; increased sugar levels in blood (diabetes); increased pressure in the eye; blurred vision	Consult doctor before use if child has heart disease, high blood pressure, kidney impairment, stomach disorders or diabetes. A low-salt diet should be followed as indicated by doctor. Notify doctor of black, tarry stools, persistent stomach pain, persistent muscle cramps, or unusual tiredness or weakness. Give with food or milk to lessen upset stomach. Avoid discontinuing abruptly after prolonged use, since adverse effects can occur (fever, weakness, dizziness, shortness of breath). Risk of ulcers is enhanced if taken with aspirin. May interfere with the effects of insulin. Consult doctor before child receives any vaccinations. Intended effects of this drug may be reduced when given with phenytoin and phenobarbital.
PROCHLORPERA-ZINE (Rx) COMPAZINE	Alleviates nausea and vomiting	Constipation; drowsiness; dizziness; dry mouth; nasal congestion	Stiffness, trembling, twisting movements, difficulty swallowing; liver damage; reduced white blood cell counts; skin rash (allergic reaction); high fever with blood-pressure changes	Consult doctor before use if child has heart disease, high blood pressure, bone marrow disorders or liver impairment. Inform doctor if child develops severe dizziness, muscle spasms, any unusual body movements, sore throat, fever, or yellowing of the whites of the eyes or the skin.
PROMETHAZINE (Rx) PHENERGAN PHENERGAN EXPECTORANT PLAIN*	Relieves runny nose, sneezing, itching and other allergic conditions; used for mild sedation	Drowsiness; dizziness; dry mouth or throat	Nightmares or unusual excitement (paradoxical effect); reduced blood cell counts; severe drowsiness; difficulty breathing; rapid heartbeat; muscle spasms, stiffness, trembling or unusual body posturing	Consult doctor before use if child has asthma or other respiratory difficulties. Notify doctor if child develops sore throat, fever or abnormal body movements.

DRUG	Intended effect	Minor side effects	Serious side effects	Special cautions
PSEUDOEPHEDRINE SUDAFED NOVAFED ACTIFED SYRUP*	Treats symptoms of common cold and sinusitis	Nervousness; sleeping difficulty; nausea; dizziness	Irregular heartbeat; hallucinations; difficulty breathing; extreme restlessness or excitement; convulsions	Consult doctor before use if child has heart disease, high blood pressure, thyroid disease or diabetes. Administer the medicine to the child several hours before bedtime to avoid insomnia. Inform doctor if symptoms do not improve within five days or if fever is present.
PYRANTEL (Rx) ANTIMINTH	Treats roundworm and pinworm infestations	Nausea; diarrhea; stomach cramps; dizziness; drowsiness	Allergic reactions, such as skin rash; twitching or muscle spasms; lightheadedness; difficulty breathing	This drug is given as a single oral dose; child may take on full or empty stomach, with or without milk or fruit juice, but entire dose must be given unless otherwise specified. All family members should be treated to ensure eradication of pinworms.
PYRVINIUM (Rx) POVAN	Treats pinworm infestations	Nausea; diarrhea; dizziness; increased sunlight sensitivity	Allergic reactions, such as skin rash	Child should take on empty stomach and avoid chewing tablets. (Swallow whole to avoid staining of teeth.) Take entire amount as a single dose unless otherwise directed. This drug will produce bright red stools for up to two days (harmless, but stain clothing). Consult doctor before use if child has stomach disorders. All household members should be treated to ensure eradication.
SODIUM FLUORIDE (Rx) PEDIAFLOR LURIDE PEDI-DENT	Prevents dental caries	Upset stomach; headache	Allergic reactions, such as skin rash; ulceration of skin of mouth and lips; discoloration of teeth with prolonged use of high amounts; excessive salivation or tearing, severe nausea, abdominal pain, vomiting or diarrhea (overdose)	Inform doctor before use if child has thyroid disorders or dental abnormalities (dental fluorosis). Notify doctor or dentist if any visible changes occur in child's teeth. Oral tablets and drops should be taken with meals to minimize stomach upset. Avoid concurrent use of milk and dairy products when swallowed. Oral solution may be given with cereal or fruit juice, or it may be added to water for use in infant formulas or other food.
SULFACETAMIDE (Ophthalmic)(Rx) SODIUM SULAMYD CETAMIDE VASOSULF*	Treats bacterial eye infections	Burning or stinging of eyes	Allergic reactions, such as itching, rash or swelling	Consult doctor before use if child has an allergy to sulfa drugs. Child should use as directed until drug is gone, even if eye feels better in a few days.
SULFISOXAZOLE (Rx) GANTRISIN	Treats inflammation of the middle ear (otitis media) and other bacterial infections	Nausea; vomiting; diarrhea; headache; appetite loss; light sensitivity	Allergic reactions, such as itching or skin rash; reduced blood cell counts; severe skin reactions; liver or kidney damage; aching muscles and joints	Do not use for infants under one month of age. Consult doctor before use if child has kidney disease, liver disease or porphyria. Child should drink plenty of fluids while taking this drug and should take as directed until drug is gone. Inform doctor if child develops sore throat, fever, bruising or bleeding, pain on urination or blood in the urine, or yellowing of the whites of the eyes or the skin. Inform doctor if symptoms worsen or if they do not improve within several days.
THEOPHYLLINE (Rx) SLO-PHYLLIN ACCURBRON THEO-DUR	Prevents and treats asthma	Nausea; nervousness; headaches; insomnia	Diarrhea, severe nausea or vomiting; stomach pain; tremors; confusion; rapid or irregular heartbeat; stomach bleeding; muscle twitching; convulsions	Consult doctor before use if child has heart, liver, thyroid or kidney disease. Notify doctor if child vomits blood or material resembling coffee grounds, develops black, tarry stools or experiences any other serious side effects. If asthma is not improved, do not increase dose without consulting doctor. Restrict caffeine-containing beverages. Take with food to lessen stomach upset. Side effects may be increased when given with erythromycin, an antibiotic. Combined use with phenytoin or carbamazepine (antiseizure drugs) may reduce effects of both drugs.

DRUG	Intended effect	Minor side effects	Serious side effects	Special cautions
THIABENDAZOLE (Rx) MINTEZOL	Treats roundworm, pinworm, thread-worm, hookworm and whipworm infestations	Nausea; appetite loss; vomiting; dizziness, bed-wetting	Blurred or yellowed vision; abnormal sensation in the eyes; ringing in the ears; tingling or numbness of hands and feet; irritability; liver damage; skin rash; muscle and joint pain; pain on urination	Consult doctor before use if child has liver or kidney disease. Take with food to minimize stomach upset. Child should chew tablets before swallowing. For pinworm infestations, all family members should be treated to ensure eradication. The drug may impart an asparagus-like odor (or other unusual odor) to the urine; this is insignificant. Child should take as directed until drug is gone.
TOLMETIN (Rx) TOLECTIN	Actions similar to IBUPROFEN			
TOLNAFTATE TINACTIN AFTATE	Treats fungal infections of the skin	Stinging; burning	Allergic reactions, such as skin rash or irritation	Avoid contact with the eyes. Clean the affected area before application unless otherwise directed. Inform doctor if irritation occurs.
TRIAMCINOLONE (Rx) AZMACORT	Treats asthma in children	Dry mouth; throat irritation; coughing; dizziness; headache; diarrhea or upset stomach; hoarseness	Lung infections, such as influenza; fungal infection inside mouth (candidiasis); potassium loss, weight gain, weakness, ulcers (prolonged use or high doses); impaired immune response; breathing difficulties; skin rash	This medication will not relieve an acute asthmatic attack. Consult doctor before use if child has any bacterial or fungal infections, heart disease or stomach disorders. If child is taking another steroid preparation, do not discontinue that medication unless advised by doctor, even if child's asthma is better with the triamcinolone. Inform doctor if child develops fever, chest pain or chills, or if white patches appear inside the mouth. Avoid abrupt discontinuation after prolonged use. Gargling and rinsing mouth after use may help prevent hoarseness, throat irritation and dry mouth.
TRIETHANOLAMINE POLYPEPTIDE OLEATE-CONDENSATE (Rx) CERUMENEX DROPS	Dissolves earwax	Ear irritation	Skin rash	Consult doctor before use if child has perforated eardrum or middle-ear inflammation.
TRIMEPRAZINE (Rx) TEMARIL	Relieves itching and other allergies; treats skin rash of poison ivy	Drowsiness; lightheadedness; dizziness; dry mouth; nausea; blurred vision	Reduced white blood cell count; severe drowsiness; difficulty breathing; muscle spasms, stiffness or unusual body movements; rapid heartbeat	Do not give to newborn or premature infants. Consult doctor before use if child has asthma or other respiratory disorders or liver disease. Notify doctor of sore throat or fever. Drowsiness and other side effects may be accentuated when given with antihistamines. Combined use with sedatives or narcotics may cause extreme drowsiness. This drug may aggravate some effects of epinephrine, a drug used to treat asthma.
TRIMETHOPRIM AND SULFAMETHOXAZOLE (Rx) SEPTRA BACTRIM	Treats middle ear infections (otitis media) and other infections; treats severe traveler's diarrhea	Nausea; vomiting; diarrhea (paradoxical effect)	Reduced blood cell counts; severe skin rash; allergic reactions, such as skin rash, itching and difficulty breathing; muscle aches and pains, liver damage; disturbed kidney function	Consult doctor before use if child has kidney disease, liver disease, or any allergies (particularly to sulfa drugs). Avoid in infants under one month of age. Child should drink plenty of fluids while taking this medication and should take as directed until drug is gone. Notify doctor if child develops sore throat, fever, weakness, bruising or bleeding.

Bibliography

BOOKS

American National Red Cross:
Advanced First Aid and Emergency Care. New York: Doubleday, 1982.
Family Health and Home Nursing. Garden City, N.Y.: Doubleday, 1979.

Arena, Jay M., M.D., and Miriam Bachar, *Child Safety Is No Accident: A Parents' Handbook of Emergencies.* Durham, N.C.: Duke University Press, 1978.

Barnard, Christiaan, M.D., ed., *Junior Body Machine: How the Human Body Works.* New York: Crown, 1983.

Behrman, Richard E., M.D., and Victor C. Vaughan III, M.D., *Nelson Textbook of Pediatrics.* Philadelphia: W. B. Saunders, 1983.

Berkow, Robert, M.D., ed., *The Merck Manual of Diagnosis and Therapy.* Rahway, N.J.: Merck & Co., 1977.

Bevan, James Stuart, M.D., *Anatomy and Physiology.* New York: Simon and Schuster, 1978.

Boston Children's Medical Center and Richard I. Feinbloom, M.D., *Child Health Encyclopedia: The Complete Guide for Parents.* New York: Dell, 1975.

Brace, Edward R., and John P. Pacanowski, M.D., *Childhood Symptoms: Every Parent's Guide to Childhood Illnesses.* New York: Harper & Row, 1985.

Columbia University College of Physicians and Surgeons, *Complete Home Medical Guide.* New York: Crown, 1985.

Crelin, Edmund S., *Functional Anatomy of the Newborn.* New Haven, Conn.: Yale University Press, 1973.

Cuthbertson, Joanne, and Susie Schevill, *Helping Your Child Sleep through the Night.* Garden City, N.Y.: Doubleday, 1985.

Dawson, Helen L., *Basic Human Anatomy.* New York: Appleton-Century-Crofts, 1974.

Eiser, Christine, *The Psychology of Childhood Illness.* New York: Springer-Verlag, 1985.

Ferber, Richard, M.D., *Solve Your Child's Sleep Problems.* New York: Simon and Schuster, 1985.

Gabel, Stewart, M.D., ed., *Behavioral Problems in Childhood: A Primary Care Approach.* New York: Grune & Stratton, 1981.

Green, Martin I., *A Sigh of Relief: The First-Aid Handbook for Childhood Emergencies.* New York: Bantam Books, 1984.

Green, Morris, M.D., and Robert J. Haggerty, M.D., *Ambulatory Pediatrics III.* Philadelphia: W. B. Saunders, 1984.

Haessler, Herbert A., M.D., Christine Harris and Raymond Harris, *How to Make Sure Your Baby is Well — and Stays That Way.* New York: Avon, 1984.

Hardin, James W., and Jay M. Arena, M.D., *Human Poisoning from Native and Cultivated Plants.* Durham, N.C.: Duke University Press, 1974.

Katz, Harvey P., M.D., *Telephone Manual of Pediatric Care.* New York: Wiley, 1982.

Kaye, Robert, M.D., Frank A. Oski, M.D., and Lewis A. Barness, M.D., *Core Textbook of Pediatrics.* Philadelphia: J. B. Lippincott, 1978.

Krugman, Saul, M.D., and Samuel L. Katz, M.D., *Infectious Diseases of Children.* St. Louis: C. V. Mosby, 1981.

Kunz, Jeffrey R. M., M.D., ed., *The American Medical Association Family Medical Guide.* New York: Random House, 1982.

Leach, Penelope, *The Child Care Encyclopedia: A Parents' Guide to the Physical and Emotional Well-Being of Children from Birth through Adolescence.* New York: Alfred A. Knopf, 1984.

Levine, Melvin D., M.D., et al., *Developmental-Behavioral Pediatrics.* Philadelphia: W. B. Saunders, 1983.

Martin, Richard, M.D., *A Parent's Guide to Childhood Symptoms: Understanding the Signals of Illness from Infancy through Adolescence.* New York: St. Martin's Press, 1982.

Meadowbrook Medical Reference Group, *The Parents' Guide to Baby & Child Medical Care.* Ed. by Terril H. Hart, M.D. Deephaven, Minn.: Meadowbrook Press, 1983.

Pantell, Robert H., M.D., James F. Fries, M.D., and Donald M. Vickery, M.D., *Taking Care of Your Child: A Parent's Guide to Medical Care.* Reading, Mass.: Addison-Wesley, 1984.

Pascoe, Delmer J., M.D., and Moses Grossman, M.D., eds., *Quick Reference to Pediatric Emergencies.* Philadelphia: J. B. Lippincott, 1978.

Petrillo, Madeline, R.N., and Sirgay Sanger, M.D., *Emotional Care of Hospitalized Children: An Environmental Approach.* Philadelphia: J. B. Lippincott, 1980.

Pomeranz, Virginia E., M.D., and Dodi Schultz, *The Mothers' and Fathers' Medical Encyclopedia.* New York: New American Library, 1977.

Pringle, Sheila M., R.N., and Brenda E. Ramsey, R.N., M.S.N., *Promoting the Health of Children: A Guide for Caretakers and Health Care Professionals.* St. Louis: C. V. Mosby, 1982.

Rosenberg, Stephen N., M.D., *The Johnson & Johnson First Aid Book.* New York: Warner, 1985.

Samuels, Mike, M.D., and Nancy Samuels, *The Well Child Book.* New York: Summit, 1982.

Schmitt, Barton D., M.D., *Pediatric Telephone Advice: Guidelines for the Health Care Provider on Telephone Triage and Office Management of Common Childhood Symptoms.* Boston: Little, Brown, 1980.

Shiller, Jack G., M.D.:
Childhood Illness: A Common Sense Approach. New York: Stein and Day, 1972.
Childhood Injury: A Common Sense Approach. New York: Stein and Day, 1977.

Spock, Benjamin, M.D., and Michael B. Rothenberg, M.D., *Baby and Child Care.* New York: Pocket Books, 1985.

West, Richard, M.D., and Richard Dodds, M.D., *The Complete Medical Guide to Children's Ailments.* New York: Exeter Books, 1983.

Your Child: A Medical Guide, by the Editors of Consumer Guide and Ira J. Chasnoff, M.D. New York: Beekman House, 1983.

PERIODICALS

Carney, Cynthia L., "Everything You Need To Know About AIDS." *Parents,* April 1986.

Centers for Disease Control, "Recommendations for Assisting in the Prevention of Perinatal Transmission of HTLV-III/LAV and AIDS." *Morbidity and Mortality Weekly Report,* December 6, 1985.

Cherskov, Myk, "MDs: Share Day-Care Health Techniques." *American Medical News,* November 8, 1985.

Hinman, Alan R., M.D., and Jeffrey P. Koplan, M.D., "Pertussis and Pertussis Vaccine: Reanalysis of Benefits, Risks, and Costs." *JAMA,* June 15, 1984.

Jaret, Peter, "Our Immune System: The Wars Within." *National Geographic,* June 1986.

"Standards of CPR and ECC." *JAMA,* June 6, 1986.

Thompson, Sharon W., and Karen R. Gietz, "Acquired Immune Deficiency Syndrome in Infants and Children." *Pediatric Nursing,* July/August 1985.

OTHER PUBLICATIONS

"Acquired Immunodeficiency Syndrome (AIDS)." Richmond: Virginia Department of Health Recommendations for Day Care Center Attendance, November 1985.

"Allergies." NIH Publication No. 81-1948. Washington: U.S. Department of Health and Human Services, September 1981.

"Bacteria: The Littlest Cells." DHEW Publication No. (NIH) 76-896. Washington: Department of Health, Education, and Welfare, 1976.

Black, Yuill, M.D., and William F. Thompson, M.D., "Patient Information: Allergy and Immunology." Unpublished ms., American Board of Allergy and Immunology, Philadelphia.

"Caring For Your Child in the Emergency Room." Washington: Association for the Care of Children's Health, 1984.

"A Child Goes to the Hospital." Washington: Association for the Care of Children's Health, 1983.

Krasinski, K., M.D., "Aids in Children." Unpublished ms., New York University Medical Center, Bellevue Hospital Center, New York.

McCarthy, Paul L., M.D., and Katharine Lustman-Findling, "Observing Your Febrile Child: The Yale Observation Scales." Department of Pediatrics, Yale University School of Medicine, Yale-

New Haven Hospital, no date.

"Miscellaneous Microbes: The Non-Conformists." DHEW Publication No. (NIH) 76-898. Washington: Department of Health, Education, and Welfare, 1976.

"Poison Ivy Allergy." NIH Publication No. 82-897. Washington: U.S. Department of Health and Human Services, March 1982.

"Poison Ivy, Poison Oak and Poison Sumac: Identification, Precautions, and Eradication." Farmer's Bulletin No. 1972. GPO stock number 001-000-03883-4. Washington: Department of Agriculture, December 1978.

"Rocky Mountain Spotted Fever." NIH Publication No. 85-400. Washington: U.S. Department of Health and Human Services, September 1985.

"Understanding the Immune System." NIH Publication No. 85-529. Washington: U.S. Department of Health and Human Services, July 1985.

"Viruses: On the Border of Life." DHEW Publication No. (NIH) 76-895. Washington: Department of Health, Education, and Welfare, 1976.

Acknowledgments and Picture Credits

The index for this book was prepared by Louise Hedberg. For their help in the preparation of this volume, the editors also wish to thank the following: Yuill Black, M.D., Washington, D.C.; Thomas R. Crock, M.D., Falls Church, Va.; Janet LaFleur, Maryland General Care, Inc., Baltimore, Md.; Joan Macdonell, Armed Forces Institutes of Pathology, Medical Museum, Washington, D.C.; Jeff Molter, Department of Communication, American Academy of Pediatrics, Elk Grove Village, Ill.; James Nolti Jr., Maryland General Care, Inc., Baltimore, Md.; Nancy O'Shea, The Fairfax Hospital, Falls Church, Va.; William Thompson, M.D., and Alan D. Woolf, Ambulatory Medicine, The Children's Hospital, Boston, Mass.

The sources for the photographs in this book are listed below, followed by the sources for the illustrations. Credits from left to right are separated by semicolons; credits from top to bottom are separated by dashes.

Photographs. Cover: Fil Hunter. 9, 43, 129: Susie Fitzhugh.

Illustrations. 4, 5: Marguerite E. Bell from photograph by Elisabeth Kupersmith. 10, 11: Bill Burrows & Associate. 12, 13: Robert Hynes. 14: Robert Hynes (6); Marguerite E. Bell from photograph by Elisabeth Kupersmith. 15: Robert Hynes. 16: Marguerite E. Bell from photographs by Elisabeth Kupersmith. 17: Marguerite E. Bell. 18: Marguerite E. Bell from photographs by Elisabeth Kupersmith. 21: Marguerite E. Bell from photograph by Elisabeth Kupersmith; Donald Gates. 22: Donald Gates from photograph by Elisabeth Kupersmith. 23: Marguerite E. Bell from photographs by Elisabeth Kupersmith. 24: Donald Gates from photographs by Elisabeth Kupersmith. 25: Marguerite E. Bell; Donald Gates from photographs by Elisabeth Kupersmith. 26: Robert Hynes; Marguerite E. Bell from photographs by Elisabeth Kupersmith. 28: Robert Hynes from photograph by Elisabeth Kupersmith. 29: Donald Gates; Marguerite E. Bell from photographs by Elisabeth Kupersmith. 30, 31: Marguerite E. Bell from photographs by Elisabeth Kupersmith. 32-39: Donald Gates from photographs by Elisabeth Kupersmith. 40, 41: Robert Hynes from photographs by Elisabeth Kupersmith. 44, 45: Robert Demarest. 49, 50: Gloria Marconi. 51: Marguerite E. Bell from photographs by Elisabeth Kupersmith. 53: Gloria Marconi. 55: Kathe Scherr from photograph by Enrico Ferorelli. 57: Gloria Marconi. 58: Peter A. Sawyer. 63: Gloria Marconi. 64, 65: Kathe Scherr from photographs by Elisabeth Kupersmith. 66: Walter Hilmers Jr. from H J Commercial Art. 69: Gloria Marconi — Marguerite E. Bell from photographs by Elisabeth Kupersmith. 70: Gloria Marconi. 71: Marguerite E. Bell from photograph by Elisabeth Kupersmith; Walter Hilmers Jr. from H J Commercial Art. 72, 73: Gloria Marconi. 76: Kathe Scherr from photographs by Elisabeth Kupersmith. 77: Marguerite E. Bell from photograph by Bruce Wells. 78: William Hennesy. 80: Marguerite E. Bell from photograph by Elisabeth Kupersmith. 81: William Hennesy. 83: Gloria Marconi. 86: Marguerite E. Bell from photograph by Elisabeth Kupersmith. 87: Jane Hurd. 88, 89: Marguerite E. Bell from photographs by Elisabeth Kupersmith. 90: Jane Hurd. 92: Marguerite E. Bell from photographs by Elisabeth Kupersmith (2) — Bill Burrows & Associate (2). 93: Bill Burrows & Associate. 94: Marguerite E. Bell from photograph by Elisabeth Kupersmith. 101-110: Gloria Marconi. 111: Marguerite E. Bell from photograph by Elisabeth Kupersmith. 112: Gloria Marconi. 114: Marguerite E. Bell from photograph by Elisabeth Kupersmith. 115, 116: Gloria Marconi. 117: Marguerite E. Bell from photograph by Elisabeth Kupersmith. 119: Maps by John Drummond, leaves by Robert Hynes. 120: Marguerite E. Bell from photograph by Elisabeth Kupersmith. 124, 125: Gloria Marconi. 130, 131: Bill Burrows & Associate. 135: Marguerite E. Bell. 138: Donald Gates from photograph by Elisabeth Kupersmith. 141: Gloria Marconi — Marguerite E. Bell from photograph by Elisabeth Kupersmith. 143-151: John Drummond.

Index

Brain, *101*
  growth in first two years of life, 101
  tumor, 102
  See also Nervous system
Breast-feeding:
  advantages of, 46, 47, 65, 98
  bowel movements of breast-fed babies, 65, 66
  and jaundice, 70
Breasts, swollen at birth, 108
Breathing, respiratory system and, *73*
Breathing difficulties, 10-11, 16-17
  after a burn, 20, 21
  apnea, 73
  asthma, 74
  choking rescue, *23*
  in cystic fibrosis, 95
  emergency treatment for acute distress, 16-17
  with hives, 116
  obstructed airway, 10, 16-17
  stridor, 16
    symptom of croup, 77-78
  symptom of:
    allergic reaction to insect sting, 12
    anaphylactic shock, 38
    bronchiolitis, 75
    bronchitis, 74-75
    in croup, 77-78
    drug allergy, 46-47
    epiglottitis, 16, 17, 78
    obstructed airway, 10, 16-17, 40
    pneumonia, 81-82
    poisoning, 36-37
    Reye syndrome, 105-106
    rheumatic fever, 82
    swallowed object, 40
  when to call the doctor, 16, 17
  See also Wheezing
Broken bones, 17-19
Broken nose, 35
Bronchioles, *73;* infection of, 75
Bronchiolitis, 75
Bronchitis, 74-75
Brown recluse spider, first aid for bite of, *13*
Bruises, 19
  to the head, 19, 32
  symptom of leukemia, 56-57
Burns, 10, 20, *21, 22*
  chemical, 20, *22*
  electrical, 20, 22, 29
  of the eye, *30*
  heat, 20-22

C

Cancer:
  Hodgkin's disease, 56
  leukemia, 56-57
  neuroblastoma, 104-105
  retinoblastoma, 89
Candidiasis, 85
Canker sore, 112
Carbon monoxide poisoning, 37
Carbuncle, 111-112
Cardiopulmonary resuscitation, 10, 16, 17
Cataracts, 90
Cavities, preventing, 141
Celiac disease, 47, 64
Cerebral palsy, 102
Chalazion, 89
Checkups, 135, 140; dental, 141
Chemicals:
  burns from, 20, *22*
  in eyes, *30*
  skin allergies to, 46
Chest:
  pain in, symptom of pneumonia, 81-82
  tightness of, symptom of:
    anaphylactic shock, 38
    asthma, 74
Chicken pox, 59
  rash, *chart* 123
  and Reye syndrome, 59, 105, 106
Chigger bites, 12

Chills, symptom of:
  blood poisoning, 99
  encephalitis, 103
  fever, 93
  influenza, 80
  meningitis, 104
  Rocky Mountain spotted fever, 121-122
  scarlet fever, 82-83
  sunburn, 21
Choking, 11, 23; rescue procedures, *23*
Chorea, 102-103
Circulatory system, *53;* problems and disorders of, 53-57
Circumcision, 109
Cleft lip, 64
Cleft palate, 64
Clubbing, of fingers, 54; symptom of cyanosis, 54-55
Clubfoot, 51
Colds, 75-76
  distinguishing from allergy, 48
  and ear infections, 80
  sinusitis and, 83
  traveling with, 85
  virus, 100
Cold sores, 100, 112-113
Colic, 65; relief from, *65*
Collarbone, *49;* fractured, 17, *18*
Colostrum, 98
Coma, 41
  diabetic, 55
Concussion, 32; checking for, *32*
Cone-shell, first aid for sting of, *15*
Confusion, symptom of:
  delirium, 27
  hypothermia, 33
Congenital heart disease, 54
Congestion, nasal, symptom of hay fever, 48
Conjunctivitis, 87-88
Consciousness, loss of. *See* Unconsciousness
Constipation, 63, 65
  and anal fissures, 64
  foods to eat while recovering, 133
  symptom of intestinal obstruction, 69-70
  during toilet training, 65
Contact dermatitis, 46; from poison ivy, oak or sumac, 119-120
Contagious diseases, 58-62. *See also specific disease;* Immunizations
Contusion, 32
Convulsions, 24, 106
  after DTP inoculation, 61
  and fever, 24, 93, 106
  first aid, *24*
  and heatstroke, 33
  from poisoning, 36
  seizure disorders, 106
  symptom of anaphylactic shock, 38
  See also Epilepsy
Copperheads, first aid for bite of, *14*
Coral snakes, first aid for bite of, *14*
Cough, 76-77
  and asthma, 77
  barking, symptom of croup, 77-78
  and choking, 23
  chronic, symptom of cystic fibrosis, 95
  dry and hacking, symptom of:
    bronchitis, 74-75
    influenza, 80
    pneumonia, 81-82
  and gagging, symptom of sinusitis, 83
  medications, 77
  productive, 75, 77
  symptom of:
    anaphylactic shock, 38
    breathing distress, 16-17
    bronchiolitis, 75
    hay fever, 48
    swallowed object, 40
    whooping cough, 62
  wet, symptom of pneumonia, 81-82
  See also Asthma; Breathing difficulties; Wheezing
CPR, 10, 16, 17

Cradle cap, 113
Cramps. *See* Abdominal pain
Cretinism, 57
Cross-eye, 88-89
Croup, 77-78
Crying:
  gauging as symptom of illness, *chart* 91
  persistent, symptom of:
    colic, 65
    DTP inoculation reaction, 61
    gas pains, 67
Cuts:
  on the ear, 28
  first aid, 25-26
  of the lip, controlling bleeding, *34*
  on the head, 32
  in the mouth, 34
  See also Bandages; Bleeding; Wounds
Cyanosis, 54-55
  symptom of:
    congenital heart defect, 54
    obstructed airway, 16-17, 40
Cystic fibrosis, 95
  pneumonia and, 82

D

Day-care centers, incidence of infections in, 98
Decongestants, 48, 77; using to equalize pressure on eardrums, 85-86
Dehydration, 63, 65-66
  fluids needed to prevent, *chart* 66
  and hypovolemic shock, 38
  preventing during illness, 93, 94
Delirium, 27; symptom of blood poisoning, 99
Dental care, 140-141
Dermatitis, 46, 113, 119-120
Diabetes, 55; mellitus, 55
Diaper rash, 113-*114*
Diaphragm, *73;* in hiccups, 79
Diarrhea, 66
  chronic, in AIDS, 98-99
  and dehydration, 94
  foods to eat while recovering, 133
  incidence of, in day-care centers, 98
  symptom of:
    food allergy, 47-48
    food poisoning, 66-67
    gastroenteritis, 68
    giardiasis, 68
    hepatitis, 68
    intestinal infection, 69
    intestinal obstruction, 69-70
    neuroblastoma, 104-105
    stomach or intestinal infection, 63
  when to call the doctor, 135
Diet:
  factor in anemia, 54
  fiber in, 64, 65
  iron in, 54
  nutritional guidelines, 63, 142
  for sick child, 133
  for strong teeth, 140
Digestive system, *63;* problems and disorders of, 63-72
Diphtheria, 59-60, 61; vaccine (DTP), 58, 59-60, 61, 62
Discharge:
  from ear, 28-29
  from eye, symptom of:
    blocked duct, 87
    conjunctivitis, 87-88
  from nose, 35
  from umbilical stump, 100
  vaginal, 108, 109
  when to call the doctor, 135
Disease:
  effect of stress on, 107
  fever and, 91
  See also specific illnesses and disorders; Immune system; Immunizations; Infection; Vaccinations
Dislocations, *17, 18;* of hip, congenital, 51
Dizziness, 78

L

Lacerations, 26
  on the ear, 28
  See also Bleeding; Cuts; Wounds
Language skills, development of, *chart* 105
Laryngitis, 77, 80
Larynx, *73*
Laxatives, 64, 66
Lazy eye (amblyopia), 88-89
Lead poisoning, 37
Legs:
  abnormalities, 50, 51
  bowlegs, 50, *51*
  injury, *17,* 19
  pain in, 51
  See also Limp
Legg-Perthes disease, 52
Leukemia, 56-57
Lice, 100, 117-118; identifying rash, *chart* 123
Ligaments, *50,* 51
  sprained, 39-40
  torn, 18
Limp, 51-52
  symptom of:
    arthritis, 50
    joint infection, 49-50, 51
    Legg-Perthes disease, 52
    rheumatic fever, 82
    toxic synovitis, 51-52
    trauma, 51
Limpness, after DTP, 61
Lips:
  cold sores, 112-113
  cuts on, *34*
  injury to, from electrical burn, 22
Liquid diet, 133
Liver, *44, 45,* 56, *63*
  function, 97
  inflammation of, in hepatitis, 68
  and levels of bilirubin in, 70
  See also Jaundice
Lockjaw. *See* Tetanus
Low blood sugar. *See* Hypoglycemia
Lump:
  in abdomen or groin, symptom of hernia, 68-69
  under skin, symptom of boil or carbuncle, 111-112
Lungs, *73*
  in asthma, 74
  of newborns, 76
  See also Breathing difficulties; Wheezing
Lymphatic system, *53, 54, 57,* 63, 97-98; cancer of (Hodgkin's disease), 56
Lymph nodes (glands), *45, 53, 57*
  in AIDS, 98-99
  See also Swollen glands

M

Marine animals, first aid for bites and stings, 12, *15*
Masturbation, 108
Measles, 60; MMR vaccine, 58, 60, 61
Meconium, 69
Medications:
  allergic reactions to, 46-47
  for coughs, 77
  drugs, *chart* 143-151
  for fever, 59, 94, 106
Medicine cabinet, supplies for, 10, *130-131*
Melanin, *110*
Meningitis, 10, 24, 60; treatment, 104
Metabolism, 53, 55, 57
  adrenals and, *44*
  See also Thyroid
Migraine, 103
Milk, cow's:
  allergy to, 47
  colic and, 65
  constipation and, 65
  factor in diarrhea, 66
  lack of iron in, 54
  PKU disorder, 96
MMR immunization, 58, 60, 61

Molds, allergy to, 48
Moles, 110, 118
Molluscum contagiosum, 118; identifying rash, *chart* 123
Mosquito bite, 12
Motion sickness, 70-71, 81
Mouth:
  dry, symptom of dehydration, 66
  electrical burns, 22
  injury, *34*
  sores in, 112
  thrush, 85
Mouth-to-mouth resuscitation, *16,* 17, *28*
Mucus:
  clearing from nose, *76*
  from colds, 76, 77
  in cystic fibrosis, 95
  in eye, symptom of blocked duct, 87
  in sinuses, *83*
Mumps, 60; MMR immunization, 58, 60, 61
Muscles:
  ache, symptom of:
    hepatitis, 68
    influenza, 80
  control, poor, symptom of cerebral palsy, 102
  pain, 52; symptom of:
    arthritis, 50
    influenza, 80
    rheumatic fever, 82
    Rocky Mountain spotted fever, 121-122
    toxic synovitis, 51-52
  strained, 39, 40
Muscular dystrophy, 96
Myelin, 101
Myopia, 89-90

N

Nausea, 71
  in motion sickness, reducing, 81
  symptom of:
    anaphylactic shock, 38
    appendicitis, 64
    brain tumor, 102
    gastroenteritis, 68
    hepatitis, 68
    hypovolemic shock, 38
    intestinal infection, 69
    sunburn, 21
  treatment of, 71
Navel, infection of umbilical cord stump, 100
Nearsightedness, 89-*90*
Neck injuries, 18
Nephritis, 84, 120; treatment, 126
Nephrosis, 126-127
Nervousness, symptom of hypoglycemia, 56
Nervous system, *101*
  disorders of, 101-107
  symptoms of neurological disorders, *chart* 105
Neuroblastoma, 104-105
Nose:
  broken, *35*
  clearing mucus from, *76*
  discharge from, symptom of:
    hay fever, 48
    sinusitis, 83
  drops, 75, 76
  injuries, *34, 35*
  nosebleed, *34, 35*
  objects in, *34,* 35
  sinuses and, *83*
  stuffed-up, symptom of cold, 75-76
  suctioning out mucus, 76

O

Orthopedic problems, 50-51
Otitis externa, 78, 79, *81,* 85
Otitis media, 78, 79, 80-*81*
Ovaries, 53, 54
Overfeeding, 69, 72

P

Pain, as symptom, when to call the doctor, 135.

See also specific part of body
Pancreas, *53,* 54, 55, 56, *63*
Parasites, in giardiasis, 68
Paregoric, 64
Pediatrician, 134, 136, 137, 140
Penicillin, 148; allergy to, 38, 46-47, 82, 99, 116
Penis, *108;* circumcision, 109
Peritonitis, 70
Pertussis. *See* Whooping cough; DTP
Petit mal seizure, 24, 106
Petroleum jelly:
  coating thermometer, 92
  removing tick with, 12, 121-122
Pharynx. *See* Throat
Phenylketonuria (PKU), 96
Pica, 71
Pigeon-toed gait, 50, *51*
Pinkeye, 88
Pinworms, 71; checking for, *71*
Pituitary gland, *53-*54, 56, *101*
Pityriasis rosea, 118; identifying rash, *chart* 123
PKU (phenylketonuria), 96
Pneumonia, 60, 81-82
Poisoning, 10, 11, 36-37
  as cause of accidental death, 36
  importance of immediate treatment, 10, 37
  prevention of, 37
  regional poison-control center, 22, 36-37
Poison ivy, 46, *119-*120; identifying rash, *chart* 123
Poison oak, 46, *119-*120; identifying rash, *chart* 123
Poison sumac, 46, *119-*120; identifying rash, *chart* 123
Polio, 61; vaccine, 58, 61
Pollen, allergy to, 46, 48
Portuguese man-of-war, first aid for sting, *15*
Postnasal drip, 77, 84
Prescription drugs, *chart* 143-151
Prickly heat. *See* Heat rash
Prophylactics, for asthma, 74
Protein, brain's need for, 101
Ptosis, 89
Pulse. *See* Heartbeat
Puncture wounds, 26-27
Purpura, *120-*121; identifying rash, *chart* 123
Pus:
  from cut or wound, symptom of infection, 100
  in eyes, symptom of conjunctivitis, 87-88
Pyloric stenosis, 71-*72*
Pylorus, *72*

R

Rabies, 13
Rash:
  common contagious, 115; identifying, *chart* 123
  diaper, 113-114
  in newborns, 118
  purple, symptom of:
    meningitis, 104
    purpura, *120-*121
  symptom of:
    arthritis, 50
    blood poisoning, 99
    chicken pox, 59
    drug allergy, 46-47
    fifth disease, 115
    food allergy, 47-48
    heat rash, 115-116
    measles, 60
    neuroblastoma, 104-105
    pityriasis rosea, 118-119
    poison ivy, oak or sumac, 119-120
    rheumatic fever, 82
    Rocky Mountain spotted fever, 12, 121-122
    roseola, 122
    rubella, 61
    scarlet fever, 82-83
    skin allergy, 46
  when to call the doctor, 135
Rattlesnake, first aid for bite, *14*
Recovery position, *24, 41*
Red blood cells, 54, 56, 70
Reproductive system, *53, 54, 108-109*